Neuroradiological Imaging of Skin Diseases and Related Conditions

Daniel Thomas Ginat
Editor

Neuroradiological Imaging of Skin Diseases and Related Conditions

Springer

Editor
Daniel Thomas Ginat
Radiology
University of Chicago
Chicago, IL
USA

ISBN 978-3-319-90929-5 ISBN 978-3-319-90931-8 (eBook)
https://doi.org/10.1007/978-3-319-90931-8

Library of Congress Control Number: 2018959113

This Springer imprint is published by the registered company Springer Nature Switzerland AG
The registered company address is: Gewerbestrasse 11, 6330 Cham, Switzerland

Foreword

One could consider the skin as the last great unexplored frontier in neuroimaging. Up until now, most MRI of the skin and its disorders has been confined to the neurocutaneous syndromes. When one looks carefully at the literature on this topic, it is easy to realize that although the lesions in the central nervous system have received considerable attention those in the skin have not. My first reaction (and I am sure that many radiologists have the same one) is, why look at the skin lesions when they are obvious to physical examination? Well, dermatology is similar to radiology in that personal experience plays a huge role in reaching a correct diagnosis and in that many lesions look similar.

In this beautifully illustrated and highly original book, Ginat and his coauthors provide radiologists with a concise but complete overview of skin lesions, many unknown to imagers. Because skin lesions occur throughout the body, this book should be helpful to all subspecialties of radiology not only neuroradiology. Appropriately, this book covers all of the traditional phakomatoses but also includes imaging of benign and malignant tumors. All entries contain clinical photographs, histology, and imaging using different modalities. Postoperative procedures including those performed for cosmetic reasons are addressed in the last chapter.

Although books such as this one are generally used as consultation sources and not completely read, this one deserves more attention than just casual perusing. Reading it cover to cover will expand the horizons of radiologists and will make us look at skin lesions differently. Instead of stating that another nonspecific skin lesion is present, after reading this book we should be able to offer a diagnosis or an intelligent differential diagnosis.

The future always lies in the previously unexplored or the insufficiently explored. Although not covered in this book, I can see a future when imaging may play an important role in the assessment of skin grafts, genetic modifications of skin lesions, and other types of therapies. But for the time being, this superb book fulfills an empty niche. I congratulate the authors for their careful work, superb illustrations, concise and informative text, and courage to venture into a new territory.

Chapel Hill, NC, USA　　　　Mauricio Castillo

Preface

When I visited my aunt's house as a child, one of my favorite activities there was perusing the vivid and dramatic photos in a skin disease atlas. Although I did not become a dermatologist, that experience has to some degree inspired me to prepare this book. The subject matter still appeals to my inner childhood imagination and is also relevant to my clinical work as a neuroradiologist.

One might wonder what skin diseases have to do with radiology. While skin lesions are readily visible on clinical exam, diagnostic imaging is useful for evaluating the depth and extent of the lesions and assessing many associated conditions that are beyond skin deep, such as neurocutaneous syndromes. Therefore, it is important to be aware of the various skin diseases and their associated systemic and neuroimaging findings. Besides the radiology findings, this book includes clinical and pathology images and descriptions, when appropriate and possible.

I hope you enjoy this first edition of ***Neuroradiological Imaging of Skin Diseases and Related Conditions***.

Chicago, IL, USA
January 2018

Daniel Thomas Ginat

Acknowledgements

Individuals:
Min Deng MD
Anisha Dua MD, MPH
Lawrence Ginsberg MD
Lawrence Gottlieb MD
Melissa Guilbeau
Rajiv Gupta MD, PhD
Amy Ho MD
Ashley Jenkins MD
Kayleen Jahangir MD
Arlene Ruiz de Luzuriaga MD
Gul Moonis MD
Veena Ramaiah MD
Ryan Salvador MD
Lohini Sundharkrishnan MD
Mark Volk MD
Fredrick Wigley MD

Companies:
Triangle Exim
Longport Inc.

Contents

Introduction: Skin Anatomy, Imaging Approaches, and Dermatology Terminology

1

Daniel Thomas Ginat and Nicole A. Cipriani

Contents

Abstract

Skin is the largest organ in the body and has an intricate structure that serves multiple important functions. The histology, imaging modalities, and normal anatomy of skin are reviewed in this chapter, along with basic dermatology terminology. Familiarity with the histology and anatomy of skin are important for understanding the corresponding imaging abnormalities discussed in subsequent chapters.

D. T. Ginat (✉)
Department of Radiology, University of Chicago, Pritzker School of Medicine, Chicago, IL, USA
e-mail: dtg1@uchicago.edu

N. A. Cipriani
Department of Pathology, University of Chicago, Chicago, IL, USA

Skin Anatomy

The skin performs several functions, including sensation, thermoregulation, protection, and synthesis of vitamin D. The skin is composed of two layers, the epidermis and dermis; the epidermal layer is composed of keratinized stratified squamous epithelium, and the dermal layer is composed of connective tissue. Several adnexal structures are present in the skin, including the hair follicles, sweat glands, sebaceous glands, and ceruminous glands, which are modified sweat glands found in the external ear. The subcutaneous layer, or hypodermis, is located beneath the dermis and attaches to muscle or bone, but is not considered part of the skin.

The epidermis is mostly composed of keratinocytes arranged in the following layers throughout most of the body: stratum corneum, which is the most superficial layer, stratum lucidum,

D. T. Ginat (ed.), *Neuroradiological Imaging of Skin Diseases and Related Conditions*,
https://doi.org/10.1007/978-3-319-90931-8_1

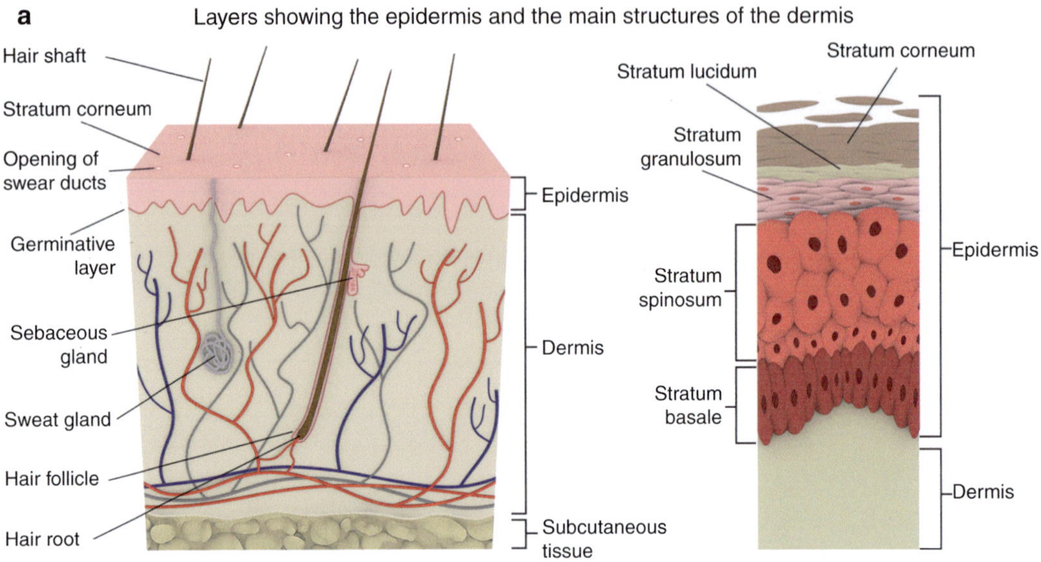

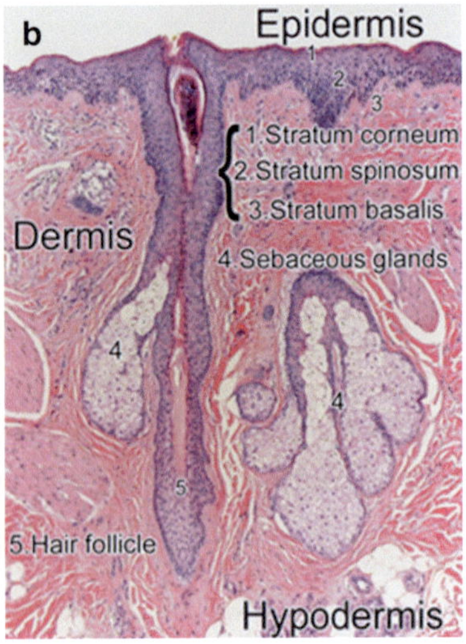

Fig. 1.1 Schematic diagrams of skin anatomy (**a**). Hematoxylin and eosin stained histopathological section of the skin shows the different layers and associated structures (**b**)

which is only present in the hands and feet, stratum granulosum, stratum spinosum, and stratum basale, which is the deepest layer (Fig. 1.1). The epidermis also contains melanocytes, which produce melanin, Langerhans cells, which are involved in the immune response, and Merkel cells, which are involved in the sensation of touch.

The dermis is composed of two layers, the reticular and papillary layers. The papillary layer contains the nerves and blood vessels that supply the epidermis. In particular, the skin blood vessels consist of a superficial arteriovenous plexus in the papillary dermis, just below the epidermis and the deep arteriovenous plexus in the subcutis, connected by vertical perforators (Fig. 1.2). The lymphatics parallel the blood vessels. The reticular layer of the dermis consists of connective tissue containing collagen and elastic fibers.

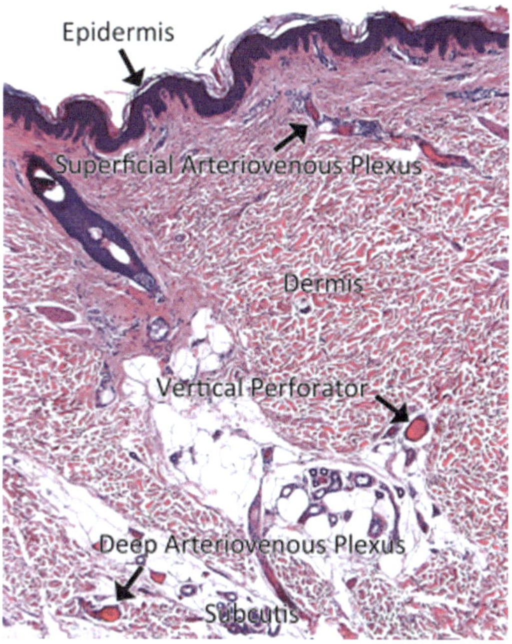

Fig. 1.2 Hematoxylin and eosin stained histopathological section of the skin shows the main types of blood vessel components

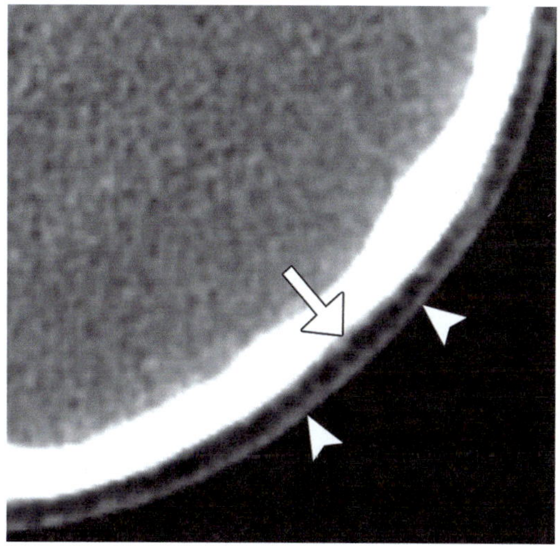

Fig. 1.3 Normal skin depicted on CT. Axial CT image of the head shows the thin soft-tissue attenuation skin (*arrowheads*), overlying the fat attenuation subcutaneous tissues (*arrow*)

Diagnostic Radiology Imaging Approaches

CT: The modality uses X-rays to create cross-sectional images that depict the different attenuation characteristics of tissues. Intravenous contrast is often administered in order to increase the conspicuity of abnormalities through enhancement. CT is suitable for characterizing of soft-tissue lesions in terms of internal mineralization and associated bone involvement, as well as the characterization of lesion vascularity, particularly via CTA. Normal skin appears as a thin soft-tissue attenuation layer over the subcutaneous fat, which has variable thickness (Fig. 1.3). The different layers of the skin are otherwise not readily discernible on routine CT.

MRI: The modality uses magnetic fields and pulses of radiofrequency energy to excite and detect the movement of protons. Variations in hydrogen density and magnetic relaxation times (T1 and T2) are responsible for creating contrast between different tissues during imaging. While standard head and neck, brain, and spine MRI protocols can be implemented for imaging of skin lesions, suplementary high-resolution MRI of the skin can be performed using microscopy coils in order to acquire submillimeter pixel size that can resolve the layers of the skin (Fig. 1.4). Applications of MRI in skin lesion imaging include morphologic assessment, such as shape, size, depth, and location, as well as the delineation of the relationship between lesions and underlying critical structures, such as periosteum, muscle, nasal cartilage, orbital septum, and lacrimal apparatus. This modality is also useful for detecting associated findings, such as perineural tumor spread and intraspinal and intracranial involvement. Contrast is routinely given in order to increase lesion conspicuity and help discern cystic from solid components. MRA, like CTA, can be helpful for delineating associated abnormal vascularity.

Ultrasound: Ultrasonography involves the detection of reflected sound waves through tissues that possess inherently different acoustic properties. In general, as the frequency of the sound waves increased, the resolution increases, while the depth decreases. With 20 MHz ultrasound, the dermis and hypodermis can be readily distinguished, but the epidermis over most of the body except on the palms and soles cannot be visualized as a separate structure because it is too thin to be resolved. Very high frequency ultrasound systems allow more detailed visualization of the upper skin layers, hair follicles, and eccrine sweat-gland ducts (Fig. 1.5). Furthermore, Doppler ultrasound is useful for detecting vascular components within lesions. Applications of cutaneous ultrasonography include differentiating between cystic and solid lesions, evaluating the inflammatory skin response in patch-test reactions, assessing the efficacy of skin-moisturizing products by objectively measuring changes in the thickness of the skin epithelium, and quantitative assessment of the extent of cutaneous radiation fibrosis after exposure to ionizing radiation.

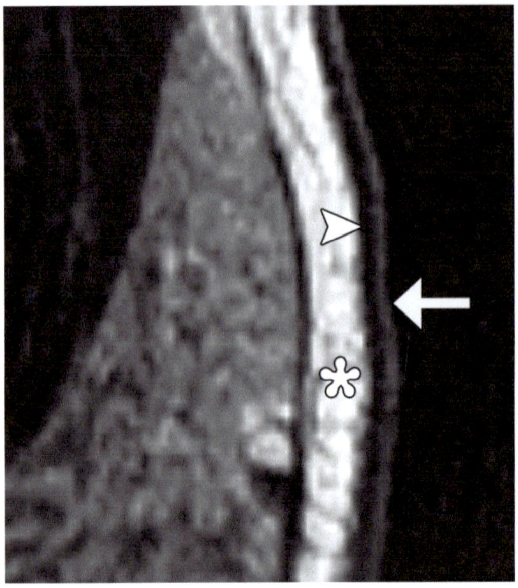

Fig. 1.4 Normal skin depicted via MRI acquired using a microscopy coil. Axial T2-weighted image of the left parotid gland region shows the epidermis (*arrow*) is hyperintense relative to the underlying dermis (*arrowhead*) and the subcutaneous fat is bright (*asterisk*) and is traverse by vessels with flow voids

FDG-PET: PET detects cellular metabolic activity based on cellular uptake of ^{18}F fluorodeoxyglucose (^{18}FDG), which can be quantitatively expressed as standardized uptake value (SUV). The images acquired must be processed in order to account for the differential attenuation of the photons produced by the decay of ^{18}F, which is much more pronounced within the body than at the skin surface. Thus, non-attenuation-corrected images will show diffusely lower level activity deep in the body compared to the skin surface than with attenuation-corrected images (Fig. 1.6). PET is often performed in conjunction with CT and can be displayed as fused PET/CT images. PET/CT has a role in the evaluation of cutaneous malignancies, such as melanoma, squamous cell carcinoma, Merkel cell carcinoma, and cutaneous lymphoma. Beside neoplasms, various infectious and inflammatory cutaneous lesions can be encountered incidental on PET.

Fig. 1.5 High-resolution ultrasound shows the various components of the skin and underlying tissues. Courtesy of Longport Inc.

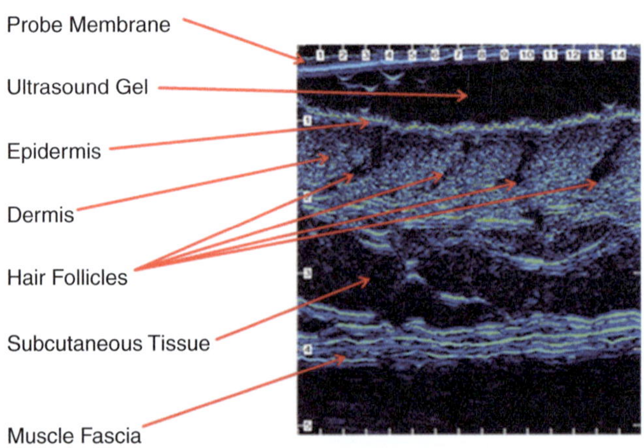

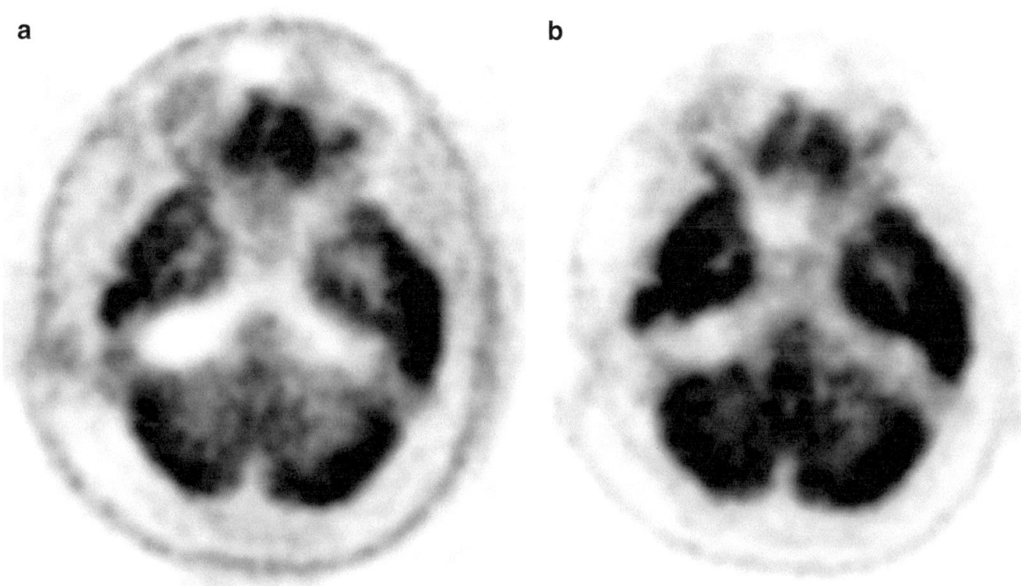

Fig. 1.6 Normal appearance of skin on [18]FDG PET. Non-attenuation-corrected PET image (**a**) shows disproportionately greater apparent metabolic activity in the skin as compared with the attenuation-corrected PET image (**b**)

Brief Dermatology Dictionary

- Abrasion: wound no deeper than the epidermis
- Abscess: localized collection of pus
- Annular: lesions grouped in a circle
- Avulsion: flap or torn skin and other tissues
- Bulla: large fluid-filled blister
- Bruise (contusion): minor hemorrhage within the skin, where disrupted vessels leak blood into the interstitial space
- Cellulitis: inflammation of the skin and subcutaneous tissues
- Crusting: rough skin surface formed from plasma exudate
- Cyst: papule or nodule that contains fluid
- Dermatitis: inflammation of the skin
- Desquamation: scaling off of skin
- Ecchymosis: A small hemorrhagic spot, larger than a petechia, in the skin or mucous membrane forming a non-elevated, rounded or irregular, blue-purple patch
- Erythema: red skin due to increased blood supply and blanch with pressure
- Fissure: thin crack in epidermis
- Fungating: large malignant tumor erupting in a mushroom morphology
- Granulation tissue: mass of new vessels and fibrous tissues in a healing wound
- Keratotic: horny scale
- Laceration: cut in the skin with jagged edges
- Lichenoid: scale tightly adherent to skin
- Macule: smooth area of color change less than 15 mm diameter
- Nodule: enlargement of a papule in three dimensions
- Papule: small palpable lesions, generally less than 5 mm in diameter
- Patch: large area of color change, with smooth surface
- Petechia: punctate focus of bleeding in the skin
- Plaque: palpable flat lesion larger than 5 mm
- Purpura: hemorrhage into the skin
- Rash: widespread eruption of lesions
- Telangiectasia: prominent cutaneous blood vessels
- Ulcer: full thickness defect in the epidermis
- Verrucous: warty
- Wheal: edematous papule or plaque

Suggested Reading

Aspres N, Egerton IB, Lim AC, Shumack SP. Imaging the skin. Australas J Dermatol. 2003;44(1):19–27.

Budak MJ, Weir-McCall JR, Yeap PM, White RD, Waugh SA, Sudarshan TA, Zealley IA. High-resolution microscopy-coil MR imaging of skin tumors: techniques and novel clinical applications. Radiographics. 2015;35(4):1077–90.

Duncan JR, Carr D, Kaffenberger BH. The utility of positron emission tomography with and without computed tomography in patients with nonmelanoma skin cancer. J Am Acad Dermatol. 2016;75(1):186–96.

Kim JH, Kim JY, Chun KA, Jee WH, Sung MS. MR imaging manifestations of skin tumors. Eur Radiol. 2008;18(11):2652–61.

Lew PP, Ngai SS, Hamidi R, Cho JK, Birnbaum RA, Peng DH, Varma RK. Imaging of disorders affecting the bone and skin. Radiographics. 2014;34(1):197–216.

McLafferty E, Hendry C, Alistair F. The integumentary system: anatomy, physiology and function of skin. Nurs Stand. 2012;27(3):35–42.

Pearl RM, Johnson D. The vascular supply to the skin: an anatomical and physiological reappraisal--part I. Ann Plast Surg. 1983;11(2):99–105.

Neuroimaging of Non-vascular Congenital Skin Lesions Unrelated to Neurocutaneous Syndromes

2

Edwina Chang, David Frim, Nicole A. Cipriani, and Daniel Thomas Ginat

Contents

E. Chang
Department of Radiology, University of Chicago, Chicago, IL, USA

D. Frim
Department of Neurosurgery, University of Chicago, Chicago, IL, USA

N. A. Cipriani
Department of Pathology, University of Chicago, Chicago, IL, USA

D. T. Ginat (✉)
Department of Radiology, University of Chicago, Pritzker School of Medicine, Chicago, IL, USA
e-mail: dtg1@uchicago.edu

Abstract

This chapter highlights cutaneous manifestations of congenital skin lesions that are non-vascular and not related to underlying neurocutaneous syndromes. These disease include aplasia cutis, branchial apparatus anomalies, epidermoid and dermoid cysts, cephaloceles, and spinal dysraphism.

D. T. Ginat (ed.), *Neuroradiological Imaging of Skin Diseases and Related Conditions*,
https://doi.org/10.1007/978-3-319-90931-8_2

Aplasia Cutis Congenita

Overview

Aplasia cutis congenita, which is also known as congenital scar and congenital absence of skin, presents as a focal absence of skin in neonates. The lesions are most commonly located in the midline scalp and may be associated with underlying calvarial and/or dural defects although they may also occur on the trunk and extremities. Although the lesions are often isolated findings, they can be associated with various syndromes, including Johanson-Blizzard syndrome, Adams-Oliver syndrome, trisomy 13, Wolf-Hirschhorn syndrome, and SCALP syndrome. The etiology of aplasia cutis is not clear, but many conditions, including intrauterine infections, teratogens, and genetic factors, have been implicated. Smaller areas of aplasia cutis congenita can heal within weeks of birth with topical treatment only. Larger areas of aplasia cutis congenita are prone to hemorrhage or infection and require surgical intervention with skin grafting.

Clinicopathologic Findings

Aplasia cutis congenita most commonly manifests as a focal absence of skin at the vertex of the scalp (Fig. 2.1). Lesions only involving the epidermal layer are usually shallow and form a scar during the perinatal period. Consequently, epidermis can grow over the affected site, but there may be persistent paucity of underlying adnexal structures (Fig. 2.2). Lesions involving the deeper layers of the skin and calvarium may appear ulcerated and are more prone to infectious and hemorrhagic complications. The depth of involvement can vary, but absence of the epidermal layer is characteristic. As the lesion heals, a thin epithelial layer with scar tissue may form.

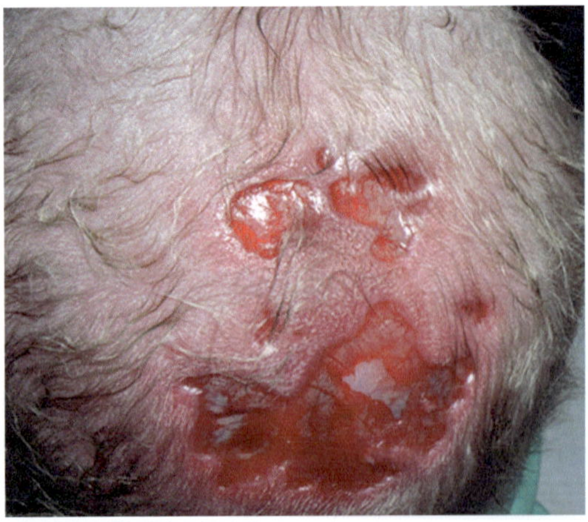

Fig. 2.1 Aplasia cutis. Photograph demonstrates focal areas with absence of skin at the vertex

Imaging Findings

CT or MRI are usually sought after a clinical diagnosis of aplasia cutis congenita in order to determine the depth of involvement and to assess for associated complications, such as meningitis, sagittal sinus thrombosis, and cerebral hemorrhage. Lesions involving just the epidermal and dermal layers can initially appear as a defect on imaging, which if not surgically repaired can eventually close via scar tissue that displays low T1 and T2 signal without other underlying findings (Fig. 2.3). Otherwise, imaging is useful for evaluating intracranial abnormalities in syndromes associated with aplasia cutis, such as white matter deficiency in Wolf-Hirschhorn syndrome (Fig. 2.4).

Branchial Apparatus Anomalies

Overview

Each of the six mesodermal branchial arches is separated by an ectoderm-lined branchial cleft and endoderm-lined branchial pouch. Branchial apparatus anomalies of the head and neck encompass a spectrum of conditions that result from abnormal embryogenesis, including cervical chondrocutaneous branchial remnants, sinus tracts, fistulas, and cysts. While branchial anomalies are often isolated findings, they may rarely be associated with congenital syndromes, such as the branchio-oto-renal and branchio-oculo-facial, Goldenhar syndrome, and Treacher-Collins syndrome.

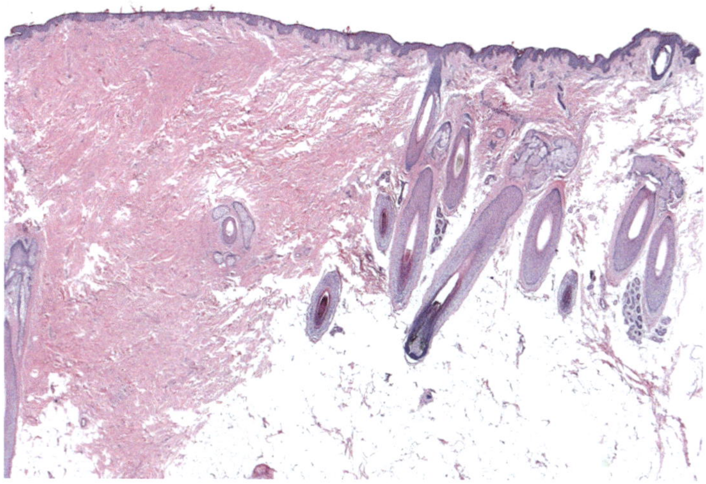

Fig. 2.2 Aplasia cutis. Low power hematoxylin and eosin stained photomicrograph shows skin with normal adnexal structures (hair follicles, sebaceous glands, eccrine glands) on the right, and almost complete absence of adnexae on the left, with the presence of dense dermal scar

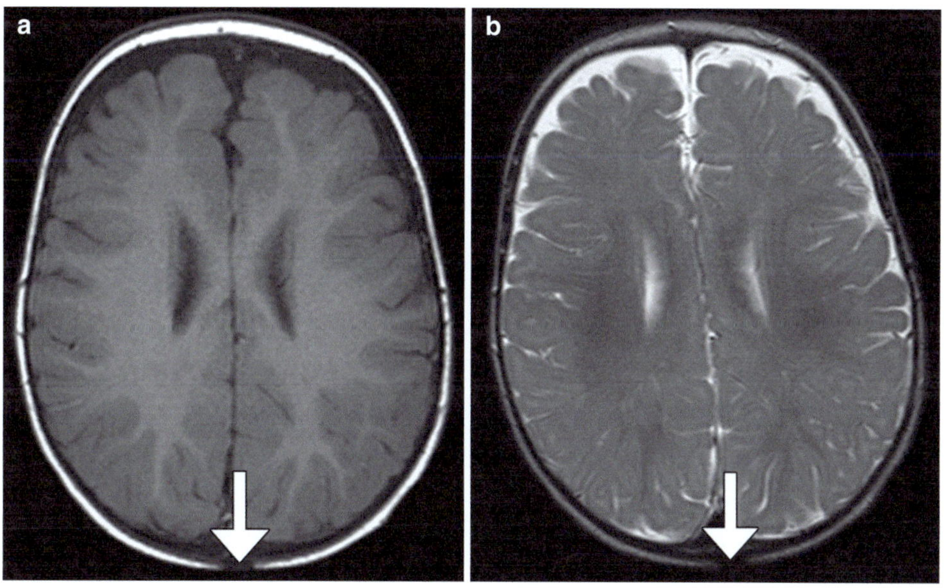

Fig. 2.3 Aplasia cutis. Axial T1-weighted (**a**) and T2-weighted (**b**) MR images show a focal area of low signal in the midline of the posterior scalp (*arrows*) attributable to scar tissue formation at the site of aplasia cutis

Clinicopathologic Findings

Branchial fistulas and sinus tracts that communicate with the skin are often apparent due to the presence of a sinus ostium and draining fluid (Fig. 2.5). Alternatively, chondrocutaneous branchial remnants and accessory tragus appear as exophytic skin projections. Infected branchial apparatus lesions may present with swelling, erythema, pain, and fever. Histologically, branchial anomalies are lined by stratified squamous or pseudostratified ciliated columnar epithelium and may contain cartilage in the case of chondrocutaneous branchial remnants (Fig. 2.6).

Imaging Findings

Diagnostic imaging via MRI, ultrasound, or CT may be performed to assess the type and extent of suspected branchial apparatus anomalies. Fistulas and sinuses are amenable to further evaluation via barium injection.

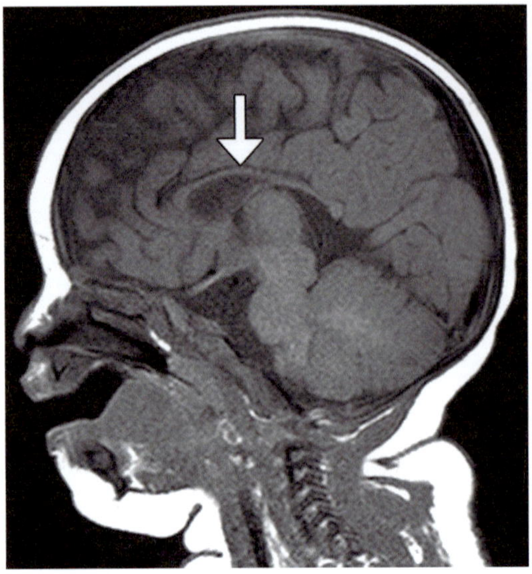

Fig. 2.4 Wolf-Hirschhorn syndrome. Sagittal T1-weighted MRI shows a paucity of white matter volume, with thinning of the corpus callosum (arrow)

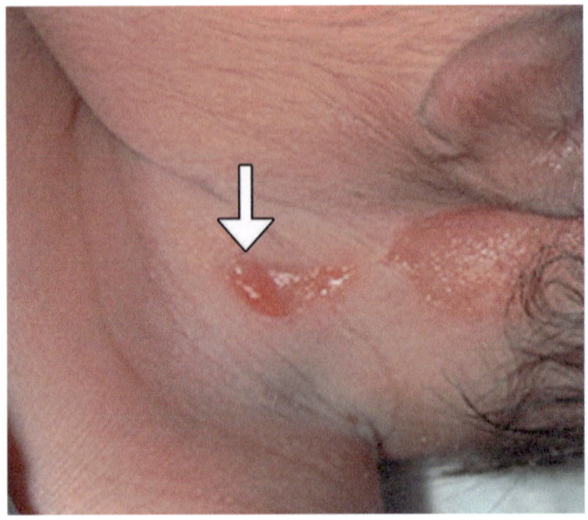

Fig. 2.5 Branchial apparatus anomaly. Photograph demonstrates an opening into a sinus tract in the left lateral neck (arrow)

Fig. 2.6 Branchial apparatus anomaly. Hematoxylin and eosin stained photomicrograph shows stratified squamous epithelium, subepithelial inflammatory cells, and cartilage (arrow)

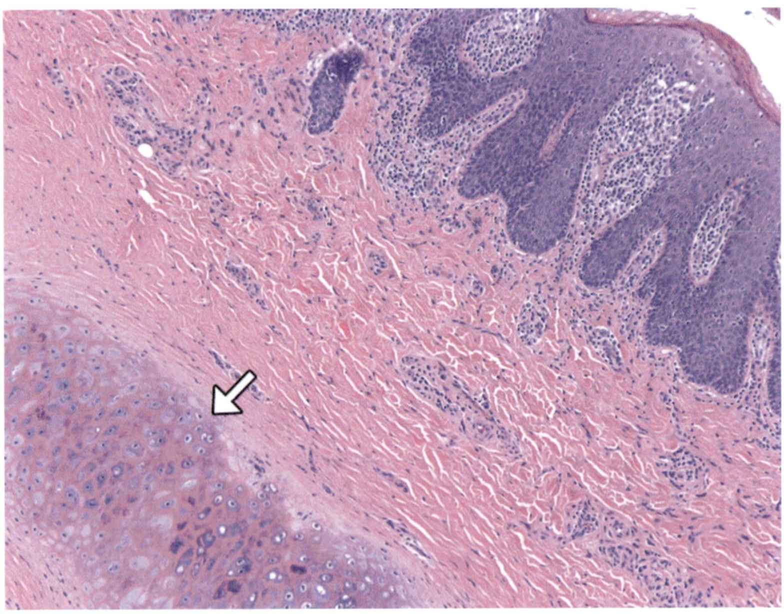

- Cervical chondrocutaneous branchial remnants appear as skin appendages with a cartilage core that appears as soft-tissue attenuation on CT and hypoechoic on ultrasound (Fig. 2.7).
- Fistulas are communications between two epithelialized surfaces and communicate with a persistent pouch and cleft. On imaging, injected contrast can be traced from the skin to the hypopharynx, for example (Fig. 2.8).
- Sinuses are blind ending tracts that connect with either the skin (branchial cleft sinus) or with the pharynx (branchial pouch sinus), which can appear as a tubular, fluid-filled structure on imaging (Fig. 2.9).
- Branchial cleft cysts are discrete fluid collections without connection to any epithelialized surface. On MRI, branchial cleft cysts can sometimes appear as high T1 and low T2

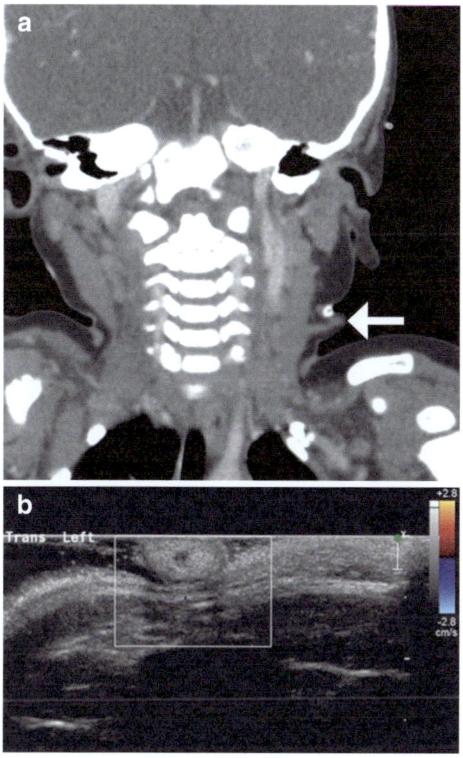

Fig. 2.7 Cervical chondrocutaneous branchial remnant. Coronal CT image (**a**) demonstrates a skin appendage in the left neck with linear soft-tissue attenuation core that corresponds to cartilage (arrow). There is an adjacent hyperattenuating marker. Ultrasound (**b**) shows the exophytic lesion in cross-section with peripheral hyperechoic subcutaneous fat and centrally hypoechoic cartilage without associated internal vascularity

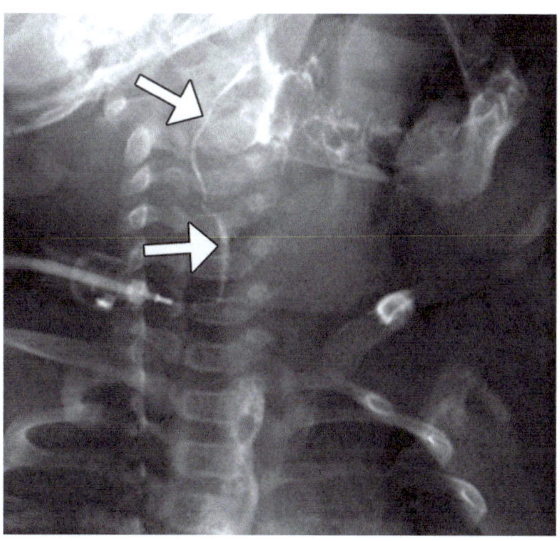

Fig. 2.8 Branchial fistula. Direct injection of contrast via a cutaneous opening in the lower anterior neck demonstrates fistula tract (arrows) extending to the apex of the piriform sinus

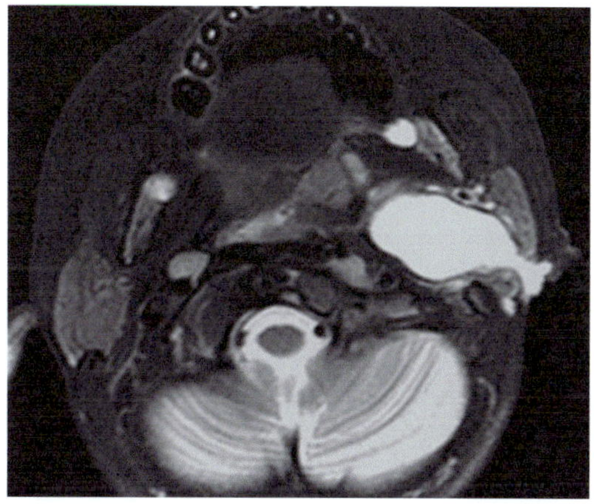

Fig. 2.9 Branchial cleft sinus. Axial T2-weighted MRI shows a left parotid space cystic lesion with a tract that extends to the skin of the external auditory canal

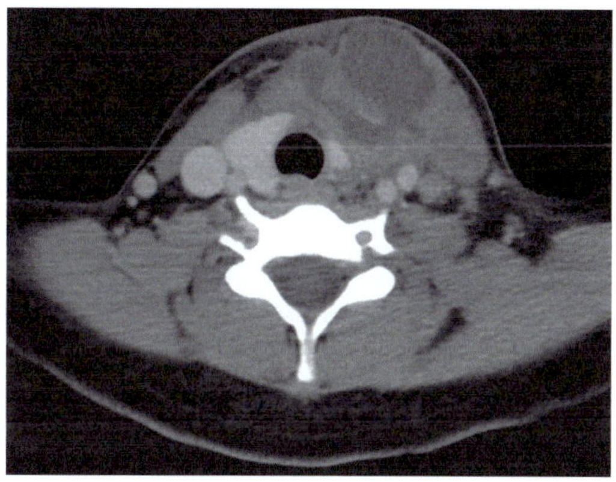

Fig. 2.10 Infected branchial cleft cyst. The patient presented with fever, cellulitis, and an enlarging left neck mass. Axial CT image shows an irregular fluid collection in the left neck with surrounding fat stranding

signal, rather than simple fluid signal, due to the presence of proteinaceous material. When infected, branchial cleft cysts can enlarge, display relatively high attenuation due to the presence of pus, and there can be surrounding fat stranding due to cellulitis (Fig. 2.10).

- Syndromes associated with branchial apparatus anomalies can present with head and neck cutaneous stigmata, such as skin tags, which can result from unfused auricular hillocks or other branchial cleft remnants. Therefore, diagnostic imaging is useful for assessing the full scope of underlying abnormalities, such as external auditory canal atresia in Treacher-Collins syndrome (Fig. 2.11).

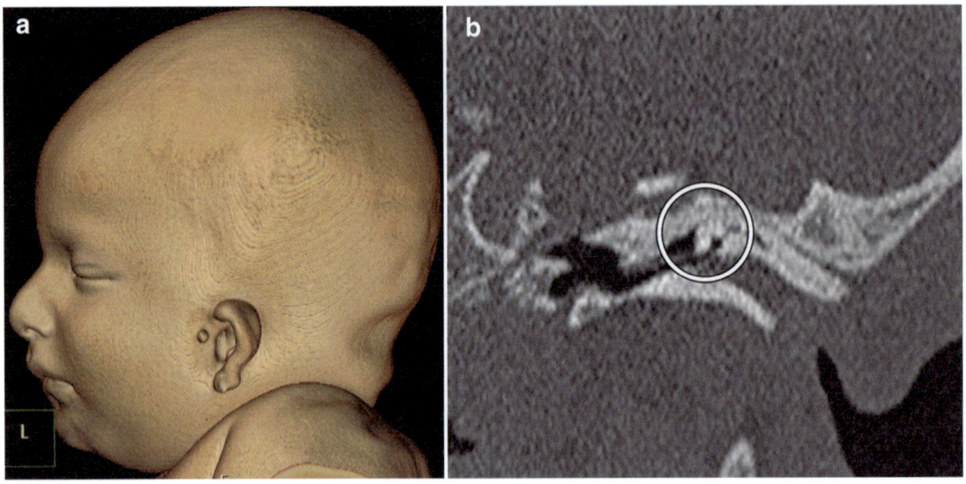

Fig. 2.11 Treacher-Collins syndrome. 3D CT image (**a**) shows a malformed auricle with a skin tag (arrow). Oblique coronal CT image (**b**) shows a narrow external auditory canal and dysmorphic ossicles fused to the epitympanic wall (encircled)

Craniofacial Dermal Sinuses and Inclusion Cysts

Overview
Among craniofacial dermal sinuses, 85% are located in the occipital protuberance, 10% in the nose, and 5% in the posterior parietal region. Dermal sinuses result from nondisjunction of the neuroectoderm and the cutaneous ectoderm and therefore can be associated with inclusion cysts, such as dermoids and epidermoids. In particular, nasal dermal sinuses result from invagination of skin components into the prenasal space, such as through the foramen cecum, along with the dural diverticulum as it regresses in the embryo.

Clinicopathologic Findings

Congenital dermal sinuses are lined by stratified squamous epithelium and may terminate at the dura, subarachnoid space, or as dermoids/epidermoids. Histologically, epidermoid cysts are lined by squamous epithelium, usually with a granular layer, and contain keratin debris (Fig. 2.12), while dermoid cysts are lined by squamous epithelium with associated skin appendages, such as hair follicles and sebaceous glands (Fig. 2.13), and are also filled with keratin debris.

Nasal dermal sinuses often present as a midline nasal pits (Fig. 2.14), without or with an associated nasal mass attributable to underlying dermoid/epidermoid cysts. Alternatively, dermoids/epidermoids can present as tumors in the subcutaneous tissues without associated skin defects (Fig. 2.15). Complete surgical excision is often performed in order to prevent infectious complications and recurrence.

Imaging Findings

Dermal sinus tracts and their potential intracranial extension are best evaluated via high-resolution, 2–3 mm section MR images, particularly T2-weighted sequences with fat suppression. These lesions typically appear as fluid signal tracts with associated cystic components, which can have a dumbbell configuration (Fig. 2.16). Ultrasound is also a reasonable option for evaluating dermal sinuses, which appear as hypoechoic, but is generally of limited utility for evaluating the intracranial contents. Associated osseous anomalies, such as a patent foramen

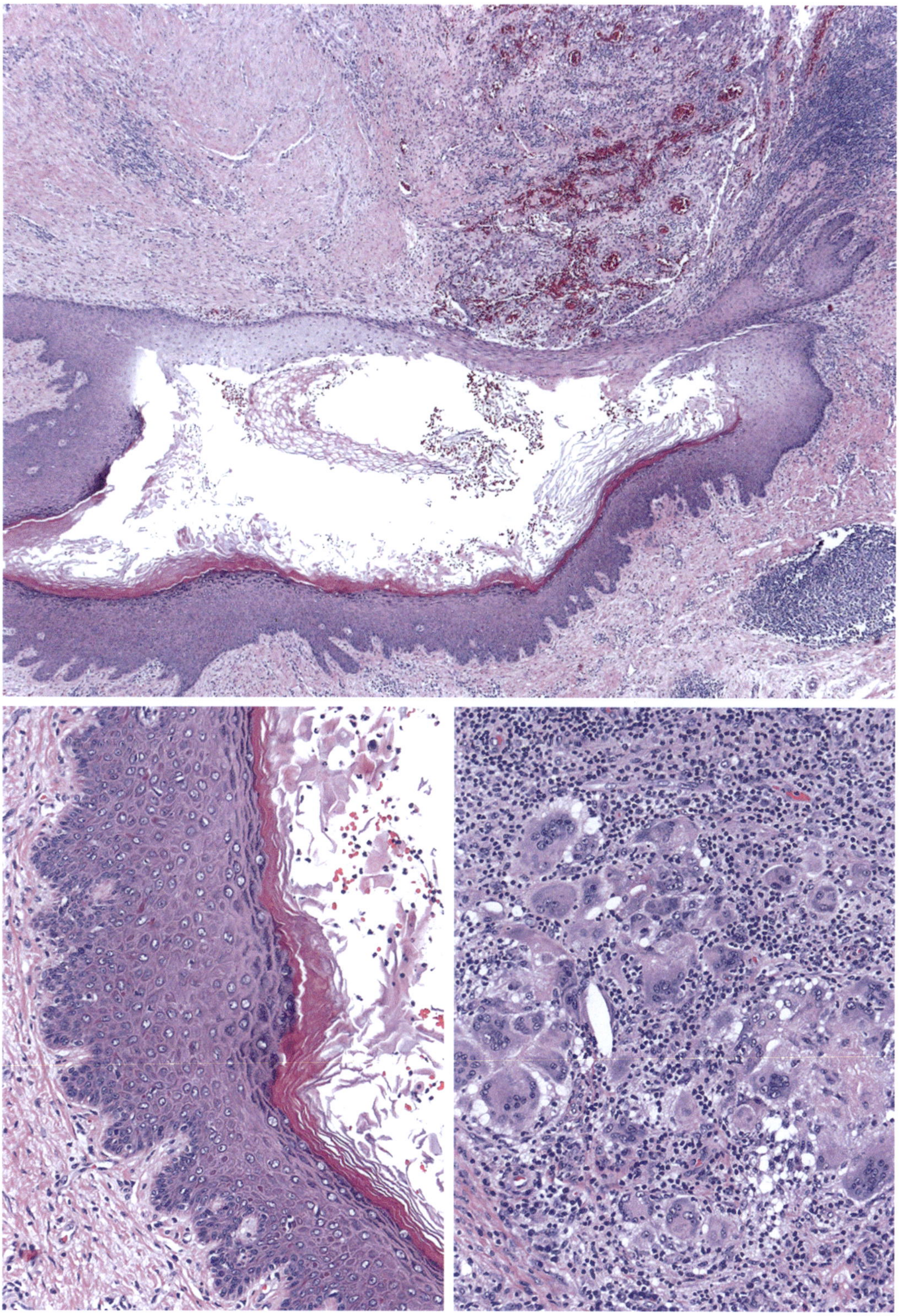

Fig. 2.12 Epidermoid cyst. Low and high power hematoxylin and eosin stained photomicrographs show a cyst lined by stratified squamous epithelium (top and bottom left) without associated skin adnexal structures. Rupture is frequent and can manifest as chronic inflammation in the wall of the cyst and foreign body giant cell reaction to keratin debris (bottom right)

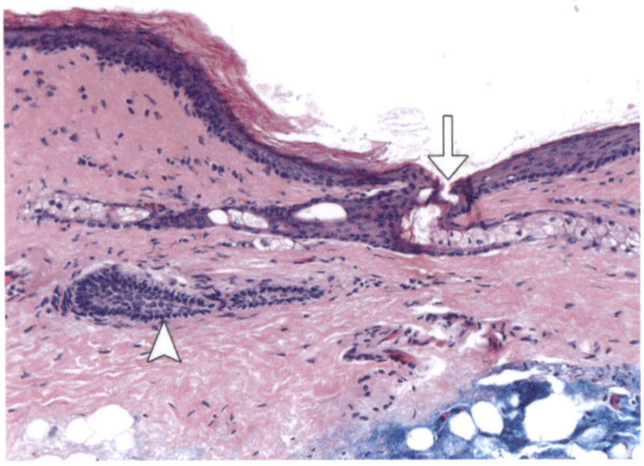

Fig. 2.13 Dermoid cyst. Hematoxylin and eosin stained photomicrograph shows a cyst wall lined by thin, keratinized, stratified squamous epithelium with sebaceous units (arrow) draining into the cyst lumen and associated hair follicles (arrowhead)

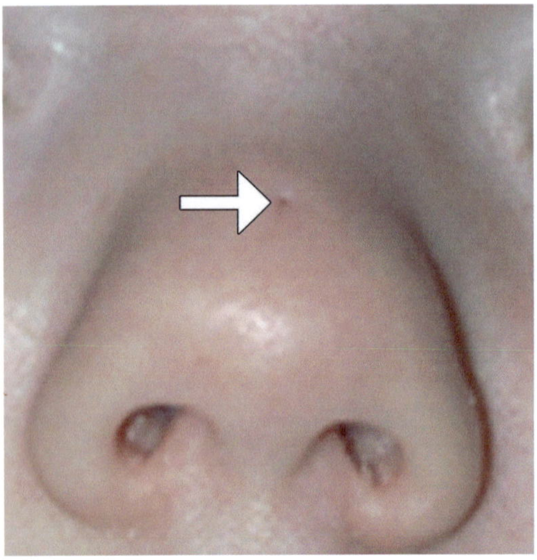

Fig. 2.14 Nasal dermal sinus. Photograph shows a punctate skin opening in the midline of the nasal dorsum (arrow)

cecum and bifid crista galli, are best depicted on CT (Fig. 2.17). The intracranial components of sinus tracts can be a portal of entry for pathogens, which can result in meningitis, abscess, and/or cerebritis (Fig. 2.18), which are best depicted on MRI, particularly post-contrast T1-weighted and T2-weighted sequences, as well as diffusion-weighted imaging.

Inclusion cysts can have varying imaging features depending upon their contents. For example, epidermoid cysts typically are fluid attenuation on CT and have fluid signal characteristics on MRI, but can have restricted diffusion. Dermoid cysts can also have these imaging features, but dermoid cysts can also have a fatty appearance (Fig. 2.19).

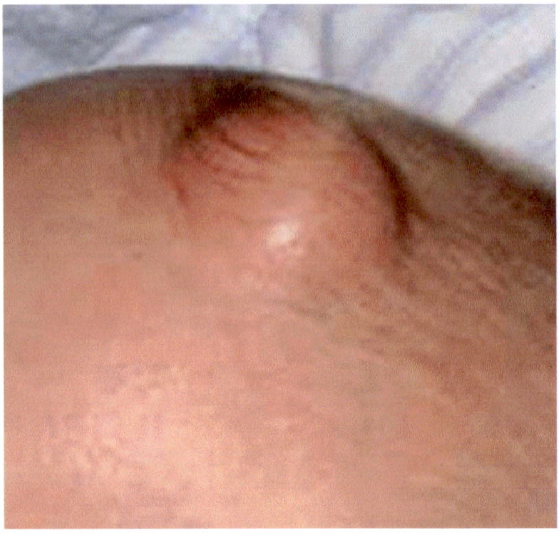

Fig. 2.15 Dermoid cyst. Photograph demonstrates a dome-shaped scalp lesion in the midline frontal region without associated skin defect

Cephaloceles

Overview

Cephaloceles represent herniations of intracranial contents through a skull defect that result from abnormal neural tube migration of cephalic neural crest cells. These can be categorized further as meningoceles, meningoencephalocele, or ventriculocele. Meningoceles contain dura and cerebrospinal fluid only, while meningoencephaloceles contain cerebrospinal fluid, dura, and brain tissue, which can be dysplastic, versus ventriculoceles, which are cystic compartments that connect to the ventricular system. The occipital region is the most common site, but cephaloceles can also occur in the sincipital, convexity, and skull base regions. Most cephaloceles occur in isolation, but some may be part of syndromes, such as frontonasal dysplasia and cerebro-oculomuscular syndrome.

Atretic cephaloceles are abortive rudimentary cephaloceles that contain meningeal and vestigeal tissues, such as neural and glial rests. These lesions are most commonly located in the midline parietal or occipital regions and can be associated with intracranial anomalies.

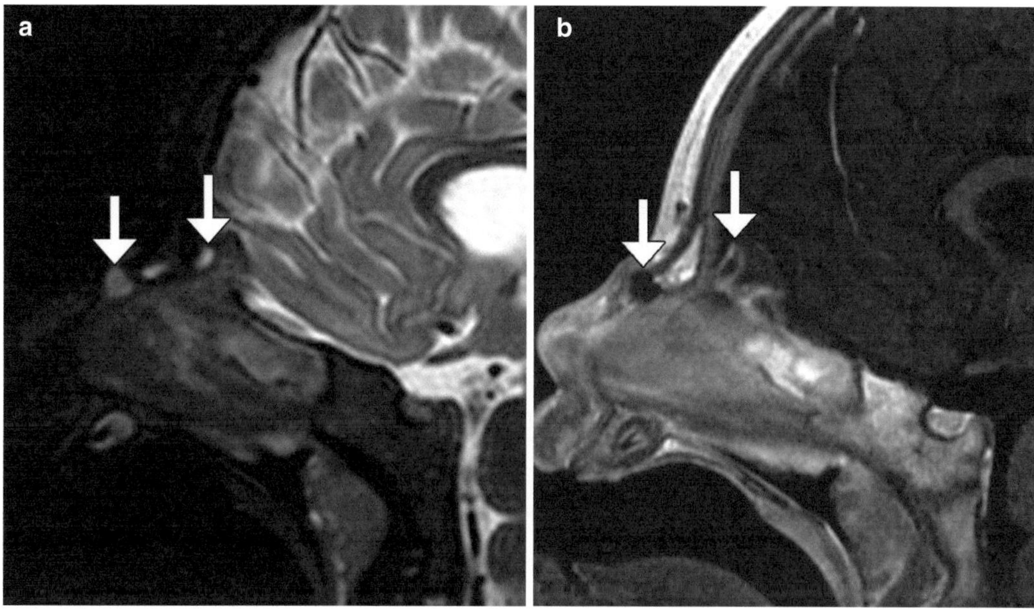

Fig. 2.16 Nasal dermal sinus. Sagittal fat-suppressed T2-weighted (**a**) and post-contrast T1-weighted (**b**) MR images show a dumbbell-shaped cystic lesion that extends from the midline nasal dorsum to anterior cranial fossa (arrows)

Fig. 2.17 Bifid crista galli. Coronal CT image shows a gap between the two halves of the crista galli, through which a dermal sinus tract passes

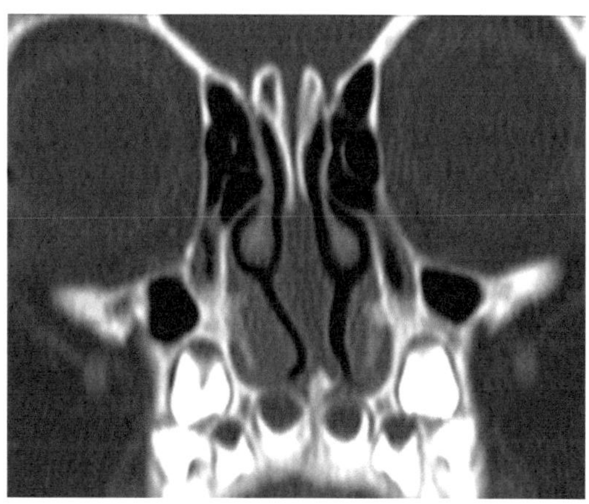

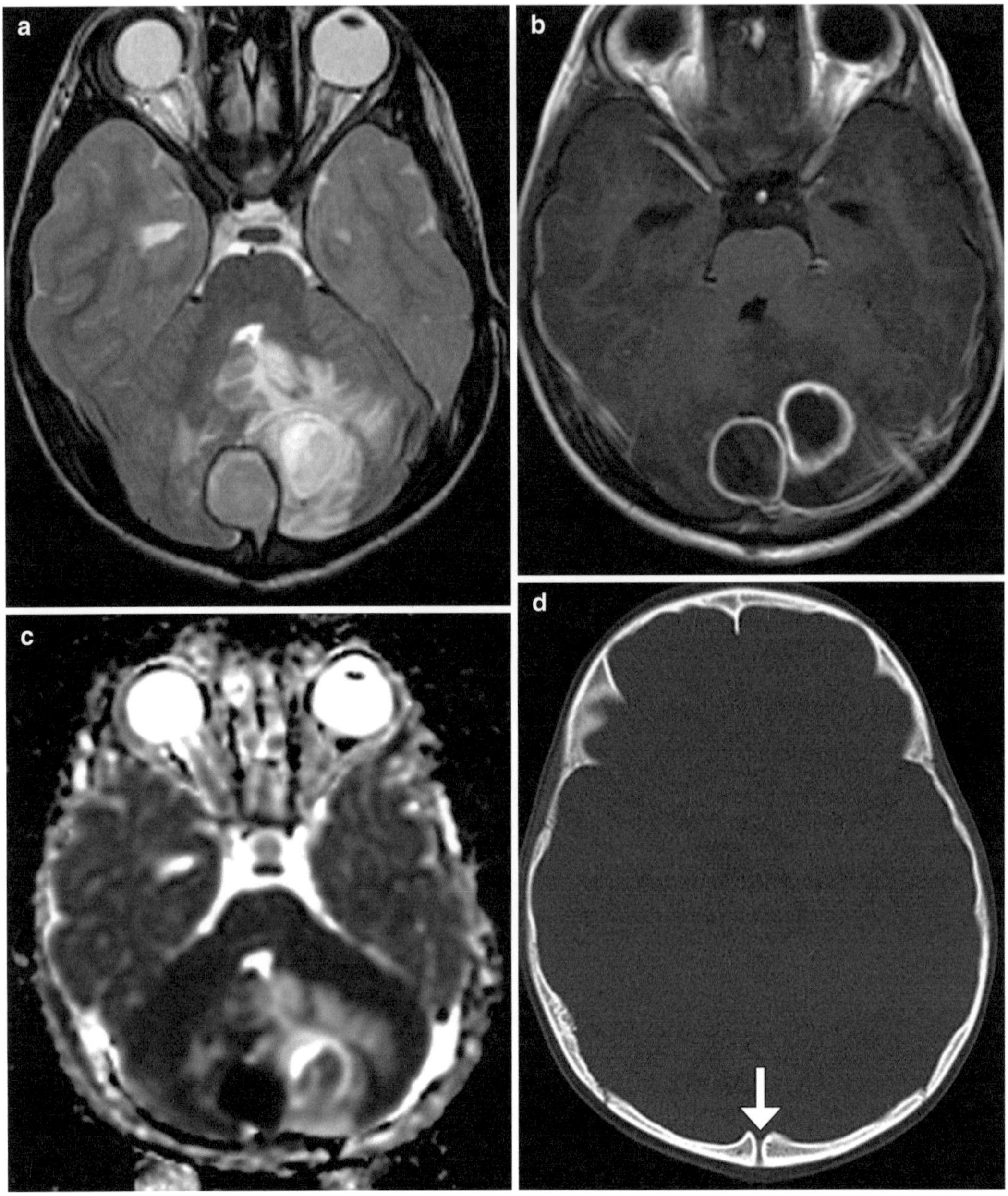

Fig. 2.18 Occipital dermal sinus with inclusion cyst and intracranial abscess. Axial T2-weighted MRI (**a**), post-contrast T1-weighted MRI (**b**), and ADC map (**c**) show a midline extra-axial posterior fossa cystic lesion with central restricted diffusion and extension into the occipital bone, as well as an adjacent left cerebellar abscess with surrounding edema. Axial CT image (**d**) shows a midline trans-occipital sinus tract (*arrow*)

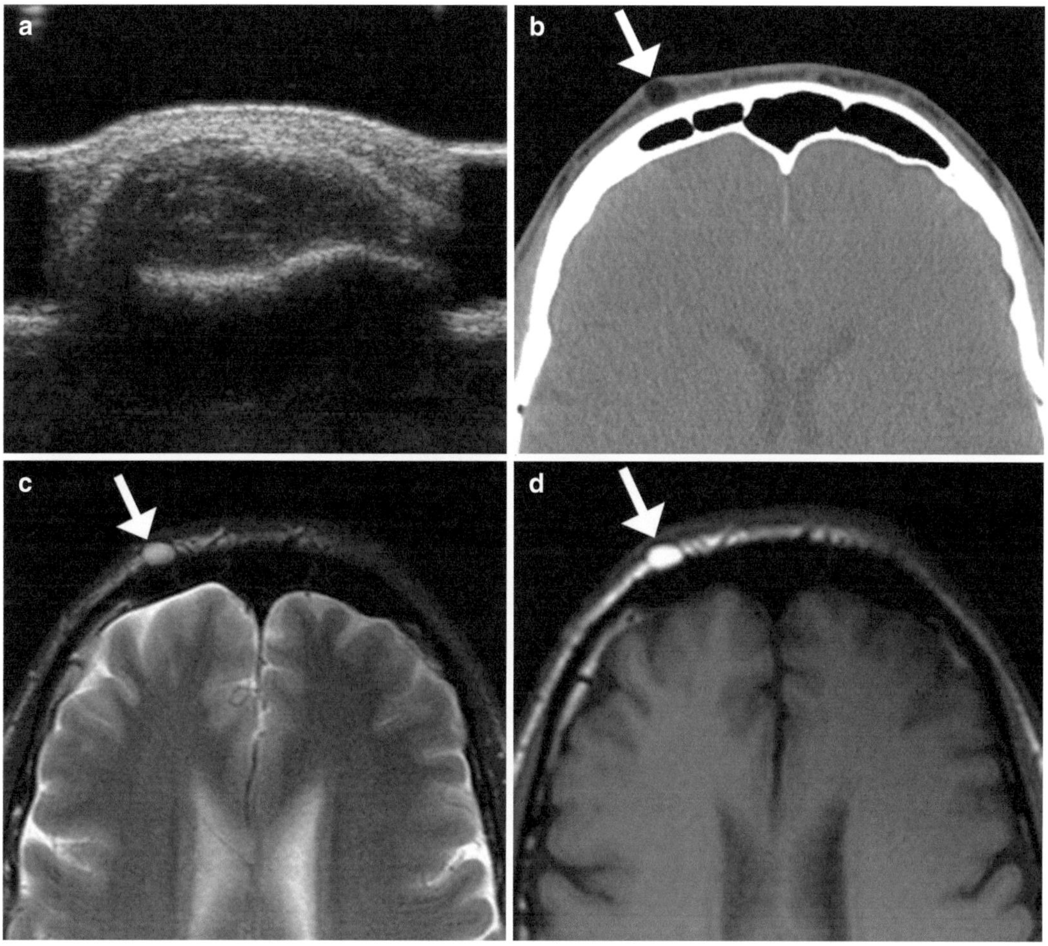

Fig. 2.19 Dermoid cyst. Ultrasound (**a**) of the right forehead demonstrates a well-defined superficial lesion that is less echogenic to adjacent subcutaneous fat. Axial CT (**b**) demonstrates a well-defined lesion anterior to the right frontal sinus of fat attenuation (*arrow*). The corresponding axial T2-weighted (**c**) and T1-weighted (**d**) MRI images show a fat signal lesion in the right frontal scalp (*arrows*)

Clinicopathologic Findings

Congenital cephaloceles may contain variable amounts of cerebrospinal fluid and intact brain or disorganized neural tissue. Clinical examination may reveal broad-based or pedunculated masses covered by skin that may be thinned, ulcerated, or infected (Fig. 2.20). Hemorrhage can occur if ulcers erode into vascular structures. The management and prognosis of cephaloceles depends upon the site, size and content, and the presence of concurrent intracranial abnormalities, such as hydrocephalus and agenesis of the corpus callosum.

Atretic cephaloceles may present as a subgaleal bulla or flat area covered by atrophic skin with alopecia or anomalous whorling of the surrounding hair (Fig. 2.21). Histologically, the lesions consist of fibrous tissue lacking cutaneous adnexal and neural tissue.

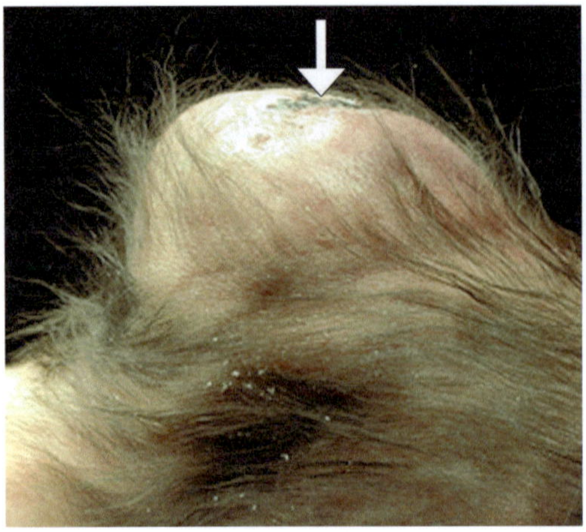

Fig. 2.20 Encephalocele. Photograph shows a large bulge in the occipital scalp with dark areas of skin necrosis (arrow)

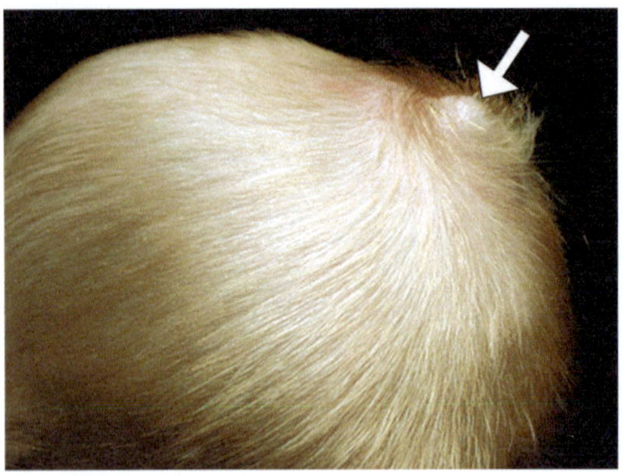

Fig. 2.21 Atretic encephalocele. Clinical photograph shows a raised area at the vertex of the head with focal alopecia (arrow)

Imaging Findings

Congenital cephaloceles may be initially discovered on a prenatal imaging or during the neonatal period. MRI is the optimal imaging modality for characterizing the contents of the cephaloceles and associated intracranial anomalies (Fig. 2.22). Contrast is generally not necessary for evaluating these lesions, unless a superimposed infection is suspected.

Atretic cephaloceles appear as nodular or flattened cystic or soft-tissue lesions in the midline parietal or occipital scalp that may be associated with fibrous stalks that extend through an open fontanelle or calvarial defect to the dura. The appearance of the atretic cephalocele can even evolve over time. There are often associated intracranial anomalies, such as porencephaly, callosal agenesis, and persistent falcine vein (Fig. 2.23). Therefore, neuroradiological evaluation of clinically occult intracranial anomalies is important for determining prognosis, rather than the presence of the scalp lesion itself.

Spinal Dysraphisms and Related Anomalies

Overview

Dysraphisms can be broadly categorized as open or closed (occult). Open spinal dysraphisms result from incomplete closure of the neuropore and manifest with a skin opening and exposure of the underlying neural tissue to the environment. Closed spinal dysraphisms result from incomplete disjunction between cutaneous and neural ectoderm, although some types may also contain interposed mesodermal elements that can account for the presence of mesenchymal components, such as with limited dorsal myeloschisis and lipomeningoceles. Closed spinal dysraphisms are covered by abnormal skin that can be associated with subcutaneous masses. Limited dorsal myeloschisis is a particular form of closed spinal dysraphism characterized by a closed midline skin defect and a fibroneural stalk that connects the skin lesion to the underlying spinal cord. Diastematomyelia, *or* "split cord malformation" consists of two hemicords that are either each contained within duplicated dural sacs separated by an osseous or fibrous septum or contained within the same dural sac. Diastematomyelia is often associated with spinal cord tethering and vertebral anomalies.

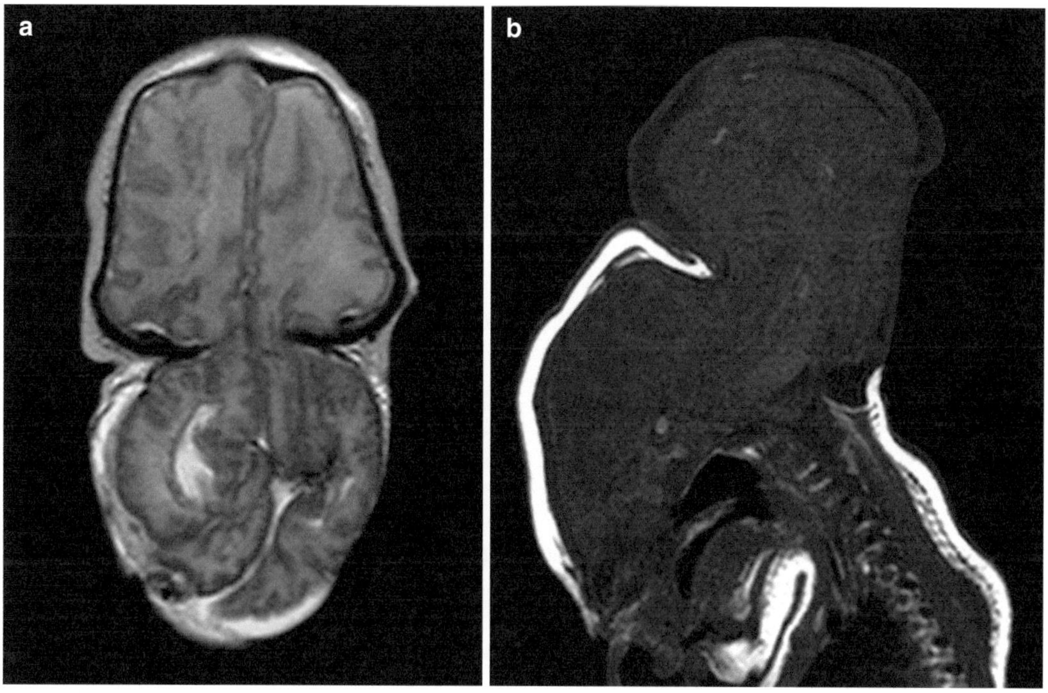

Fig. 2.22 Cephalocele. Axial T2-weighted (**a**) and sagittal T1-weighted (**b**) MR images demonstrate a large amount of herniated brain tissue along with a portion of the ventricular system through a midline defect in the occipito-cervical region

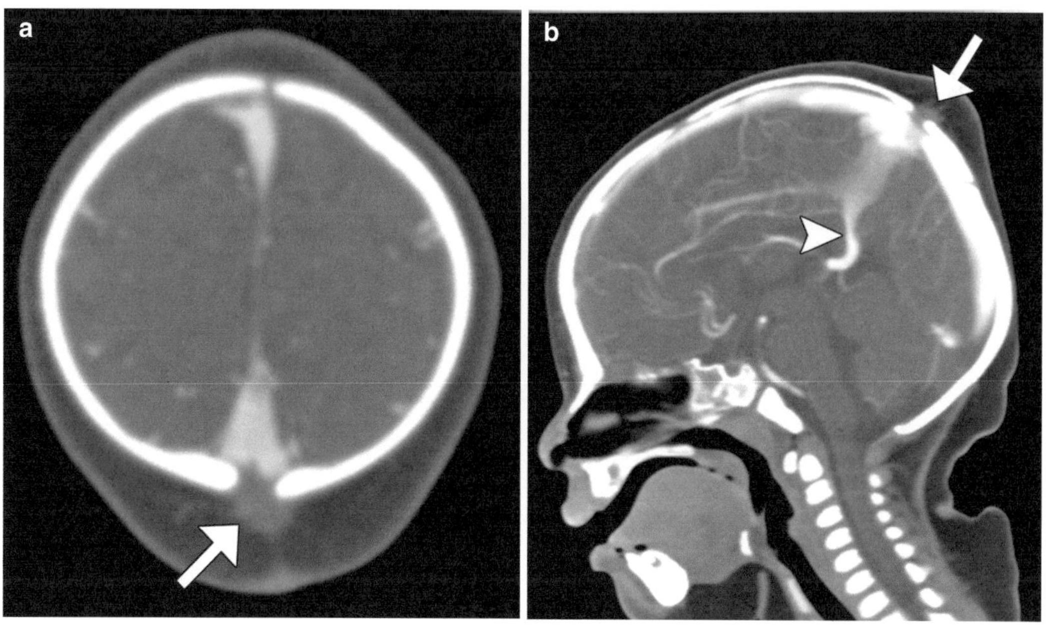

Fig. 2.23 Atretic cephalocele. Axial (a) and sagittal (b) CTV images show a soft-tissue lesion (arrows) in the scalp overlying the posterior fontanelle in an infant. There is also a falcine sinus (arrowhead)

Clinicopathologic Findings

Open dysraphisms (spina bifida aperta) includes myelomeningoceles and myloceles. The neural placode protrudes the skin surface with a myelomeningocele, but is flush with the skin surface with a myelocele. Myelomeningoceles are the most common form of open spinal dysraphisms and appear as openings in the skin with extrusion and exposure of neural tissues to the environment (Fig. 2.24).

Closed dysraphisms (spina bifida occulta) can present with a variety of cutaneous stigmata that can occur at almost any level of the neuraxis although most are located in the midline lumbosacral region. These abnormalities result from incomplete disjunction between the ectoderm and neural tube, although some types may also contain interposed mesodermal elements that can account for the presence of mesenchymal components, such as with limited dorsal myeloschisis and lipomeningoceles. Cutaneous stigmata include hemangiomas, hairy patches/faun tail, skin tags or vestigial tails, dimples, subcutaneous masses, cigarette burn marks, hyperpigmentation, aplasia cutis congenital, dermal sinus tracts, and deviated gluteal clefts (Fig. 2.25).

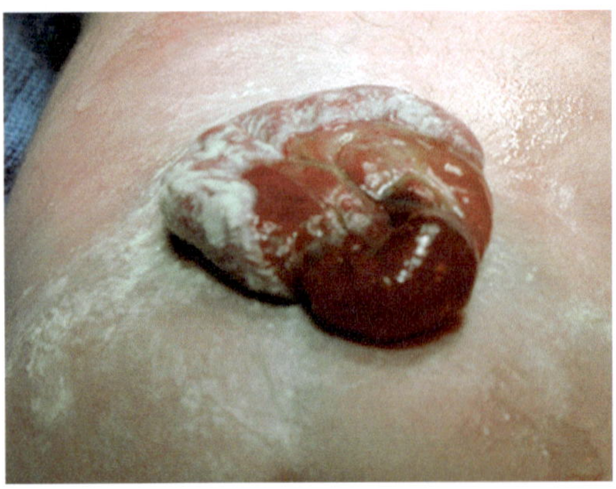

Fig. 2.24 Open spinal dysraphisms: myelomeningocele. The photograph shows herniation of neural tissue in the midline of the lower back with a lack of overlying skin

Imaging Findings

Open spinal dysraphisms can be diagnosed on prenatal imaging or are clinically evident at birth. MRI can demonstrate a posterior defect with a sac that contains cerebrospinal fluid and/or neural tissues with a lack of overlying skin covering in the setting of myelomeningoceles (Fig. 2.26). In terms of prenatal imaging, MRI can often provide additional anatomic information beyond that available with ultrasound, particularly intracranial abnormalities, such as hydrocephalus, Chiari type 2 malformation, holoprosencephaly, lipomas, and cephaloceles. Furthermore, there can be associated musculoskeletal, genitourinary, and gastrointestinal malformations. This additional information is relevant for counseling and early surgical planning.

Patients with suspected closed spinal dysraphisms may undergo imaging in order to characterize the type and extent of underlying spine anomaly. MRI is generally the modality of choice due to the excellent soft-tissue contrast capabilities. Alternatively, CT can be used to better delineate the osseous structural abnormalities, if needed. The imaging findings for the various types of dysraphism are described and depicted in the following sections:

- *Unfused spinous process*. This is a relatively mild form of dysraphism and may be encountered incidentally on imaging, but may be associated with other segmentation anomalies. The defect is best depicted on radiographs or CT and appears as an isolated gap in the spinous process without herniation of the spinal canal contents (Fig. 2.27).
- *Lipomyelomeningoceles and lipomyeloceles*. With lipomyelomeningoceles, there is a posterior spinal canal defect with lipomatous tissue covered by skin, such that the neural placode-lipoma interface lies outside the spinal canal due to expansion of subarachnoid space

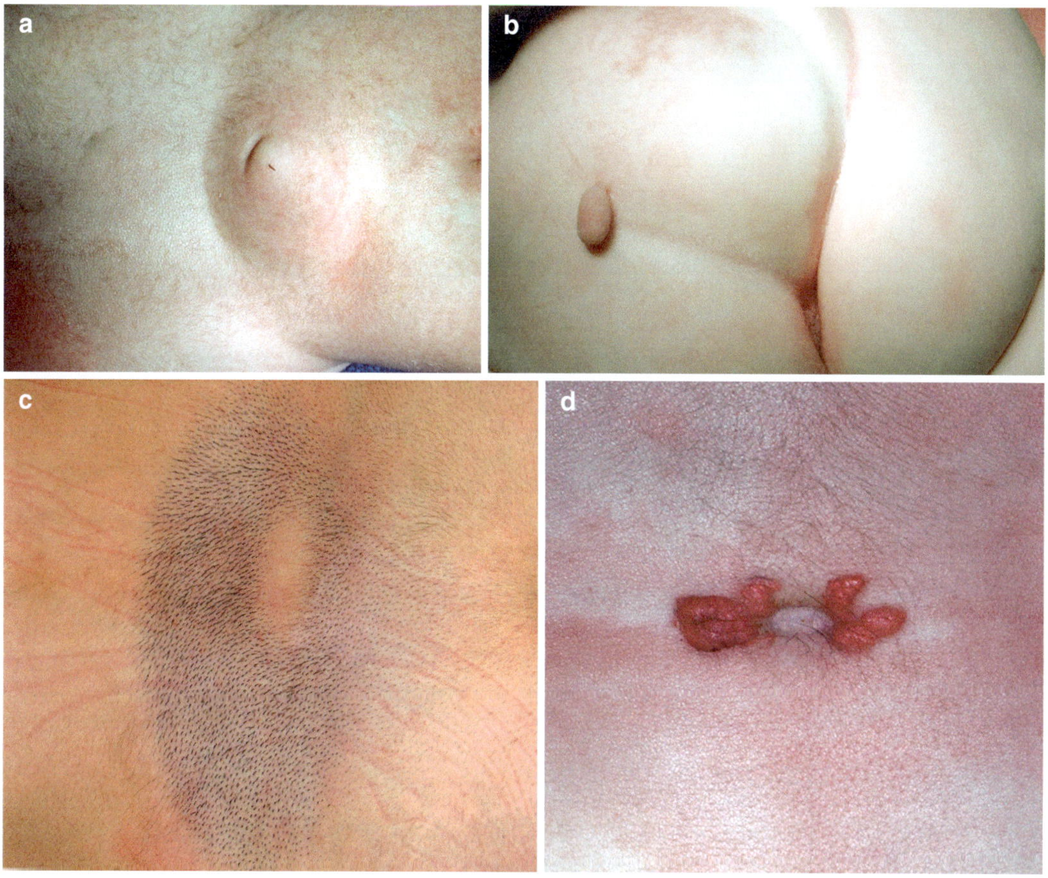

Fig. 2.25 Cutaneous stigmata related to closed spinal dysraphisms in different patients. Spinal dermal sinus and inclusion cyst: the photograph shows a midline back skin dimple associated with a subcutaneous mass (**a**). Subcutaneous lipoma and polypoid lesion: the photograph shows a subcutaneous mass in the lumbosacral region with an associated skin tag (**b**). Hairy patch: the photograph shows a patchy area of hypertrichosis in the lower back, which has been shaved down to the skin (**c**). Capillary hemangioma: the photograph shows a ring-shaped, flat, reddish vascular lesion in the midline of the lower back surrounding a circular area of skin depression (**d**)

(Fig. 2.28). With lipomyeloceles, there is also a spinal defect covered by skin and scattered lipomatous tissue, but the neural placode-lipoma interface lies within the spinal canal or at its edge without expansion of the subarachnoid space (Fig. 2.29). Both lipomyelomeningoceles and lipomyeloceles are often associated with a tethered low-lying spinal cord and/or syrinx.

- *Limited dorsal myeloschisis*. The solid, predominantly fibrous tract appears as a thin low signal linear band in the subcutaneous tissues of the back on MRI. The intrathecal portion of the tract typically attaches to the posterior spinal cord, just above the conus medullaris. MRI can also reveal a low-lying and fixed spinal cord, without or with an associated filar fibrolipoma (Fig. 2.30). However, conven-

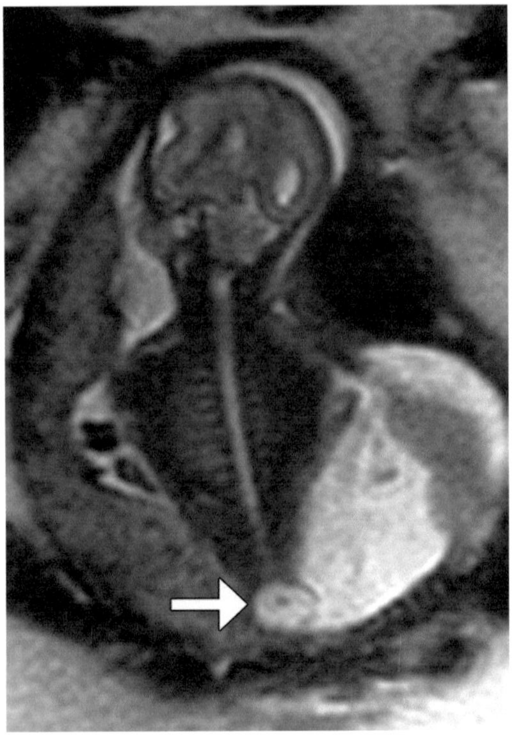

Fig. 2.26 Myelomeningocele. The fetal T2-weighted MRI shows a sac containing herniated neural elements in the lower spine (arrow)

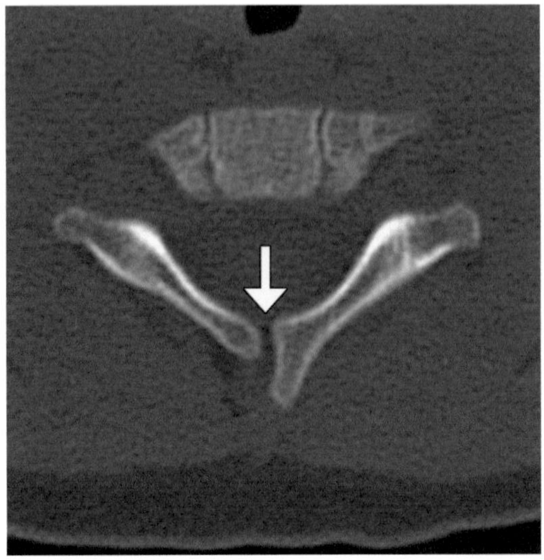

Fig. 2.27 Unfused spinous process. Axial CT image of a lower cervical vertebral body shows a cleft in the spinous process (arrow)

tional MRI sequences do not reliably depict the intradural extent of the tract. Administration of intravenous contrast and high-resolution cisternography-type MRI sequences can increase the sensitivity of MRI for detection of sinus tracts.

- *Spinal dermal sinus*. The fibrous walls of the dermal sinuses appear as relatively low T1 and T2 signal on MRI and may contain fluid, particularly if there is superimposed infection. The spinal dermal sinuses can have variable sites of intrathecal attachment and are often associated with inclusion cysts, which can even be intramedullary (Fig. 2.31). Although conventional MRI sequences are specific for the diagnosis of an inclusion cyst, the sensitivity is relatively limited. The use of high-resolution cisternography-type MRI sequences can increase the rate of inclusion cyst detection. Due to the heightened risk of infection, spinal dermal sinuses and associated anomalies require urgent surgical intervention.
- *Diastematomyelia*. Diagnostic imaging can be used to assess the severity of diastematomyelia, which consists of a longitudinally spit spinal cord. The two hemicords can be located in separate dural sacs, separated by fibrous or osseous spurs, or may be contained in a single dural sac (Fig. 2.32). CT can best depict the bony spur and associated vertebral defects, while MRI can best depict the extent of the spinal cord and dural abnormality.

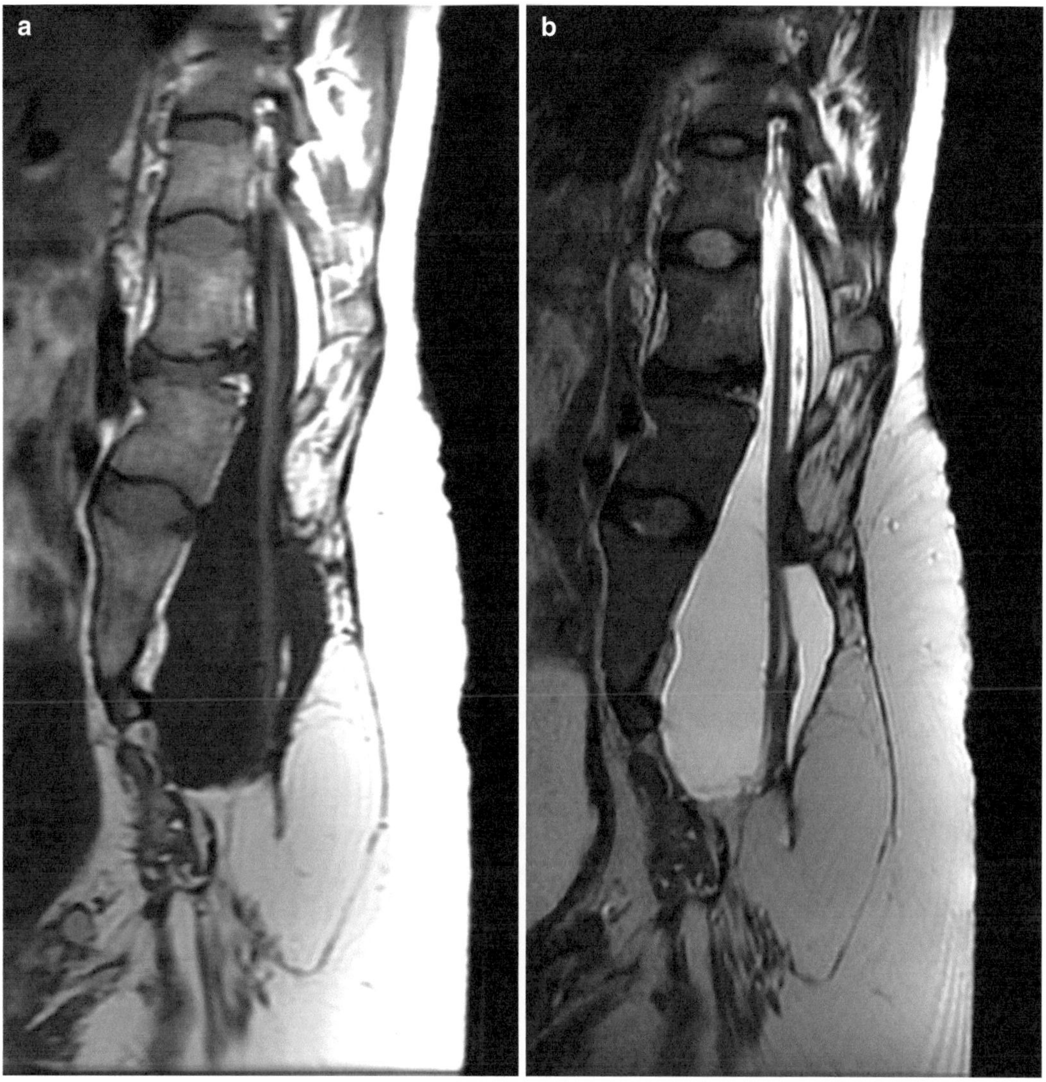

Fig. 2.28 Lipomyelomeningocele. Sagittal T1-weighted (**a**) and T2-weighted (**b**) MR images demonstrate a neural placode-lipoma complex contiguous with subcutaneous fat at the L5 through S3 vertebral levels. The lipoma is attached to and tethers the spinal cord

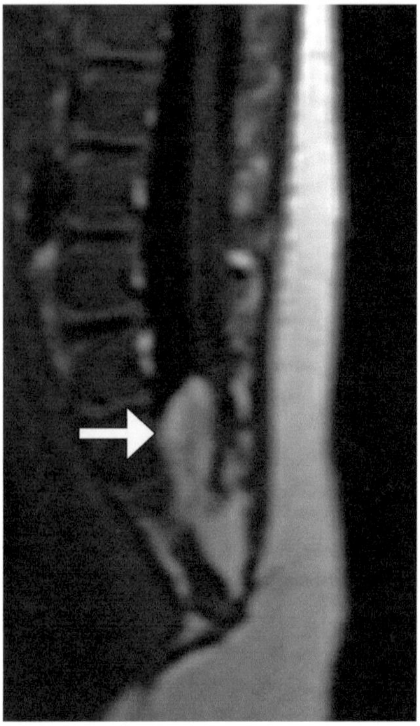

Fig. 2.29 Lipomyelocele. Sagittal T1-weighted MRI shows a lipomatous mass (arrow) in the lower spinal canal with overlying defect in the posterior vertebrae

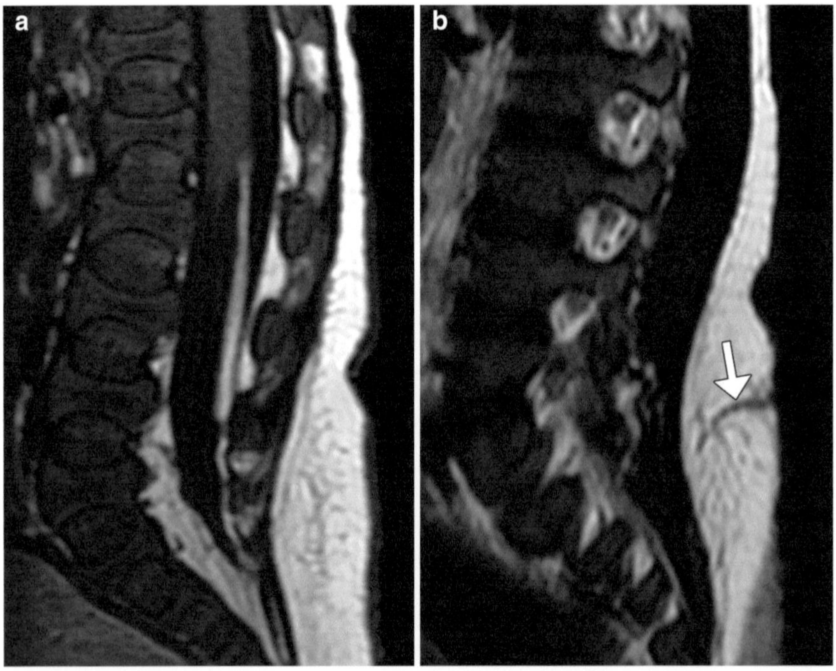

Fig. 2.30 Limited dorsal myeloschisis with tethered cord. Sagittal T1-weighted MR images (**a** and **b**) shows a filum terminale lipoma in a patient with tethered cord and a dorsal sinus tract (arrow)

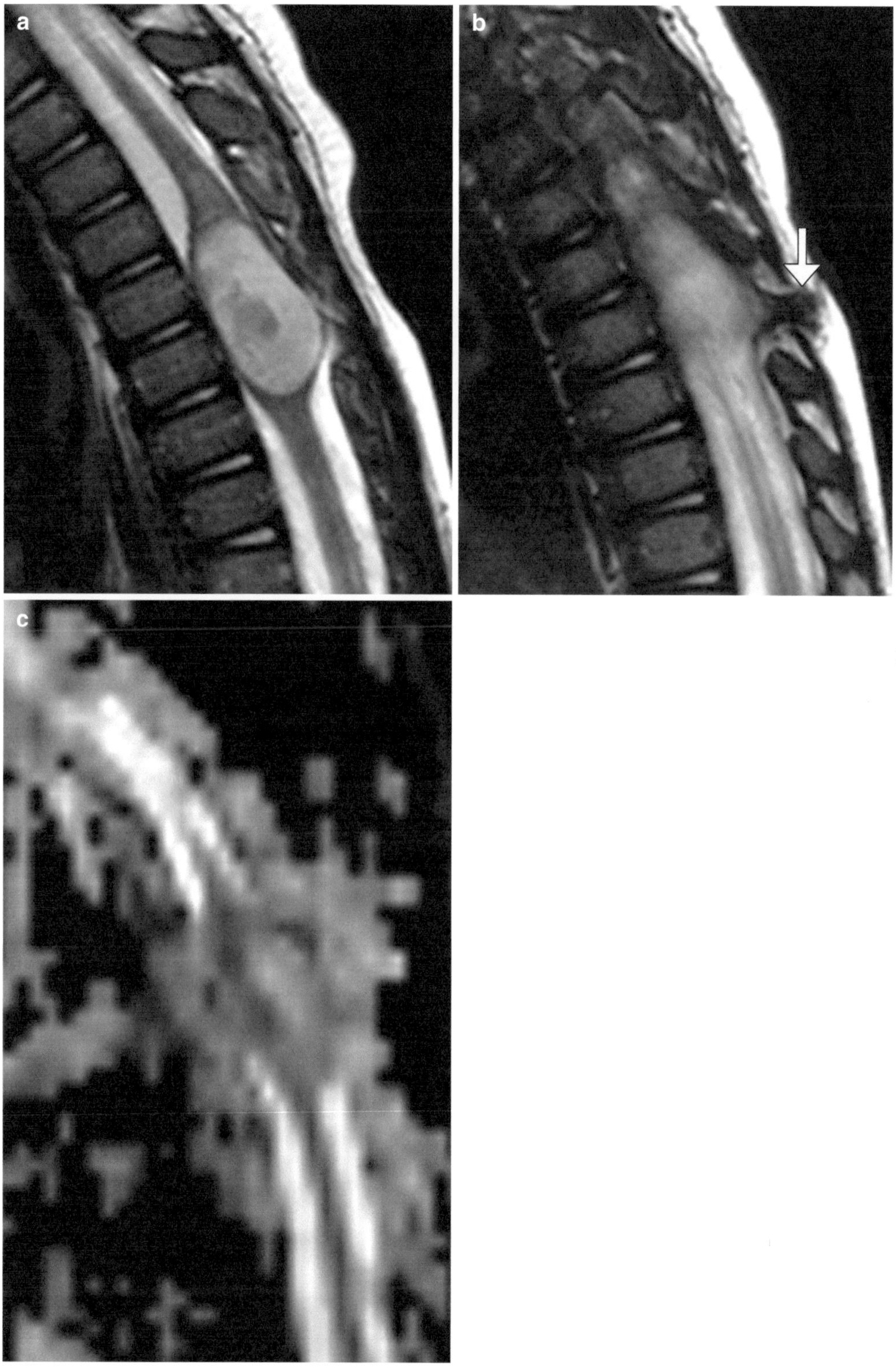

Fig. 2.31 Spinal dorsal dermal sinus with inclusion cyst. Sagittal T2-weighted MR images (**a** and **b**) show an intramedullary lesion connected to a dorsal dermal sinus tract that extends to the skin surface (arrow). The intramedullary lesion displays restricted diffusion on the ADC map (**c**) and represents an epidermoid cyst

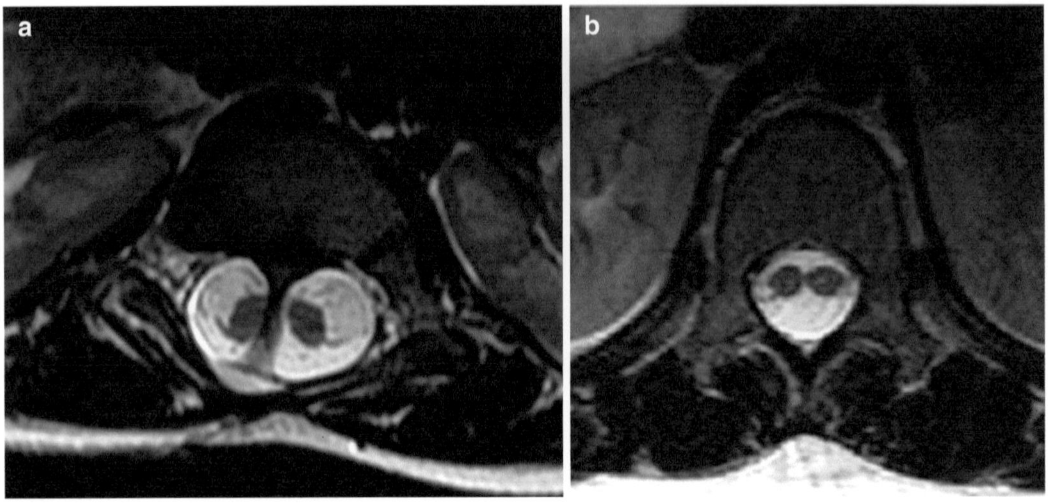

Fig. 2.32 Diastematomyelia. Axial T2-weighted MRI (**a**) shows a split spinal cord separated by a bony spur. Axial T2-weighted MRI in a different patient (**b**) shows two hemicords within a single thecal sac

Suggested Reading

Aaronson OS, Hernanz-Schulman M, Bruner JP, Reed GW, Tulipan NB. Myelomeningocele: prenatal evaluation--comparison between transabdominal US and MR imaging. Radiology. 2003;227(3):839–43.

Abbo O, Bieth E, Ballouhey Q, Vaysse F, Just W, Galinier P. Branchi-oculo-facial syndrome: a case report to highlight recent genetic considerations. J Plast Reconstr Aesthet Surg. 2012;65(11):1573–5.

Adams A, Mankad K, Offiah C, Childs L. Branchial cleft anomalies: a pictorial review of embryological development and spectrum of imaging findings. Insights Imaging. 2016;7(1):69–76.

Atlan G, Egerszegi EP, Brochu P, Caouette-Laberge L, Bortoluzzi P. Cervical chrondrocutaneous branchial remnants. Plast Reconstr Surg. 1997;100(1):32–9.

Bahrani B, Khachemoune A. Review of accessory tragus with highlights of its associated syndromes. Int J Dermatol. 2014;53(12):1442–6.

Barkovich AJ, Edwards MSB, Cogen PH MR evaluation of spinal dermal sinus tracts in children. AJNR Am J Neuroradiol. 12:123–9, January/February 1991; AJR. 156: April 1991.

Benson MT, Dalen K, Mancuso AA, Kerr HH, Cacciarelli AA, Mafee MF. Congenital anomalies of the branchial apparatus: embryology and pathologic anatomy. Radiographics. 1992;12:943–60.

Bromley B, Miller WA, Mansour R, Benacerraf BR. Prenatal findings of branchio-oculo-facial syndrome. J Ultrasound Med. 1998;17:475–7.

Brzezinski P, Chiriac AE, Chiriac A, Pinteala T, Foia L. Aplasia cutis congenita of the scalp - what are the steps to be followed? Case report and review of the literature. An Bras Dermatol. 2015;90(1):100–3.

Carter MT, Blaser S, Papsin B, Meschino W, Reardon W, Klatt R, Babul-Hirji R, Milunsky J, Chitayat D. Middle and inner ear malformations in mutation-proven branchio-oculo-facial (BOF) syndrome: case series and review of the literature. Am J Med Genet A. 2012;158A(8):1977–81.

Dias M, Partington M. Congenital brain and spinal cord malformations and their associated cutaneous markers. Pediatrics. 2015;136(4):e1105–19.

Drolet BA, Clowry L, McTigue MK, Esterly NB. The hair collar sign: marker for cranial dysraphism. Pediatrics. 1995;96(2 Pt 1):309–13.

Ginat DT, Johnson DN, Shogan A, Cipriani NA. Cervical chondrocutaneous branchial remnants. Head Neck Pathol. 2018;12(2):244–6.

Ginat DT, Robson CD. Diagnostic imaging features of congenital nose and nasal cavity lesions. Clin Neuroradiol. 2015;25:3–11.

Glass RB, Fernbach SK, Norton KI, Choi PS, Naidich TP. The infant skull: a vault of information. Radiographics. 2004;24(2):507–22.

Johnson JM, Moonis G, Green GE, Carmody R, Burbank HN. Syndromes of the first and second branchial arches, part 1: embryology and characteristic defects. AJNR Am J Neuroradiol. 2011a;32(1):14–9.

Johnson JM, Moonis G, Green GE, Carmody R, Burbank HN. Syndromes of the first and second branchial arches, part 2: syndromes. AJNR Am J Neuroradiol. 2011b;32(2):230–7.

Kaplan SB, Kemp SS, Oh KS. Radiographic manifestations of congenital anomalies of the skull. Radiol Clin N Am. 1991;29(2):195–218.

Koeller KK, Alamo L, Adair CF, Smirniotopoulos JG. From the archives of the AFIP: congenital cystic masses of the neck: radiologic-pathologic correlation. Radiographics. 1999;19:121–46.

Lam S, Barry J, Dauser RC. Dermal sinus tract: clinical presentation and imaging findings. Pediatr Neurol. 2014;51(5):747–8.

Lee SM, Cheon JE, Choi YH, Kim IO, Kim WS, Cho HH, Lee JY, Wang KC. Limited dorsal myeloschisis and congenital dermal sinus: comparison of clinical and MR imaging features. AJNR Am J Neuroradiol. 2017;38(1):176–82.

Morón FE, Morriss MC, Jones JJ, Hunter JV. Lumps and bumps on the head in children: use of CT and MR imaging in solving the clinical diagnostic dilemma. Radiographics. 2004;24(6):1655–74.

Naderi S, Nejat F, Shahjouei S, El Khashab M. Cranial dermal sinus: presentation, complications and management. Pediatr Neurosurg. 2012;48(2):86–92.

Naidich TP, Altman NR, Braffman BH, McLone DG, Zimmerman RA. Cephaloceles and related malformations. AJNR Am J Neuroradiol. 1992;13(2):655–90.

O'Neill BR, Gallegos D, Herron A, Palmer C, Stence NV, Hankinson TC, Corbett Wilkinson C, Handler MH. Use of magnetic resonance imaging to detect occult spinal dysraphism in infants. J Neurosurg Pediatr. 2017;19(2):217–26.

Pang D, Zovickian J, Wong ST, Hou YJ, Moes GS. Limited dorsal myeloschisis: a not-so-rare form of primary neurulation defect. Childs Nerv Syst. 2013;29(9):1459–84.

Perlyn CA, Schmelzer R, Govier D, Marsh JL. Congenital scalp and calvarial deficiencies: principles for classification and surgical management. Plast Reconstr Surg. 2005;115(4):1129–41.

Radmanesh F, Nejat F, El Khashab M. Dermal sinus tract of the spine. Childs Nerv Syst. 2010;26(3):349–57.

Raveh E, Papsin BC, Forte V. Branchio-oculo-facial syndrome. Int J Pediatr Otorhinolaryngol. 2000;53(2):149–56.

Rufener SL, Ibrahim M, Raybaud CA, Parmar HA. Congenital spine and spinal cord malformations - pictoral review. AJR Am J Roentgenol. 2010;194:S26–37.

Sewell MJ, Chiu YE, Drolet BA. Neural tube dysraphism: review of cutaneous markers and imaging. Pediatr Dermatol. 2015;32(2):161–70.

Singh I, Rohilla S, Kumar P, Sharma S. Spinal dorsal dermal sinus tract: an experience of 21 cases. Surg Neurol Int. 2015;6(Suppl 17):S429–34.

Siverino RO, Guarrera V, Attinà G, Chiaramonte R, Milone P, Chiaramonte I. Parietal atretic cephalocele: associated cerebral anomalies identified by CT and MR imaging. Neuroradiol J. 2015;28(2):217–21.

Smirniotopoulos JG, Chiechi MV. From the archives of the AFIP: teratomas, dermoids, and epidermoids of the head and neck. Radiographics. 1995;15:1437–55.

Tubbs RS, Wellons JC 3rd, Iskandar BJ, Oakes WJ. Isolated flat capillary midline lumbosacral hemangiomas as indicators of occult spinal dysraphism. J Neurosurg. 2004;100(2 Suppl Pediatrics):86–9.

Imaging of Neurocutaneous Diseases

3

James Tonsgard, Annie Xiao, and Daniel Thomas Ginat

Contents

J. Tonsgard
Department of Neurology, University of Chicago, Chicago, IL, USA

A. Xiao
Pritzker School of Medicine, University of Chicago, Chicago, IL, USA

D. T. Ginat (✉)
Department of Radiology, University of Chicago, Pritzker School of Medicine, Chicago, IL, USA
e-mail: dtg1@uchicago.edu

D. T. Ginat (ed.), *Neuroradiological Imaging of Skin Diseases and Related Conditions*,
https://doi.org/10.1007/978-3-319-90931-8_3

Abstract

This chapter reviews the clinical and imaging features of selected neurocutaneous diseases. The following conditions are included: Neurofibromatosis type 1, Neurofibromatosis type 2, Tuberous sclerosis complex, Sturge-Weber syndrome, Neurocutaneous melanosis, Basal cell nevus syndrome, Incontinentia pigmenti, Gardner syndrome, McCune Albright syndrome, Waardenburg syndrome, Oculocutaneous albinism, Marfan syndrome, Menkes disease, Sjogren-Larsson syndrome, and Ataxia-telangiectasia. Additional neurocutaneous syndromes are included in Chap. 7.

Neurofibromatosis Type 1

Overview

Neurofibromatosis type 1 (von Recklinghausen's disease) is the most common neurocutaneous disease with an estimated incidence of 1 in 3000 live births. Half of cases are familial, and the other half arise from de novo mutations. Neurofibromatosis type 1 is an autosomal dominant disorder due to a mutation on the long arm of chromosome 17, 17q11.2, encoding the protein neurofibromin, a RAS GTP activating protein.

Defects in neurofibromin result in overstimulation of RAS and results in abnormalities in cell growth and proliferation, including tumor formation. Since neurofibromin functions as a tumor suppressor gene, individuals with Neurofibromatosis type 1 develop various benign and malignant tumors.

Diagnosis

(1) Genetic testing is accurate in 95% of patients.
(2) Clinical Criteria (requires two or more of the following):

- At least six café-au-lait macules; greater than 5 mm in size prepubertal patients or greater than 15 mm in size in postpubertal patients
- At least two cutaneous neurofibromas or one plexiform neurofibroma
- Axillary or inguinal freckling
- At least two iris Lisch nodules
- Optic glioma
- Characteristic bony lesion (dystrophic scoliosis, pseudarthrosis, sphenoid dysplasia)
- A first-degree relative with Neurofibromatosis type 1

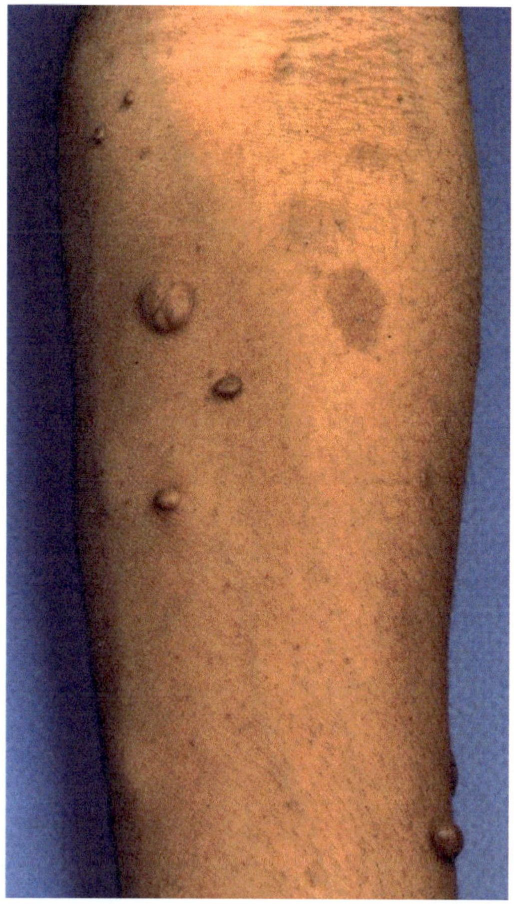

Fig. 3.1 Neurofibromatosis type 1. Photograph shows several hyperpigmented patches with smooth margins compatible with café-au-lait spots and multiple nodules that represent neurofibromas

Clinical Findings

The classic skin manifestations of Neurofibromatosis type 1 consist of café-au-lait macules and neurofibromas (Fig. 3.1). Café-au-lait spots often arise within the first year of life and increase in size and number over the first several years of life. Axillary or inguinal freckling often manifests later, by age 3–8 years. Cutaneous or dermal neurofibromas initially appear as purple or reddish, depressible macules and later as dome-shaped nodules (Fig. 3.1). Cutaneous neurofibromas usually do not become apparent until puberty and may continue to increase in size and number throughout adulthood. Plexiform neurofibromas have a variety of appearances: diffuse infiltrative lesions involving the surface of the skin, as well as deeper tissue, discrete enlargements of nerves or nerve roots, or thickened nerves with multiple nodular growths resembling grape-like clusters of lesions. Optic gliomas occur in 15% of patients and are grade I astrocytomas causing enlargement or thickening of the optic nerve or chiasm. The tumors are asymptomatic in more than half of patients. If visual compromise occurs, it is most likely between 18 months and 10 years of age. The vasculopathy in Neurofibromatosis type 1 is congenital and includes both aneurysms and steno-occlusive lesions.

Key Clinical Features: (1) Cutaneous Neurofibromas, 98%, (2) Cafe au Lait spots, 99%, (3) Plexiform neuofibromas, 50%, (4) Optic glioma, 15%, (5) Scoliosis, 25–50%, (6) Learning problems, 50–60%, (7) Epilepsy, 12%, (8) Malignant peripheral nerve sheath tumors, 9%.

Imaging Findings

Neuroimaging, including CT, MRI, and angiography, can demonstrate a variety of intracranial lesions associated with Neurofibromatosis type 1. These include neurofibromas, plexiform neurofibromas, optic pathway gliomas, central nervous system neoplasms, the so-called unknown bright objects (UBOs), vascular abnormalities, skeletal abnormalities including sphenoid wing hypoplasia, Chiari type I malformation, kyphoscoliosis, and dural ectasia. Selected lesions related to Neurofibromatosis type 1 are discussed further as follows:

- Localized neurofibromas can appear as enhancing nodules on MRI, but are most conspicuous on STIR sequences (Fig. 3.2). These tumors sometimes display a target-sign appearance, which appear as central low signal, but peripheral high signal intensity on T2-weighted sequences and is highly indicative their peripheral nerve sheath origin (Fig. 3.3).

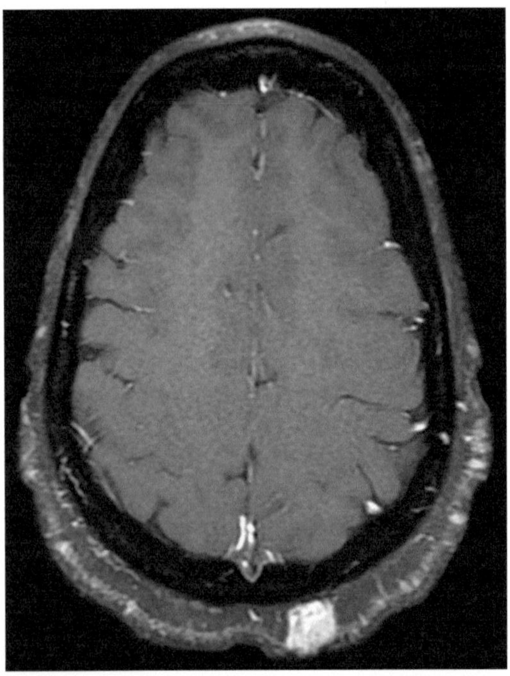

Fig. 3.2 Neurofibromatosis type 1. Axial fat-suppressed post-contrast T1-weighted MRI shows multiple enhancing scalp neurofibromas

- Diffuse neurofibromas involve the full thickness of the skin and appear as plaque-like or infiltrative enhancing lesions (Fig. 3.4).
- Plexiform neurofibromas have a variety of appearances. They may appear as enlargement of a dorsal spinal root often extending into the spinal canal with potential spinal cord compression, particularly in the high cervical spine and the lumbosacral region. Plexiform neurofibromas may also appear as beads along small peripheral nerves or as bulky tumors with a "bag of worms" appearance along major nerves (Figs. 3.5 and 3.6).
- Malignant transformation of plexiform neurofibromas and diffuse neurofibromas occurs in 9% of patients. Malignant transformation results in a Malignant Peripheral Nerve Sheath Tumor (MPNST). ^{18}FDG-PET/CT is useful for differentiating malignant peripheral nerve sheath tumors or neurogenic tumors with high risk for progression from benign neurogenic lesions in patients with Neurofibromatosis type 1 (Fig. 3.7).
- Optic pathway tumors typically appear as diffuse enlargement of the affected optic nerve, chiasm, and/or optic tract with high T2 signal on MRI (Fig. 3.8). The tumors may or may not demonstrate enhancement. There may be

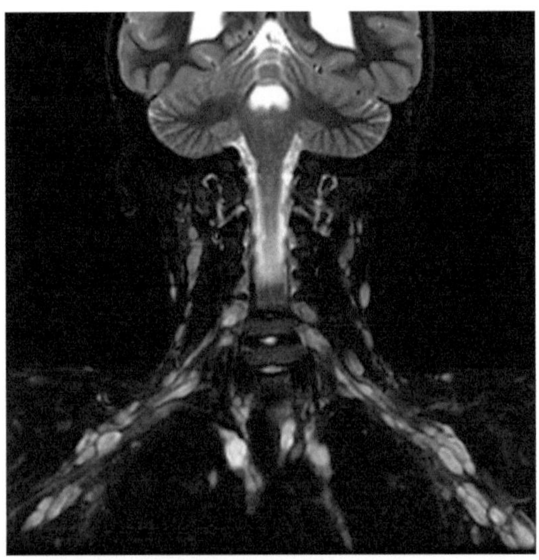

Fig. 3.3 Neurofibromatosis type 1. Coronal STIR image shows multiple hyperintense brachial plexus neurofibromas bilaterally

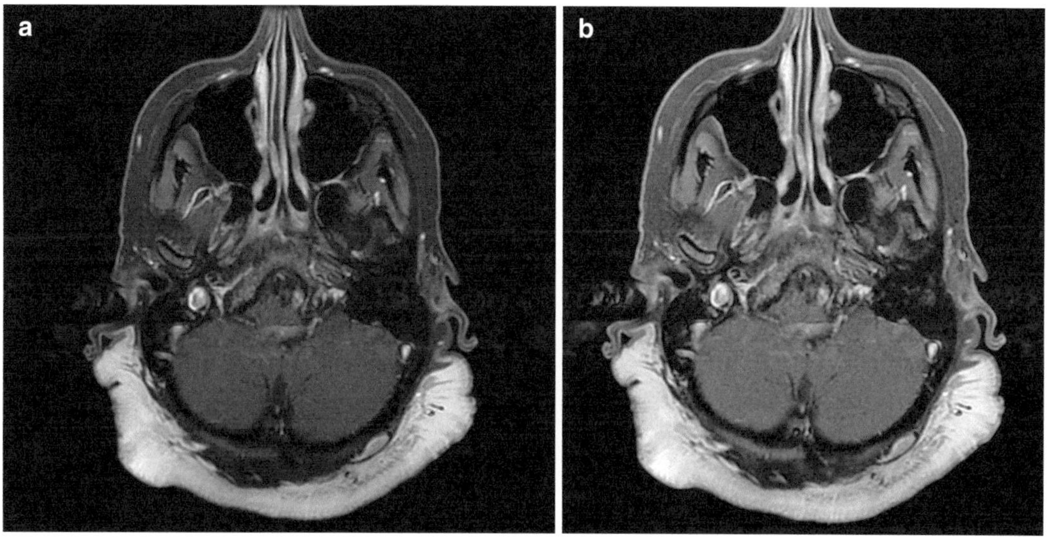

Fig. 3.4 Neurofibromatosis type 1. Axial T1-weighted (**a**) and fat-suppressed post-contrast T1-weighted (**b**) MR images show an infiltrative enhancing mass in the posterior scalp, which corresponds to a diffuse neurofibroma

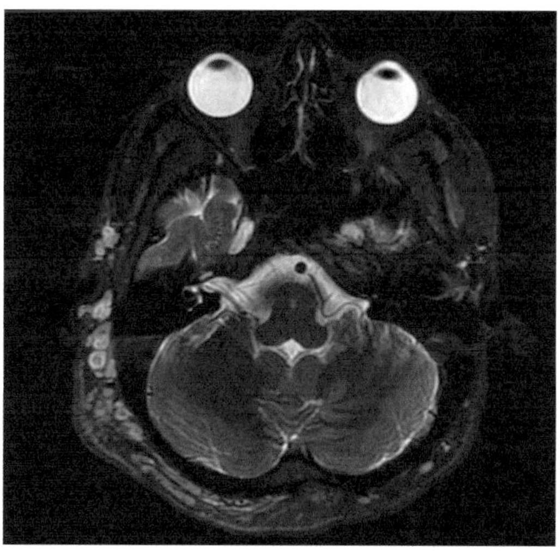

Fig. 3.5 Neurofibromatosis type 1. Axial fat-suppressed T2-weighted MRI shows an infiltrative and nodular right scalp mass, which represents a plexiform neurofibroma

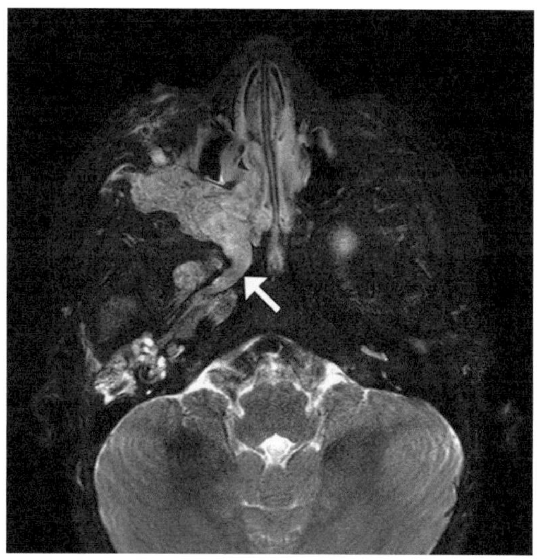

Fig. 3.6 Neurofibromatosis type 1. Axial STIR image shows a bulky mass in the right pterygopalatine fossa with a "bag of worms" appearance and extension along the right Vidian nerve (*arrow*)

associated tortuosity of the affected orbital portions of the optic nerves, prominence of the optic nerve sheaths, cystic components within the tumors, and variable degrees of contrast enhancement. Contrast enhancement is not predictive of growth or visual impairment. Besides optic pathway tumors, other parenchymal brain neoplasms occur in about 5% of patients with Neurofibromatosis type 1.

- Focal areas of increased signal intensity (FASI) or unknown bright objects (UBOs) are often apparent in the basal ganglia, cerebellum, and brainstem in pediatric and adolescent patients

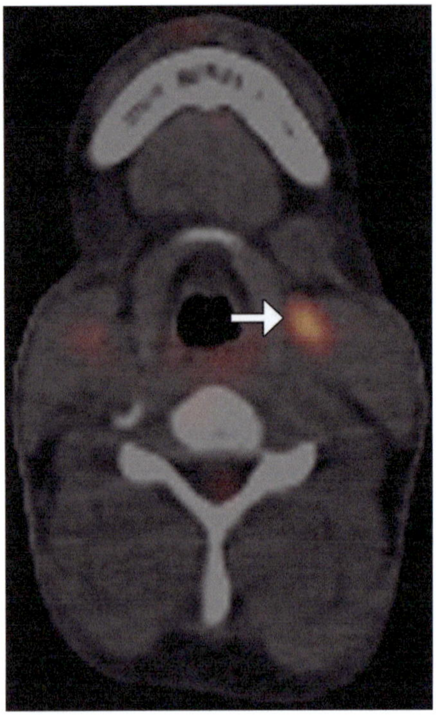

Fig. 3.7 Neurofibromatosis type 1. Fused ^{18}FDG-PET/CT image shows a hypermetabolic nodule in the left neck with an SUV of 7 that is consistent with a malignant peripheral nerve sheath tumor (*arrow*)

with Neurofibromatosis type 1. The lesions are hyperintense on T2-weighted sequences and do not enhance (Fig. 3.9). During childhood, UBOs can increase in size and number, but generally regress by adulthood.

- Vasculopathy in Neurofibromatosis type 1 can manifest as dolichoectasia and aneurysms, as well as steno-occlusive disease with development of basilar collateral vessels with a moyamoya appearance on angiographic imaging (Fig. 3.10). Perfusion studies are helpful in identifying the proliferation of small collateral vessels that can be a sign of amenability to surgical bypass procedures. Intracranial steno-occlusive disease is more frequent in patients who have other systemic vascular disease, such as renal artery stenosis or mesenteric artery or aortic disease.
- Sphenoid wing dysplasia consists of deformity and dehiscence of the sphenoid bone with expansion of the middle cranial fossa, which is best delineated on CT (Fig. 3.11). This can lead to herniation of intracranial contents into the orbit, resulting in proptosis. There is often an associated orbital plexiform neurofibroma.

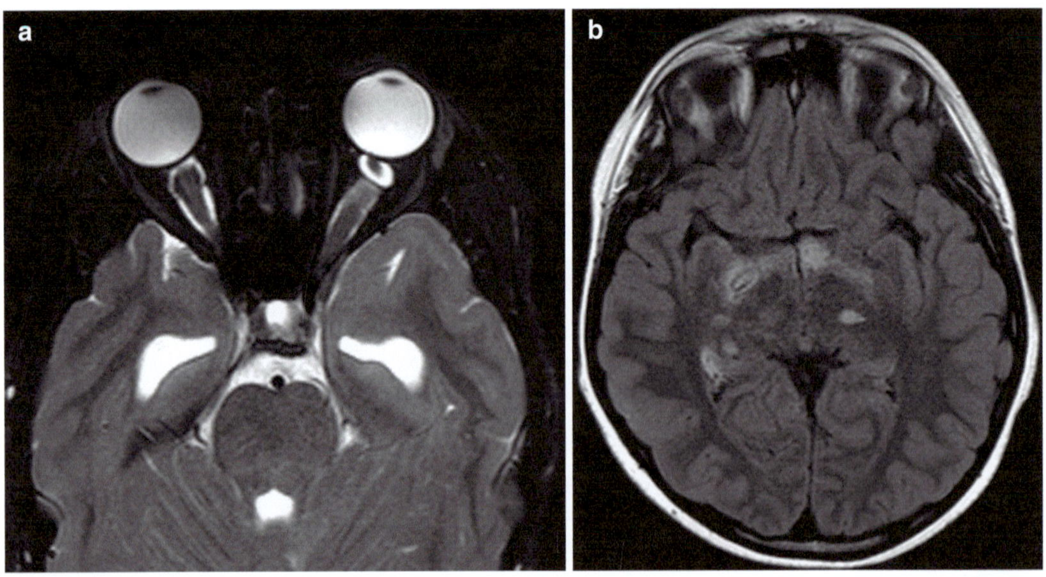

Fig. 3.8 Neurofibromatosis type 1. Axial T2-weighted MRI (**a**) shows diffuse enlargement and tortuosity of both optic nerves due to optic nerve gliomas. There is associated with prominence of the optic nerve sheath cerebrospinal fluid. Axial T2-weighted FLAIR MRI (**b**) in a different patient shows diffuse areas of signal abnormality along the bilateral optic pathways

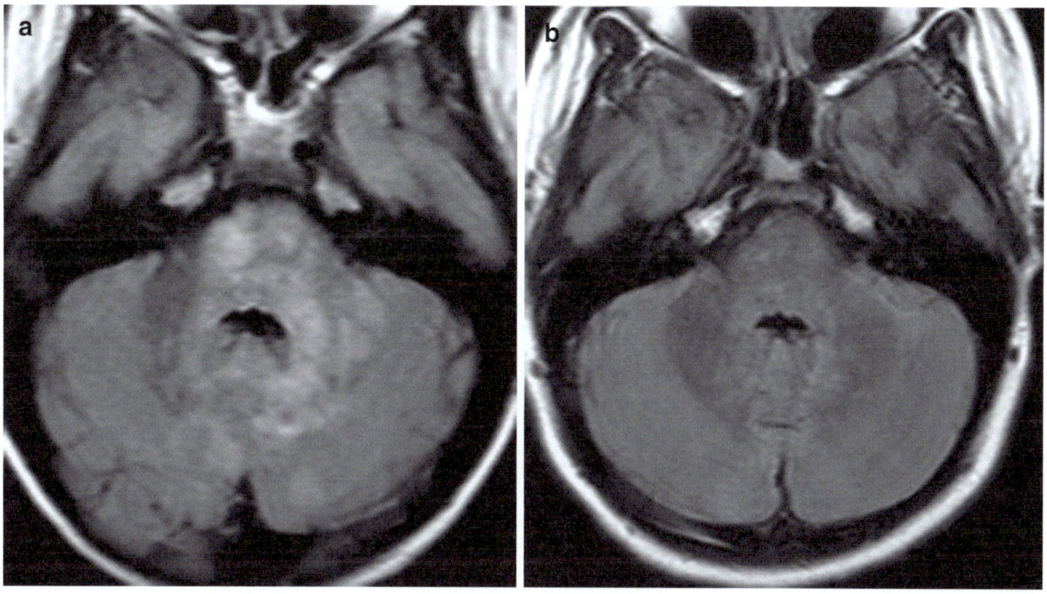

Fig. 3.9 Neurofibromatosis type 1. Axial T2-weighted FLAIR MRI (**a**) shows extensive patchy areas of high signal in the cerebellum and pons, consistent with UBOs. Axial T2-weighted FLAIR MRI (**b**) obtained approximately 5 years later shows substantial regression of the lesions

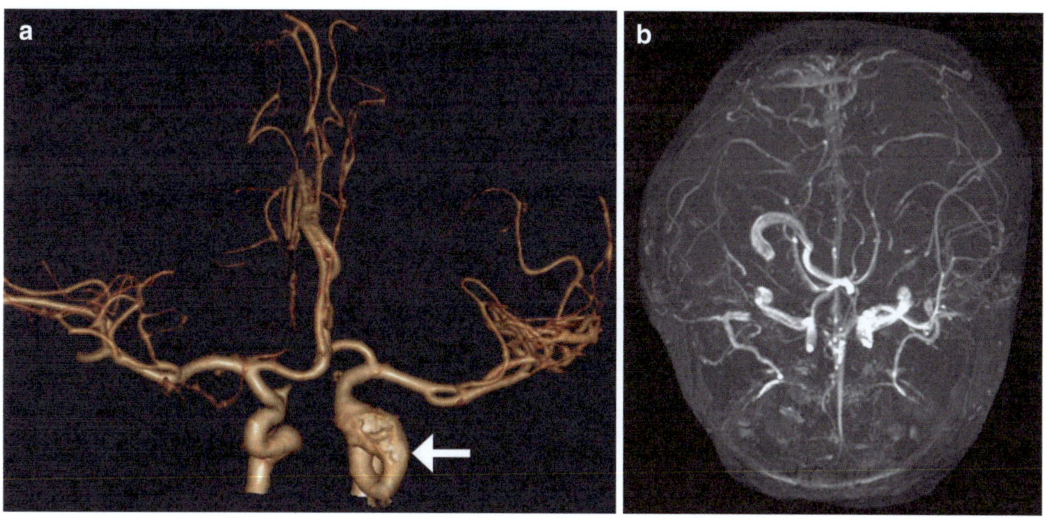

Fig. 3.10 Neurofibromatosis type 1. 3D CTA image (**a**) demonstrates a fusiform aneurysm of the cavernous segment of the left internal carotid artery (*arrow*). 3D MRA MIP image (**b**) in a different patient shows multiple steno-occlusive cerebrovascular lesions

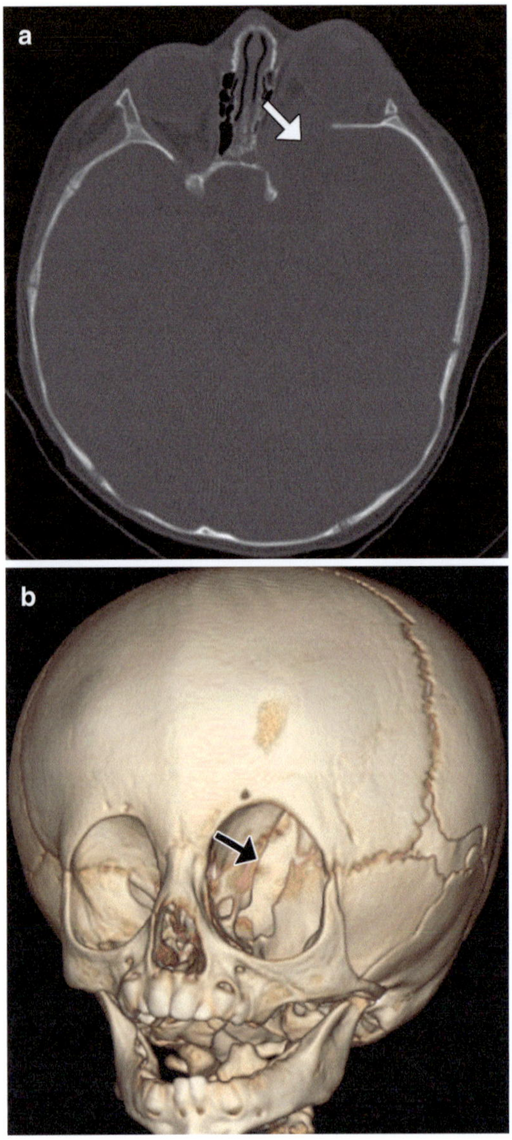

Fig. 3.11 Neurofibromatosis type 1. Axial CT (**a**) and 3D CT (**b**) images show left sphenoid wing dysplasia associated with widening of the superior orbital fissure (*arrows*) and proptosis

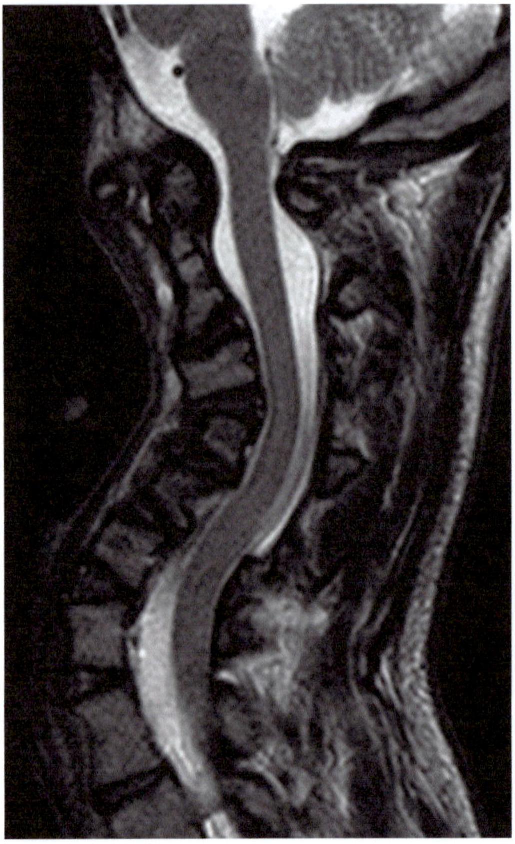

Fig. 3.12 Neurofibromatosis type 1. Sagittal T2-weighted MRI shows cervical kyphoscoliosis and dysplastic vertebrae

- Scoliosis is a common finding in Neurofibromatosis type 1 and may be due to idiopathic adolescent scoliosis, paraspinal tumor with vertebral erosion, or dystrophic scoliosis with abnormal vertebrae frequently associated with dural ectasia (Fig. 3.12). With dystrophic scoliosis, there may be associated vertebral subluxation, spinal cord impingement, or anterior meningocele formation.

Neurofibromatosis Type 2

Overview

Neurofibromatosis type 2 is an autosomal dominant disorder caused by a defect in chromosome 22q12 encoding the Merlin protein, which is a cell adhesion protein and tumor suppressor gene involved in the Hippo YAP pathway. The disease has a prevalence of 1 in 25,000 individuals and is characterized by multiple meningiomas, schwannomas, and ependymomas (MISME syndrome). Half of all cases are spontaneous mutations and a third of the new mutations are mosaicisms. There is substantial overlap between Neurofibromatosis type 2 and Schwannomatosis.

Diagnosis

(1) Genetic testing in blood or tumor samples positive in many. (2) Clinical diagnosis is based on any of of the following:

- Bilateral vestibular schwannomas before age 70 or a unilateral vestibular schwannoma with a first-degree relative with Neurofibromatosis type 2.
- Two of the following: meningioma, non-vestibular schwannoma, neurofibroma, cerebral calcification, or cataract, and either a first-degree relative with NF2 or a unilateral vestibular schwannoma and negative testing for Schwannomatosis (LZTR1 and SMARCB2) testing.
- Multiple meningiomas and a unilateral vestibular schwannoma OR multiple meningiomas and any two of the following: non-vestibular schwannoma, neurofibroma, glioma, cerebral calcification, or cataract.
- Pathogenic NF2 gene mutation in the blood or the identification of an identical mutation from two separate tumors in the same individual.

Clincal Findings

Adult patients with Neurofibromatosis type 2 generally present with hearing loss, vertigo, tinnitus, or symptoms referable to the brainstem. On the other hand, children tend to present with seizures due to meningioma, visual problems due to cataracts, or cranial nerve schwannomas, or rarely retinal hamartomas. Skin lesions occur in roughly two-thirds of patients. These can be subtle plaques, cutaneous tumors, or subcutaneous tumors (Fig. 3.13).

Key Clinical Features: (1) Vestibular Schwannoma, 95%, (2) Cranial meningioma, 50%, (3) Extramedullary spinal tumors (Schwannoma or meningioma), 80%, (4) Intramedullary spinal cord or brainstem tumors (ependymomas), 33%, (5) Cataracts and retinal hamartoma, 80%, (6) Skin tumors, 70%, (7) Seizures, (8) Cranial nerve palsies.

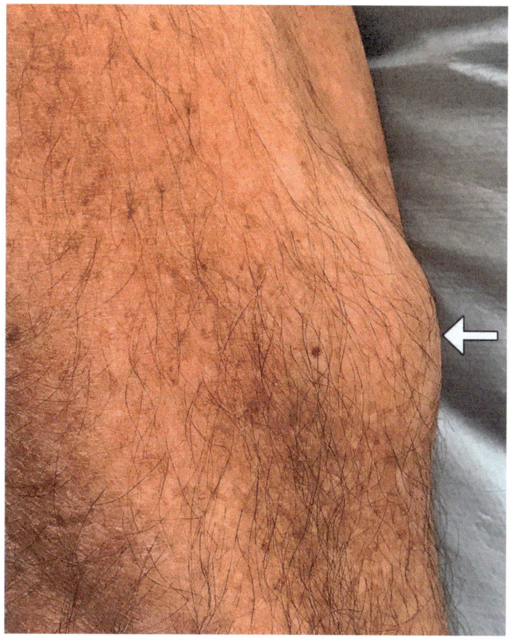

Fig. 3.13 Neurofibromatosis type 2. Photograph shows a subcutaneous mass without skin discoloration in the forearm (*arrow*), which corresponds to a peripheral nerve sheath tumor

Imaging Findings

Patients with suspected Neurofibromatosis type 2 should undergo high-resolution MRI of the internal auditory canals and brain with and without contrast. Patients diagnosed with Neurofibromatosis type 2 should also have an MRI of the entire spine with and without contrast. Surveillance imaging of the brain should be at 1–2 year intervals depending on the location and size of tumors. Surveillance imaging of the spine should be performed every 3 years depending on the presence of tumors.

Schwannomas usually appear as well-defined enhancing tumors on MRI (Fig. 3.14). The growth rate of vestibular schwannomas is quite variable, but the tumors often remain static for prolonged periods. Skin lesions in patients with Neurofibromatosis type 2 are also often schwannomas, which can appear as nodular or plaque-like enhancing tumors (Fig. 3.15).

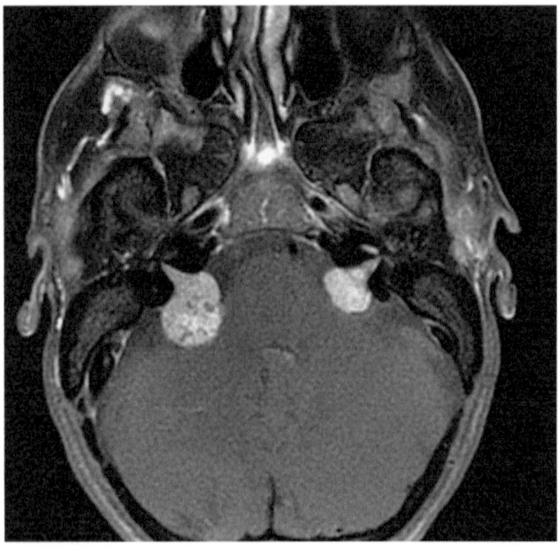

Fig. 3.14 Neurofibromatosis type 2. Axial fat-suppressed post-contrast T1-weighted MRI shows bilateral enhancing vestibular schwannomas

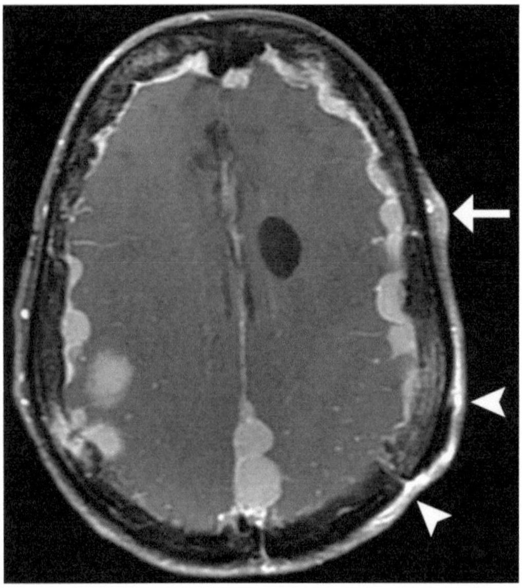

Fig. 3.15 Neurofibromatosis type 2. Axial fat-suppressed post-contrast T1-weighted MRI shows a nodular enhancing lesion (*arrows*) and a plaque-like enhancing lesion (*arrowhead*) in the left scalp. There are also extensive intracranial meningiomas

Meningiomas in Neurofibromatosis type 2 are found anywhere along the dura, including the optic nerve sheath and the thecal sac. On MRI, meningiomas typically appear as plaque-like or dome-shaped enhancing tumors with dural tails (Figs. 3.15 and 3.16).

Ependymomas in Neurofibromatosis type 2 are most commonly located in the cervicomedullary region, but can occur anywhere along the spinal cord and can be multifocal. On MRI, these tumors tend to appear T2 hyperintense with or without cystic areas, can be expansile, and show enhancement (Fig. 3.17).

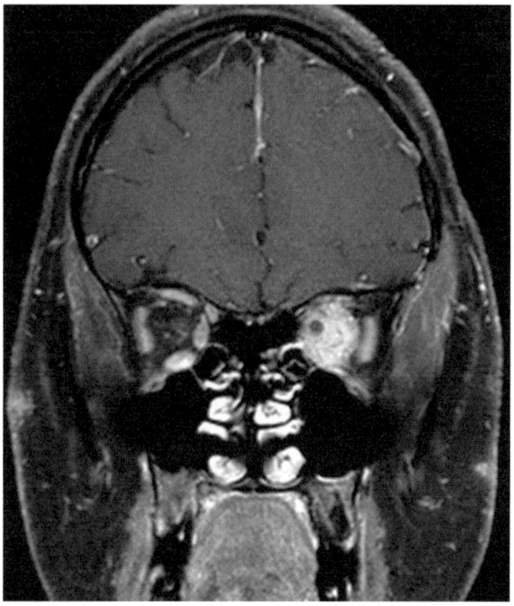

Fig. 3.16 Neurofibromatosis type 2. Coronal post-contrast T1-weighted MRI shows an enhancing mass surrounding the left optic nerve, which corresponds to an optic nerve sheath meningioma. There are also enhancing nodules in the facial subcutaneous tissues bilaterally

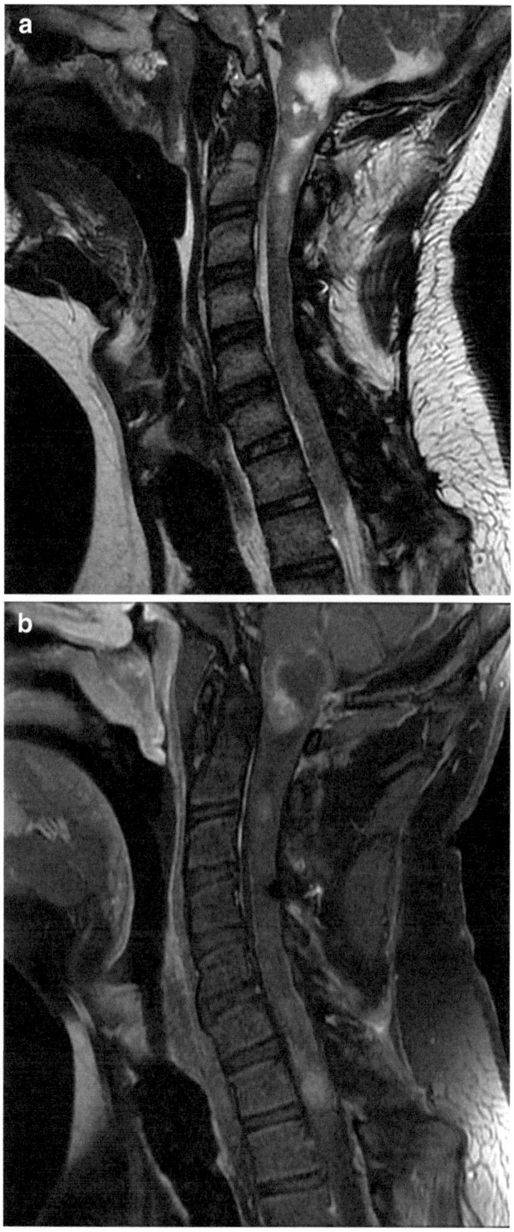

Fig. 3.17 Neurofibromatosis type 2. Sagittal T2-weighted (**a**) and sagittal fat-suppressed post-contrast T1-weighted (**b**) MR images show expansile enhancing tumors throughout the brainstem and upper spinal cord, which represent ependymomas

Tuberous Sclerosis Complex

Overview

Tuberous sclerosis complex, or Bourneville disease, is a progressive autosomal dominant disorder with an estimated incidence as high as 1 in 6800 live births. Tuberous sclerosis complex is caused by mutations in either the TSC1 gene on chromosome 9 or the TSC2 gene on chromosome 16, encoding the proteins hamartin and tuberin. These proteins are expressed in the brain and other tissues and function as a heterodimeric signaling complex. Expression is prominent in the embryo and is important in brain development and cellular organization. Hamartin interacts with ERM proteins, like in NF2, and regulates cytoskeleton-mediated processes, while tuberin appears to be a GTPase activating protein. The hamartin/tuberin complex is an important negative regulator of mTOR. The incidence of tuberous sclerosis complex is estimated to be between 1 in 6800 and 1 in 17,300 live births. The severity and presentation of TSC is highly variable between individuals and between affected families. In general, patients with mutations in the TSC 2 gene have more severe manifestations.

Diagnosis

(1) Genetic testing positive in 85–90%, (2) Clinical Criteria (two major or one major and two minor): Major criteria include facial angiofibroma, ungual fibroma, Shagreen patch, hypopigmented spots, cortical tubers, subependymal nodules, SEGA, retinal hamartoma, cardiac rhabdomyoma, renal angiolipoma, pulmonary

leiomyoma. Minor criteria include dental enamel pits, hamartomas, gingival fibroma, confetti skin lesion, renal cysts.

- Shagreen patches are thick, slightly elevated flesh colored macules that are usually located in the lumbosacral region.

Clinical Findings

Tuberous sclerosis complex can involve multiple organs including the brain, kidney, heart, lungs, and skin. Seizures occur in almost all patients and mental retardation affects slightly more than half of patients. A variety of skin lesions are associated with tuberous sclerosis complex, including the following:

- Cortical tubers in 60–90%, Subependymal giant cell astrocytoma (SEGA) in 15%, Subependymal nodules, 50%, Epilepsy, 60–90%, Mental retardation, 45%, Rhabdomyoma of heart, 50%, angiomyolipoma of kidneys, 70–80%. Hypomelanotic macules (ash leaf spots) are present in 60–90% of patients.
- Multiple small clustered hypomelanotic macules ("confetti" spots) are present in half of patients.
- Adenoma sebaceum are small red-pink flat topped lesions that are distributed in a butterfly-like distribution on the face (Fig. 3.18). These lesions appear during late childhood in 70% of patients. Fibrous plaques are similar, usually appearing in late childhood or adult years in 19%. Both adenoma sebaceum and fibrous plaques are angiofibromas characterized by a proliferation of connective tissue and vascular tissue.
- Ungual fibromas of the nail bed are also angiofibromas and appear in late adolescence (Fig. 3.19).

Imaging Findings

Characteristic tuberous sclerosis complex brain lesions include cortical tubers, subependymal nodules, and subependymal giant cell astrocytomas (SEGAs):

- Tubers, which consist of abnormal neurons and glia with disorganization of the corticaal layers, appear as T2 hyperintense lesions in the cortical and subcortical region with blurring of the gray-white matter junction (Fig. 3.20). These are often multiple and supratentorial. Tubers occasionally contain calcifications and enhance.
- Subependymal nodules are one of the earliest radiologic manifestations of tuberous sclerosis complex. The nodules are typically subcentimeter, often enhance, and are often calcified (Figs. 3.21 and 3.22).
- Subependymal giant cell astrocytomas appear as enhancing tumors typically located at the caudothalamic groove, adjacent to the foramen of Monro (Fig. 3.23). Besides the classic location, a cutoff size ranging between 5 and 10 mm may be used to differentiate subependymal giant cell astrocytomas (SEGAs) from subependymal nodules. Patients should have brain imaging performed every 1–3 years to look for subependymal giant cell astrocytomas.

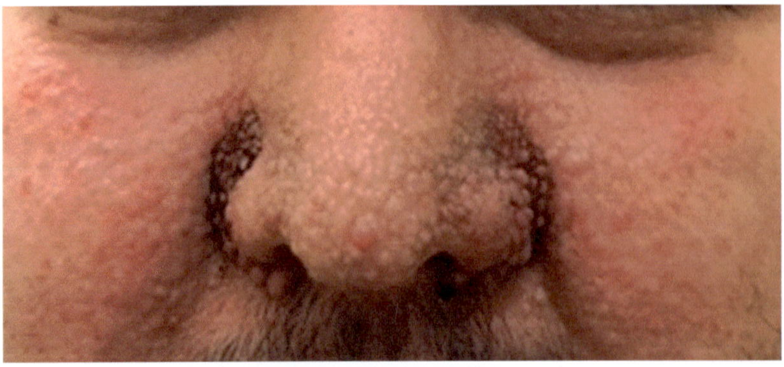

Fig. 3.18 Tuberous sclerosis complex. Photograph shows multiple papules in the midface that represent angiofibromas

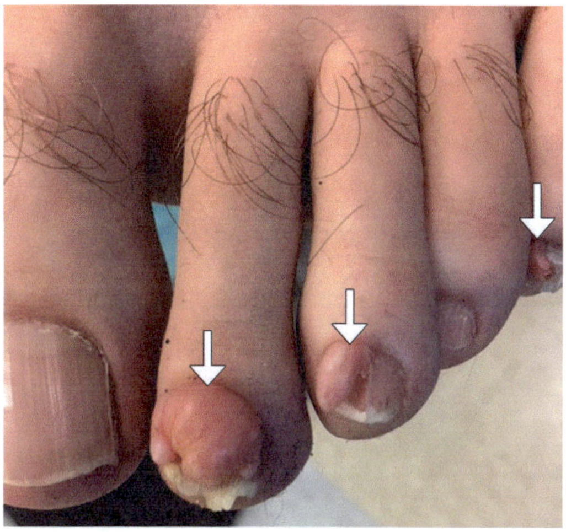

Fig. 3.19 Tuberous sclerosis complex. Photograph shows multiple periungual fibromas (*arrows*)

- Although facial angiofibromas may not be discernible on neuroimaging, patients sometimes have hamartomas in the scalp, which may contain fat (Fig. 3.22).

Sturge-Weber Syndrome

Overview

Sturge-Weber syndrome (encephalotrigeminal angiomatosis) is a sporadic disorder with an incidence of 1 in 50,000 live births. While the cause of Sturge-Weber syndrome is unknown, a developmental defect of the embryonic vascular plexus in the cephalic mesenchyme adjacent to the telencephalic vesicle is postulated. It is hypothesized that abnormal regulation of blood vessels and extracellular matrix expression produces tortuous vessels in the leptomeninges with sluggish flow that results in progressive ischemia of the underlying cortex. The hallmark feature of Sturge-Weber syndrome is a facial cutaneous venous malformation, known as nevus flammeus or port-wine stain (which is sometimes absent). The defining feature of the syndrome is the leptomeningeal angioma.

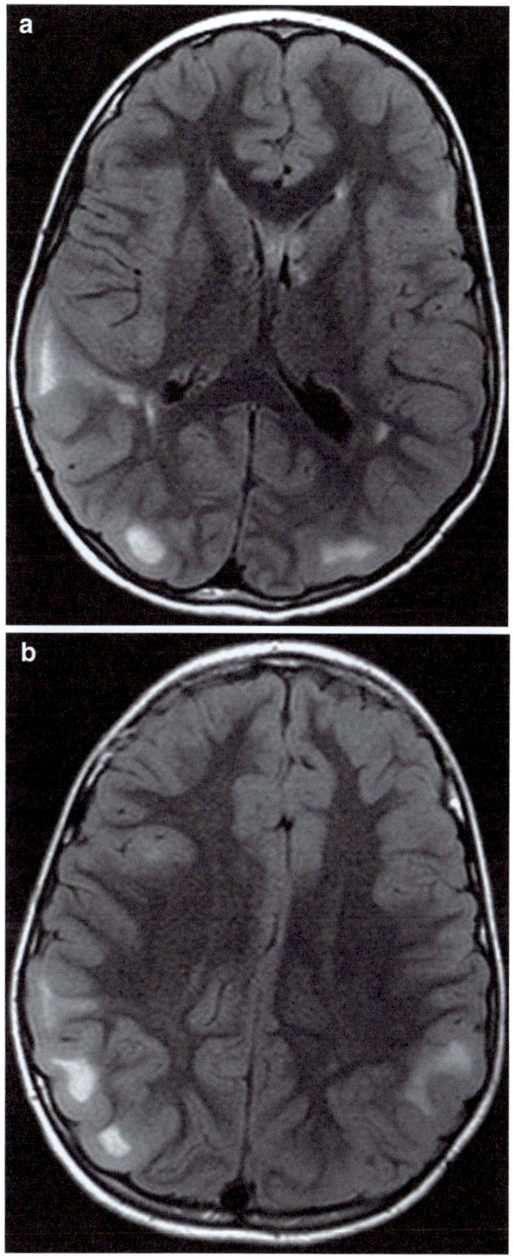

Fig. 3.20 Tuberous sclerosis complex. Axial T2-weighted FLAIR MR images (**a** and **b**) show multiple hyperintense cortical and subcortical tubers in the brain, some of which demonstrate linear extensions directed towards the ventricles

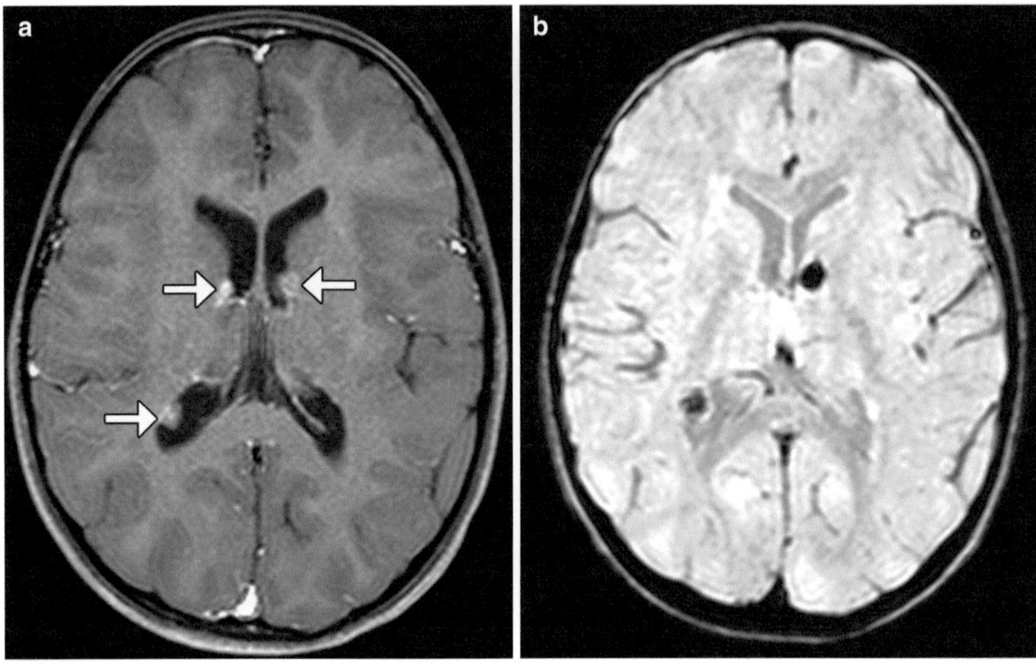

Fig. 3.21 Tuberous sclerosis complex. Axial post-contrast T1-weighted MRI (**a**) shows enhancing subependymal nodules along the margins of the lateral ventricles bilaterally (*arrows*). The corresponding SWI sequence (**b**) shows low signal in some of the nodules related to the presence of calcifications

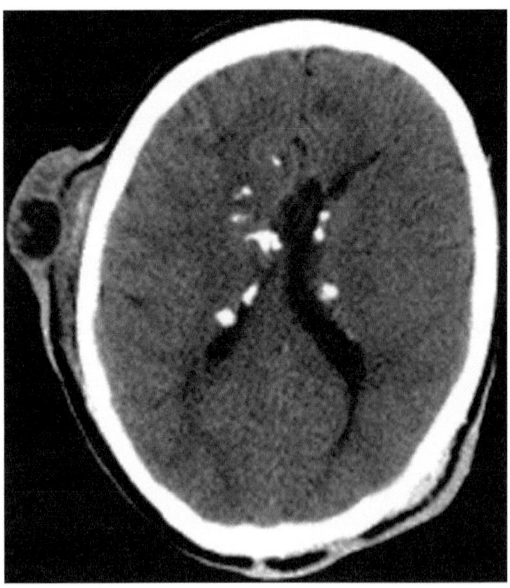

Fig. 3.22 Tuberous sclerosis complex. Axial CT image shows numerous calcified subependymal nodules. There is also a heterogeneous right scalp mass that represents a hamartoma

Diagnosis

The Diagnosis is made on the basis of the cortical leptomeningeal angioma.

Clinical Findings

- Facial capillary cutaneous angioma (port-wine stain), which is usually unilateral and involves at least the ophthalmic division of the trigeminal nerve dermatome distribution (Fig. 3.24).
- Hemiplegia contralateral to the leptomeningeal angioma due to progressive ischemia of the underlying cortex.
- Epilepsy.
- Variable degrees of mental retardation.
- Choroidal vascular malformations, which are on the same side as the facial capillary malformation in 70% of patients with Sturge-Weber syndrome.
- Glaucoma.

Imaging Findings

Dystrophic gyriform calcifications related to chronic ischemia results in the so-called tram-track sign visible on CT or even radiographs (Fig. 3.25). However, calcifications are not present in most patients younger than 2 years of age. Contrast-enhanced MRI is useful to depict abnor-

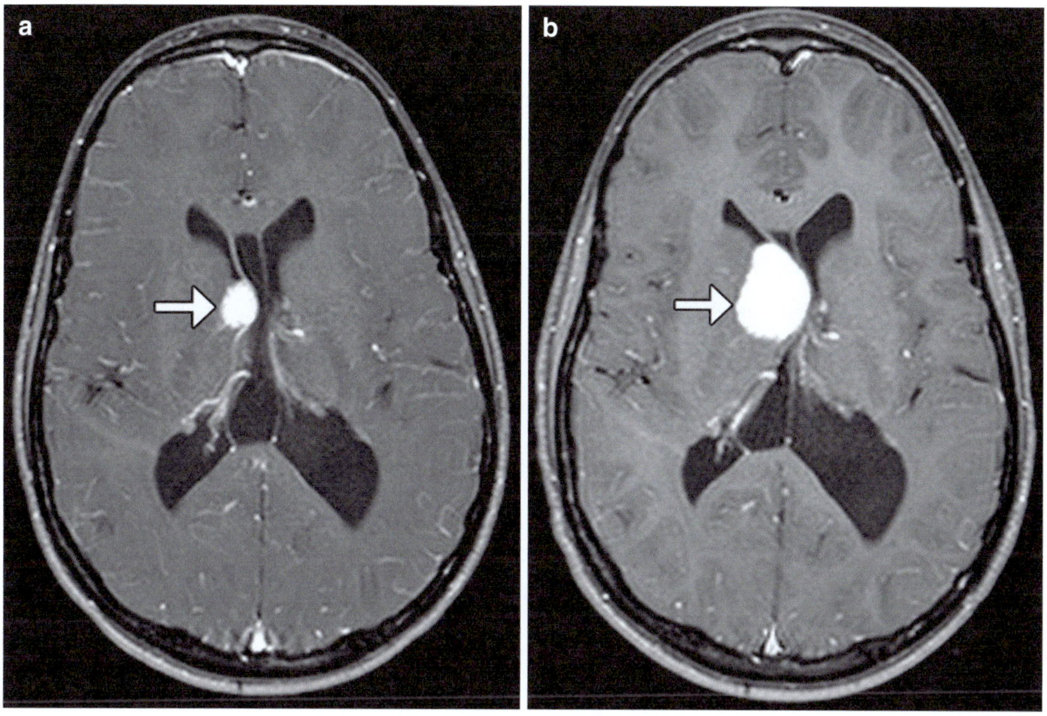

Fig. 3.23 Tuberous sclerosis complex. Initial axial post-contrast T1-weighted MRI (**a**) shows an enhancing mass at the right foramen of Monro (*arrow*). Follow-up axial post-contrast T1-weighted MRI (**b**) shows interval enlargement of the tumor (*arrow*), which proved to be a subependymal giant cell astrocytoma

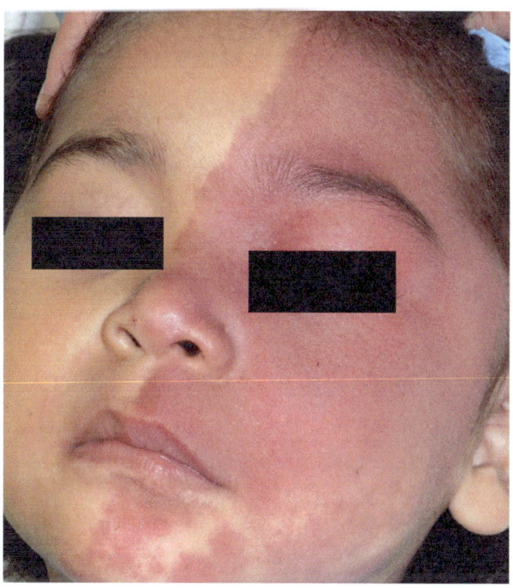

Fig. 3.24 Sturge-Weber syndrome. Photograph shows a left facial port-wine stain in the distribution of the trigeminal nerves

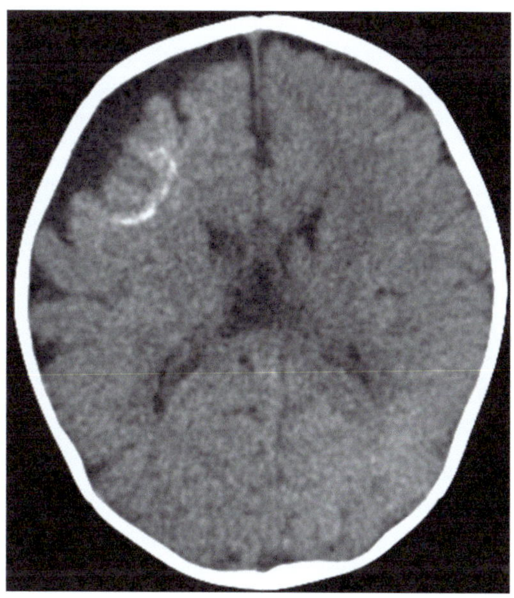

Fig. 3.25 Sturge-Weber syndrome. Axial CT image shows gyriform calcification in the right frontal lobe, which is atrophic

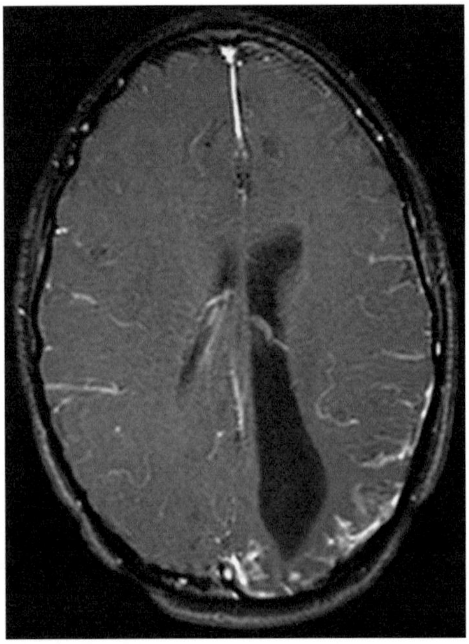

Fig. 3.26 Sturge-Weber syndrome. Axial post-contrast T1-weighted MRI shows diffuse leptomeningeal enhancement related to angiomatosis and associated underlying brain volume loss in the posterior left cerebral hemisphere

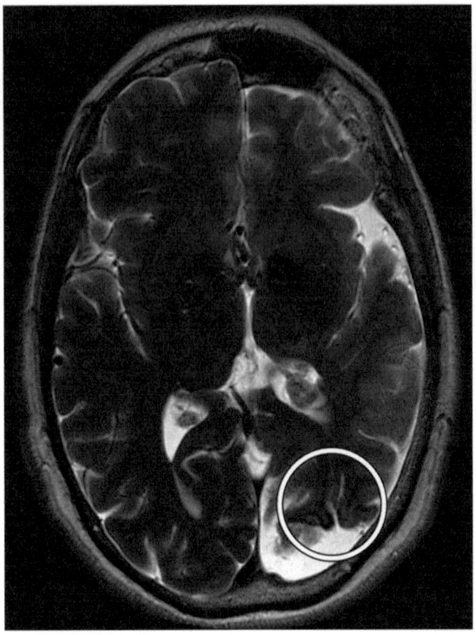

Fig. 3.27 Sturge-Weber syndrome. Axial T2-weighted MRI shows diffuse left cerebral atrophy with overlying calvarial expansion and asymmetric prominence of the left frontal sinus. There is also gyriform low signal in the left occipital lobe related to the presence of calcifications (encircled)

mal enhancement associated with leptomeningeal angiomas (Fig. 3.26). The occipital pole is most commonly involved, but the entire hemisphere or rarely even both hemispheres can be involved. Other findings on neuroimaging may include prominent deep medullary and subependymal veins, developmental venous anomalies, and enlarged globes. The cerebral atrophy present in infancy can be associated with Dyke-Davidoff-Masson syndrome, in which there is calvarial and/or paranasal sinus expansion (Fig. 3.27).

Neurocutaneous Melanosis

Overview

Neurocutaneous melanosis (NCM) is a rare sporadic congenital disorder characterized by the presence of congenital melanocytic nevi on the skin and melanocytic tumors in the neuraxis and variable involvement of the liver. The disease is caused by mosaic somatic mutations in the NRAS gene on chromosome 1p13.

Diagnosis

Presence of meningeal melanosis in patients with large or multiple (>3) congenital nevi without evidence of cutaneous melanomas.

Clinical Findings

Patient with neurocutaneous melanosis tend to have large melanocytic nevi, which are proliferations of benign melanocytes that appear as hyperpigmented, hairy patches, often involving the trunk (Fig. 3.28). Leptomeningeal deposits of melanin in the brain can be associated with seizure, obstructive hydrocephalus, and developmental delay. However, the involvement and clinical findings are variable and a large portion of patients with neurocutaneous melanosis are neurologically asymptomatic. Transformation to malignant melanoma occurs in some patients.

Imaging Findings

Melanin in the brain can be identified on MRI as focal T1 hyperintense lesions, most commonly located in the amygdala (Fig. 3.29), but the thalamus and cerebellum are also sites of predilection. Alternatively, neurocutaneous melanosis can manifest with diffuse leptomeningeal involvement and associated hydrocephalus (Fig. 3.30). When enhancement, edema, necrosis, and progressive enlargement are observed, superimposed malignant melanomas should be considered. Some studies suggest that foci of melanocytes are more difficult to detect on MRI with increasing age.

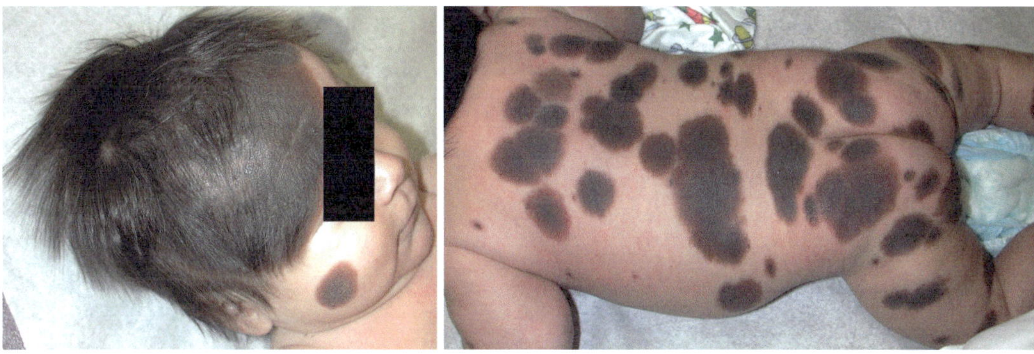

Fig. 3.28 Neurocutaneous melanosis. Photographs show numerous dark melanocytic nevi on the face and body

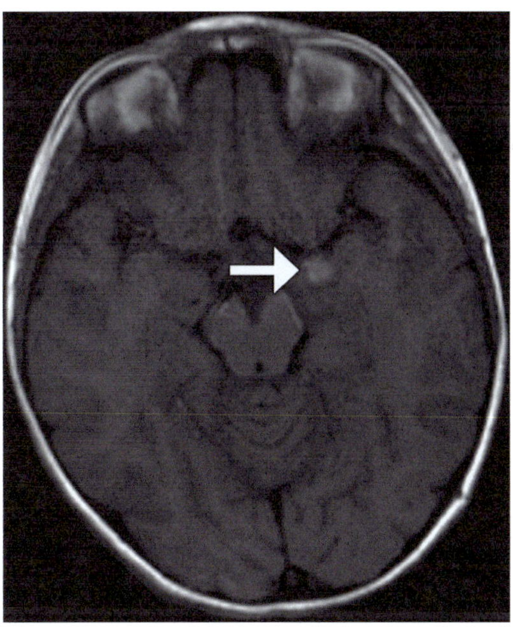

Fig. 3.29 Neurocutaneous melanosis. Axial T1-weighted MRI shows a hyperintense focus in the left amygdala (*arrow*)

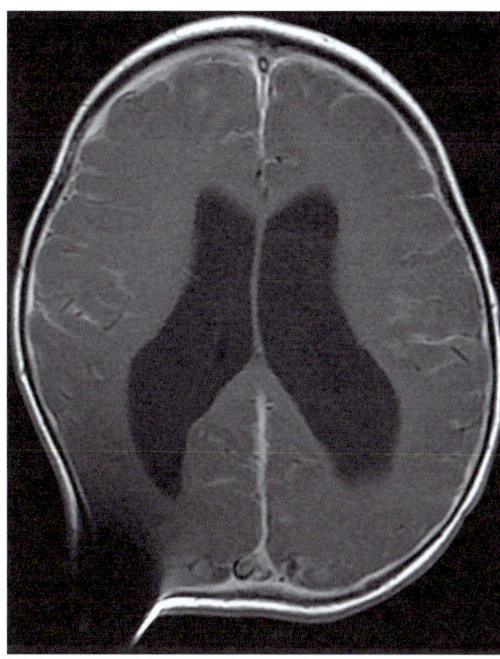

Fig. 3.30 Neurocutaneous melanosis. Axial post-contrast MRI shows diffuse leptomeningeal enhancement and hydrocephalus. There is also diffuse dural enhancement and a shunt reservoir

Incontinentia Pigmenti

Overview

Incontinentia pigmenti is a rare X-linked disorder that affects the skin, hair, teeth, nails, and central nervous system. The disease is caused by mutations in NEMO/IKK-gamma, a regulatory component responsible for NF-kappaB pathway activation, which is critical for immune and inflammatory processes. Incontinentia pigmenti is lethal prenatally in males and presents with highly variable severity in females. After the skin, the central nervous system is the second-most affected system, with neurologic manifestations present in 10–40% of patients.

Diagnosis

In patients without a family history of incontinentia pigmenti, one major criteria is required (typical neonatal rash with erythema, vesicals, and eosinophilia; typical hyperpigmentation, mainly on the trunk, following the lines of Blaschko, fading in adolescence; linear atrophic hairless lesions. In patients with a family history of incontinentia pigmenti the presence of one criterion: Suggestive history of typical rash, vertex alopeccia, dental anomalies, retinal disease, multiple male miscarriages.

Clinical Findings

The dermatological findings of incontinentia pigmenti occur in four phases, following the lines of Blaschko, which are lines of normal development of skin that trace the migration of embryonic cells. Patients do not necessarily have all four stages and the cutaneous lesions can occur at different sites at different stages (Fig. 3.31).

- Stage 1: vesicles on an erythematous base within the first 2 weeks of life.
- Stage 2: verrucous papules or plaques on the extremities that appear within the second and 6th weeks of life.
- Stage 3: whorls or streaks of brown or gray hyperpigmentation on the trunk or extremities that begin between 12 and 26 weeks of life and persist for several decades. Skin biopsy of stage 3 incontinentia pigmenti lesions reveals loss of melanin from the basal cells in the epidermis with collection of melanin in the dermis as free pigment or aggregates of melanophages.
- Stage 4: hypochromic atrophic lesions.

Other frequently encountered dermatological abnormalities include alopecia and dystrophic nails.

Neurologic manifestations of incontinentia pigmenti include infantile spasms in 13%, spasticity in 11%, microcephaly in 5%, optic nerve atrophy in 4%, and developmental delay.

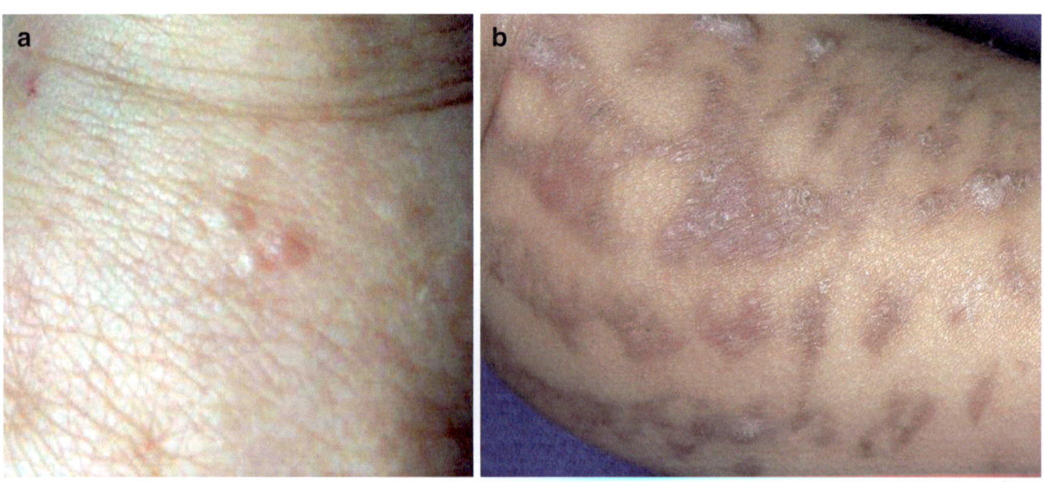

Fig. 3.31 Incontinentia pigmenti. Photograph (**a**) of the hand of a newborn shows vesicles with an erythematous base. Photograph (**b**) of the leg in an infant shows crusted nodules of the early verrucous stage and hyperpigmented streaks

Imaging Findings

Neuroimaging findings in patients with incontinentia pigmenti may include periventricular and subcortical white matter lesions due to ischemia and/or inflammation (Fig. 3.32), hemorrhages, and cerebral and cerebellar volume loss. MRI may also be able to demonstrate retinal detachment, optic atrophy, and microphthalmia (Fig. 3.33).

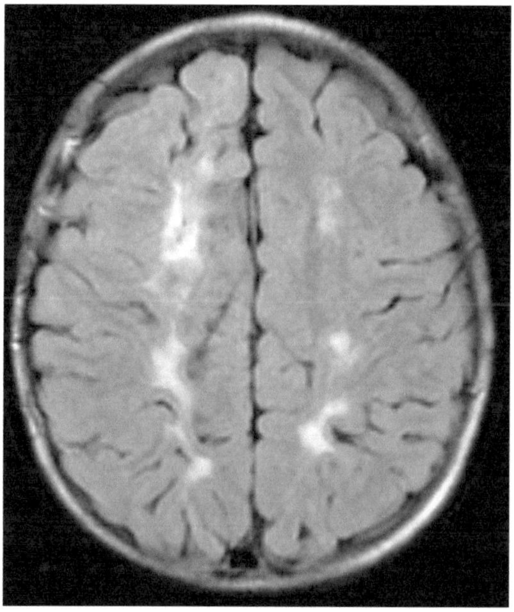

Fig. 3.32 Incontinentia pigmenti. Axial T2-weighted FLAIR MRI shows multiple areas of high T2 signal in the bilateral cerebral watershed zones related to prior infarcts

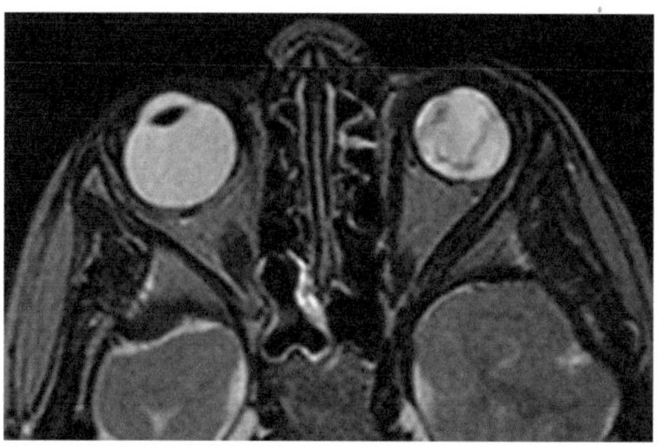

Fig. 3.33 Incontinentia pigmenti. Axial T2-weighted MRI shows left microphthalmia and retinal detachment

Gardner Syndrome

Overview
Gardner syndrome is an autosomal dominant disorder that consists of familial adenomatous polyposis and a variety of extra-intestinal lesions including congenital hypertrophy of the retinal epithelium, skin lesions, dental anomalies, osteomas, sarcomas, Marfan syndrome phenotype, medulloblastoma, papillary thyroid cancer, and desmoid tumors. Gardner syndrome results from mutations in the adenomatous polyposis coli (APC) gene and the estimated overall prevalence ranges from 1 in 6850 to 1 in 31,250 individuals. The severity correlates with the type and site of the mutation within the APC gene, as well as somatic mutations in other genes. Patients with an APC gene mutation between codons 697 and 1224 are at a 13-fold increased risk of developing medulloblastoma.

Diagnosis

(1) Genetic testing for mutation in APC gene, (2) Adenomatous polyposis and a variety of extra-intestinal manifestations:

Clinical Findings

Clinical manifestations of Gardner syndrome in the head and neck region may include the following:

- Dental abnormalities: supernumerary teeth, compound odontomas, hypodontia, and abnormal tooth morphology.
- Cutaneous lesions: epidermoid cysts are the most prevalent dermatologic finding in Gardner syndrome and tend to develop before puberty, can range in size from a few millimeters to several centimeters, tend to be multiple, and sometimes become inflamed and pruritic. Fibromas, lipomas, and pilomatrixomas involving the skin and subcutaneous tissues also have an increased incidence in patients

with Gardner syndrome. Furthermore, craniofacial osteomas may present as palpable lumps.

- Thyroid cancer: well-differentiated papillary cancer is the most common thyroid cancer associated with Gardner syndrome. Multicentric thyroid cancer is significantly more common in Gardner syndrome compared to sporadically occurring thyroid cancer.
- Medulloblastoma

Imaging Findings

Neuroimaging of patients with Gardner syndrome demonstrates osteomas. These lesions commonly occur in the skull and mandible and are best depicted on CT as focal dome-shaped cortical bone excrescences (Fig. 3.34). The osteomas associated with Gardner syndrome are often multiple, manifest before colonic polyposis, and continue to grow throughout life. Imaging of the head and neck may also be performed to evaluate skin and subcutaneous tumors, such as epidermoid cysts and pilomatrixomas. The general imaging features of these lesions are discussed in Chaps. 2 and 5. Otherwise, ultrasound is useful for periodic screening of patients with Gardner syndrome for papillary thyroid cancer (Fig. 3.35).

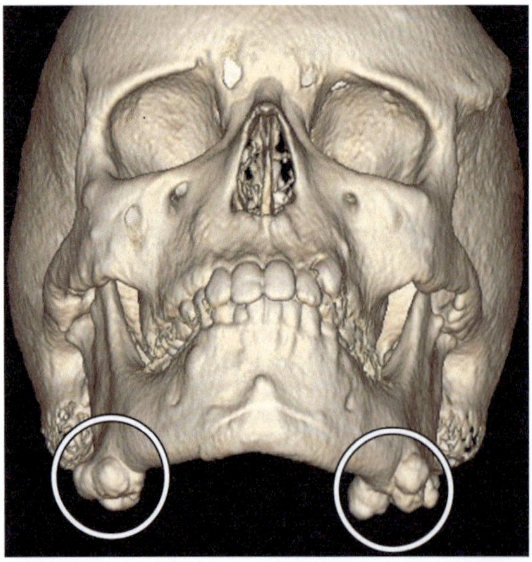

Fig. 3.34 Gardner syndrome. 3D CT image shows multiple bilateral lobulated bony excrescences (encircled), which represent osteomas

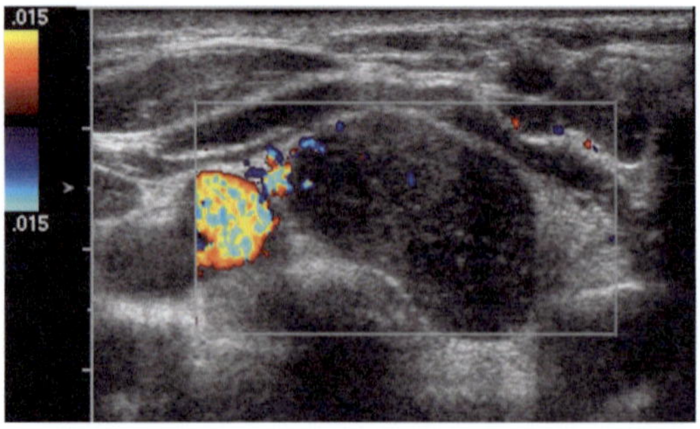

Fig. 3.35 Gardner syndrome. Ultrasound image shows a hypoechoic mass in the thyroid, which proved to be a papillary thyroid carcinoma

McCune Albright Syndrome

Overview

McCune Albright syndrome is characterized by a triad of irregular café-au-lait macules, polyostotic fibrous dysplasia, and precocious puberty. The condition is caused by a somatic mutation in *GNAS1*, which encodes the G protein alpha subunit responsible for activating adenylyl cyclase.

Diagnosis

(1) Somatic mutation in GNAS1, (2) Clinical triad of cafe-au-lait spots, fibrous dysplasia, and precocious puberty.

Clinical Findings

The earliest manifestation of McCune Albright syndrome is the formation of café-au-lait macules, which arise shortly after birth. These macules are often unilateral, tend to follow the Blaschko lines and respect the midline, and have a jagged "coast of Maine" appearance in contrast to the café-au-lait spots in neurofibromatosis type 1, which tend to be oval, smooth bordered, and bilateral. Patients can also develop oral mucosal lentigines, but these often do not appear until later in life.

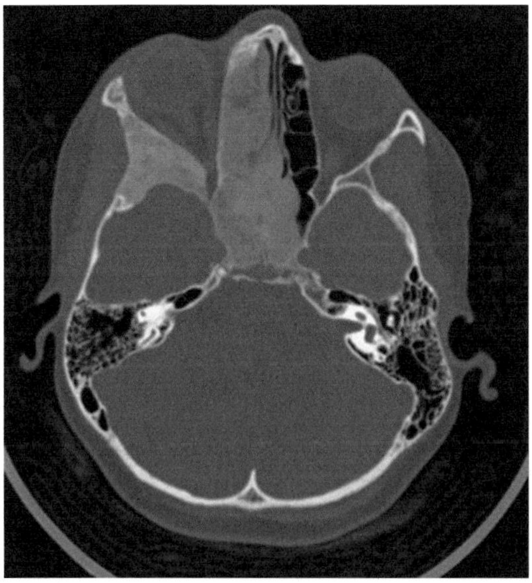

Fig. 3.36 McCune Albright syndrome. Axial CT image shows diffuse, expansile ground-glass lesions involving the right craniofacial skeleton

Imaging Findings

In polyostotic fibrous dysplasia, the bone lesions are typically asymmetric, particularly when the facial and skull bones are involved, but can affect any part of the skeleton. CT is useful for delineating the extent of craniofacial fibrous dysplasia, which characteristically appears as ground-glass attenuation (Fig. 3.36). Pathologic fractures or narrowing of cranial foramina resulting in cranial nerve deficits have also been described.

Basal Cell Nevus Syndrome

Overview

Basal cell nevus syndrome, which is also known as Gorlin-Goltz syndrome, Gorlin syndrome, and nevoid basal cell carcinoma syndrome is characterized by the development of basal cell carcinoma (3rd decade or older), odontogenic keratocystic tumors (2nd and 3rd decades), and other anomalies. The syndrome is an autosomal dominant disorder caused by mutations in the PTCH1 gene on chromosome 9q22, the PTCH2 gene on chromosome 1p32, and the SUFU gene on chromosome 10q24-q25. The PTCH1 gene may act as a tumor suppressor and that the variety of clinical abnormalities is attributable to a second hit in a somatic gene. The product of the PTCH genes is a transmembrane receptor for the secreted ligand sonic hedgehog protein, which is essential for cerebellar development. Patients with the BCNS are unusually sensitive to radiotherapeutic doses of ionizing radiation. There is high penetrance, but variable expression of the disease. The estimated prevalence of the disease ranges from 1 in 55,600 to 1 in 256,000 individuals.

Diagnosis

Diagnosis is based on the presence of two major or one major and two minor criteria. The major criteria include (1) More than two basal cell carcinomas or one under the age of 20 years, (2) Odontogenic keratocysts of the jaw, (3) Three or more palmar or plantar pits, (4) Bilamellar calcification of the falx cerebri, (5) Bifid, fused, or splayed ribs, (6) First degree relative with BCNS. Minor criteria include: (a) Macrocephaly, (b) Congenital malformations (cleft lip or palate, frontal bossing, coarse face, hypertelorism, (c) Skeletal abnormalities (Sprengel deformity, pectus, syndactyly), (d) Radiologic abnormalities, including bridging of sella turcica, vertebral anomalies, and flamed shaped lucencies of hands and feet. (e) Ovarian fibroma, (f) Medulloblastoma.

Clinical Findings

The following abnormalities can be associated with basal cell nevus syndrome:

- Multiple nevoid basal cell carcinomas, 97% over age 40
- Brain tumors, 5%

- Odontogenic keratocysts, 74%
- Vertebral abnormalities, 19%
- Bifid ribs, 26%
- Frontal and parietal bossing, 26%
- Hypertelorism, 10%
- Sprengel's deformity, 11%
- Ectopic calcification of the falx cerebri, 65%
- Plantar and/or palmar pits, 87%
- Cleft lip and palate, 5%
- Ovarian fibroma, 24%

Of note, medulloblastomas are reported in 5% of patients with Gorlin syndrome. Medulloblastomas associated with Gorlin syndrome tend to be the desmoplastic medulloblastoma variant, which has an average age of onset of around 2 years.

There is also an increased incidence of meningiomas and astrocytomas.

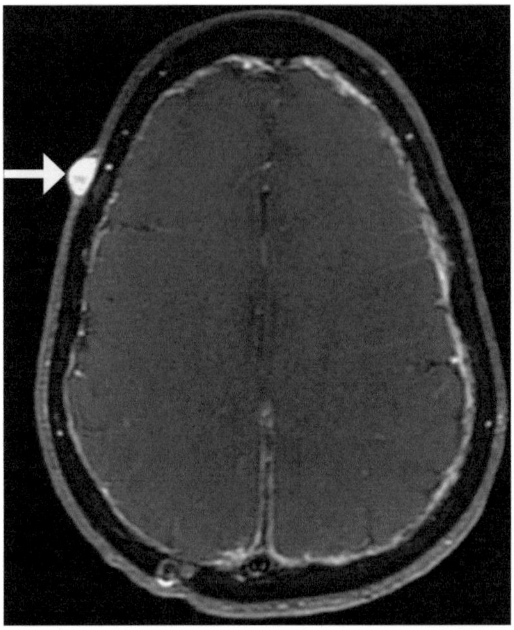

Fig. 3.37 Basal cell nevus syndrome. Axial fat-suppressed post-contrast T1-weighted MRI shows an enhancing mass in the right frontal scalp that represents a basal cell carcinoma (*arrow*)

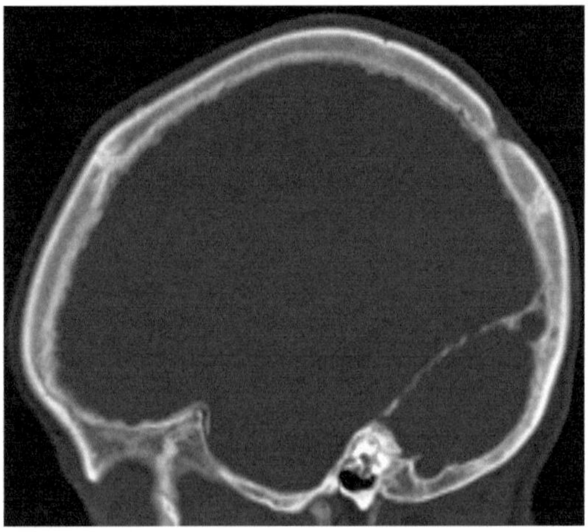

Fig. 3.38 Basal cell nevus syndrome. Sagittal CT image shows diffuse thin dural calcifications

Imaging Findings

Diagnostic imaging can be useful for the early detection and assessment of abnormalities related to Gorlin syndrome. Examination of infants at risk can demonstrate enlarged head, cleft lip/palate, and plain X-rays can demonstrate skeletal abnormalities. MRI and/or CT are useful for evaluating the extent of skin basal cell carcinomas in the head and neck region, which can appear as nodular enhancing tumors (Fig. 3.37). The imaging of basal cell carcinomas is otherwise discussed further in Chap. 6.

CT is best suited for depicting dural calcifications, which tend to be more diffuse than those sporadically enountered in normal individuals (Fig. 3.38). In particular, the dural calcifications are most common along the falx cerebri, but also frequently involve the tentorium cerebelli, petroclinoid ligament, and diaphragma sellae. There can also be osseous bridging of the sella turcica.

Dental radiographs or maxillofacial CT with 3D reconstructions are useful for depicting keratocystic odontogenic tumors, which appear as either unilocular or multilocular with an anteroposterior orientation (Fig. 3.39). These lesions are most commonly located in the mandible molar-ramus region, but can also be present in other parts of the mandible and can involve the maxilla as well. Maxillofacial CT is also appropriate for imaging cleft palate in patients with Gorlin syndrome if surgery is considered.

MRI is suitable for evaluating medulloblastomas and other brain tumors. Of note, desmoplastic medulloblastoma is often more laterally situated within the cerebellar hemispheres than the other types of medulloblastomas and can be

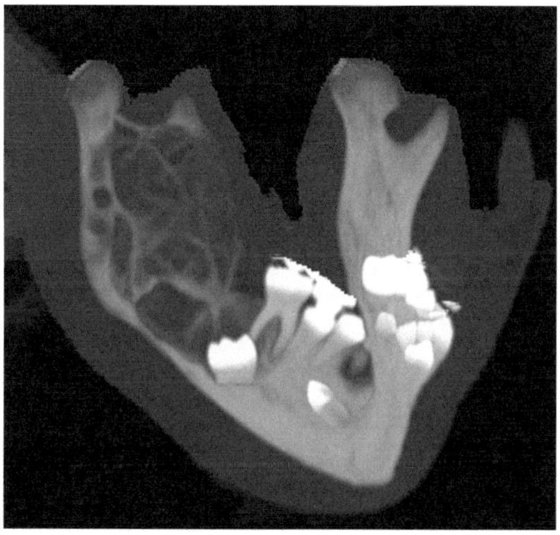

Fig. 3.39 Basal cell nevus syndrome. 3D CT image of the mandible shows a multicystic lesion in the mandible, which represents a keratocystic odontogenic tumor

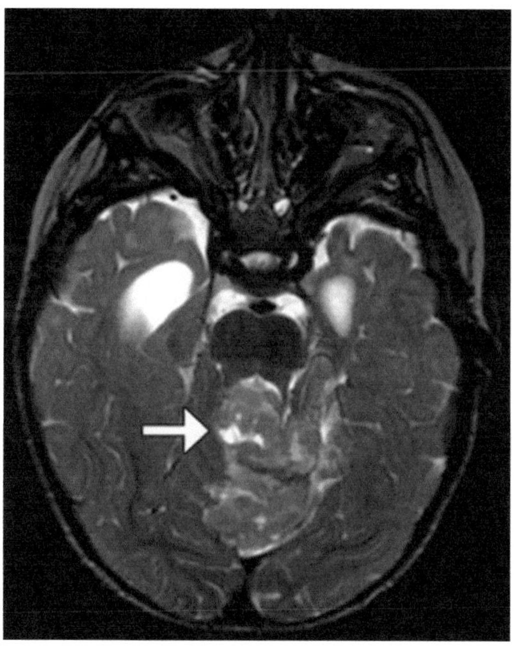

Fig. 3.40 Basal cell nevus syndrome. Axial T2-weighted MRI shows a heterogeneous mass involving the vermis and left cerebellar hemisphere (*arrow*), which represents a medulloblastoma. There is associated obstructive hydrocephalus, as evidenced by dilatation of the bilateral temporal horns

associated with meningeal infiltration. Another important complication of these posterior fossa tumors that should be identified on imaging is the presence of obstructive hydrocephalus (Fig. 3.40).

Oculocutaneous Albinism

Overview

Oculocutaneous albinism is characterized by partial or complete reduction of melanin in the eyes, skin, and the hair. Oculocutaneous albinism is an autosomal recessive disease with four subtypes caused by four distinct genes. These genes play essential roles in the production of melanin in melanocytes in the skin, hair follicles, irises, and retina. The prevalence of all forms of ocular albinism varies considerably worldwide and has been estimated at approximately 1 per 17,000 of the population.

Diagnosis

The diagnosis is established clinically on the presence of decreased or absent pigmentation in the hair, skin, and eyes. Abnormalities in the eye and optic system are specific and necessary for the diagnosis and include decreased pigmentation of the iris and retina, decreased visual acuity, misrouting of the optic nerves at the chiasm, and nystagmus.

Clinical Findings

There are four types of oculocutaneous albinism:

- Oculocutaneous albinism type 1 (OCA1) is characterized by an inability to produce melanin in the skin, hair, and eyes resulting in white hair, pale or pink skin, and blue eyes. OCA1 also causes significant ocular problems including vision impairment, nystagmus, and photophobia.
- Oculocutaneous albinism type 2 (OCA2) is associated with the same vision problems that occur in OCA1, but individuals with OCA2 also exhibit a wide range of skin pigmentation that is partially dependent on their genetic background and the mutations present.
- Individuals affected with oculocutaneous albinism type 3 (OCA3) have red to reddish-brown skin, ginger or reddish hair, and hazel or brown eyes.

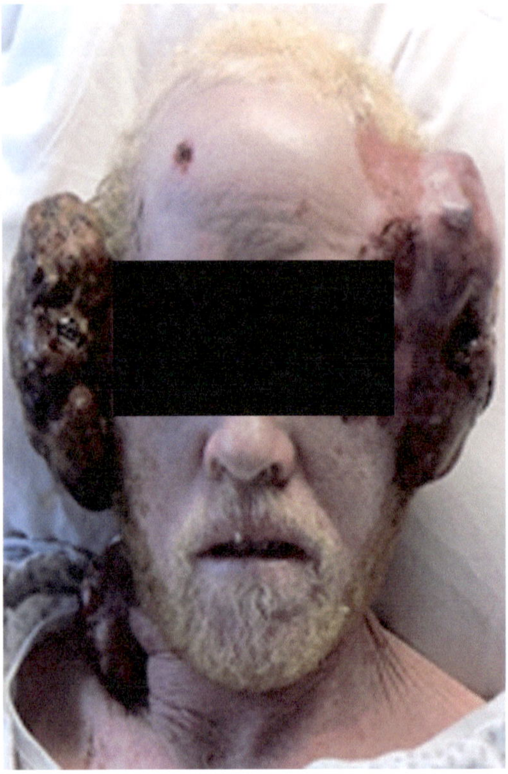

Fig. 3.41 Oculocutaneous albinism. Photograph shows an albino with multiple bulky head and neck tumors that represent squamous cell carcinomas. Courtesy of Jason Johnson MD

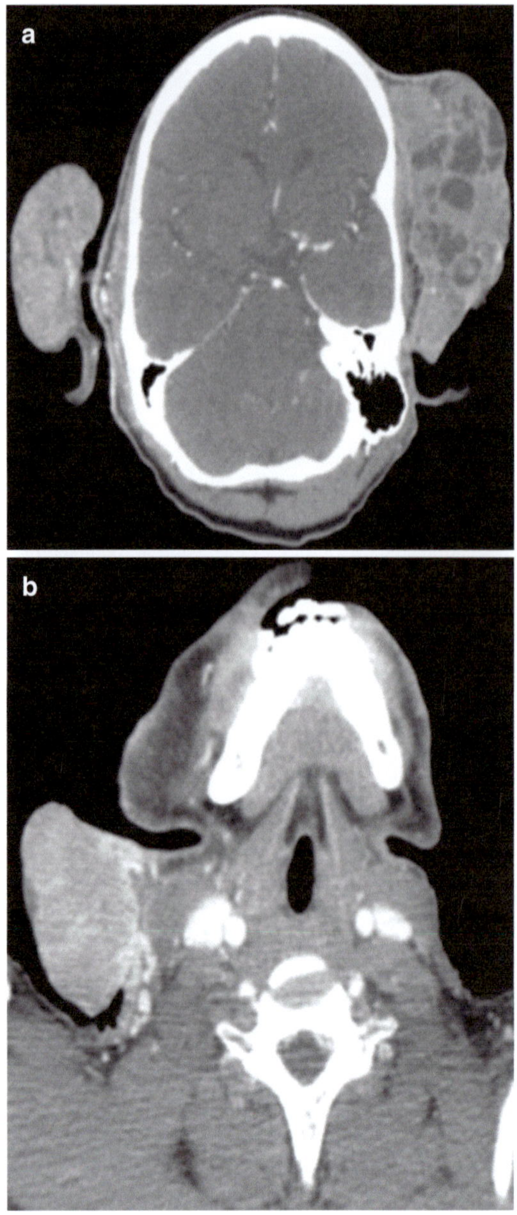

Fig. 3.42 Oculocutaneous albinism. Axial CT images (**a** and **b**) show multiple head and neck skin tumors that represent squamous carcinomas in the same patient as shown in Fig. 3.41. Courtesy of Jason Johnson MD

- Oculocutaneous albinism type 4 (OCA4) is characterized by physical features that are similar to those of OCA2 and is more common among East Asians. The hair color of affected individuals with OCA4 ranges from yellow to brown and the visual acuity deficits vary in severity.

Due to the inability of melanocytes to produce photo-protective melanin pigment, individuals with oculocutaneous albinism are at increased risk of cancers, especially squamous cell carcinoma, basal cell carcinoma, and melanoma (Fig. 3.41). Individuals with albinism have an over 1000× higher risk for developing skin squamous cell carcinoma than ordinary individuals.

Imaging Findings

CT or MRI can be used to evaluate head and neck skin cancers, which are often multiple (Fig. 3.42). The imaging features of skin cancers are otherwise described in more detail in Chap. 6. In addition, neuroimaging can demonstrate abnormally thin optic nerves, chiasm and tracts in patients with oculocutaneous albinism. This is attributed to the abnormal crossing of optic fibers and the relative paucity of retinal ganglion cells.

Marfan Syndrome

Overview
Marfan syndrome is an autosomal dominant disorder with an incidence of 1 in 3000–5000 individuals. MFS typically arises from a mutation in the fibrillin-1 gene (FBN1), although absence of this gene mutation has been described in less than 10% of affected patients. Fibrillin-1 is an important matrix protein and a defect in this protein results in multisystemic abnormalities.

Diagnosis

Diagnosis is based on the revised Ghent criteria. The cardinal features of Marfan of aortic root aneurysm/dissection and ectopia lentis should be sufficient to make the diagnosis in most cases, with confirmation with testing the blood for FBN1 mutations. When aortic disease is present but ectopia lentis is not, the Ghent criteria include a complex scoring system where the presence of 7 or more points indicates systemic disease. The scoring system is: wrist and thumb sign—3 points, pectus carinatum deformity—2 points, hindfoot deformity—2 points, pneumothorax—2 points, dural ectasia—2 points, protusio acetabulum—2 points, reduced US/LS and increased arm/height and no severe scoliosis—1 point, scoliosis—1 point, reduced arm extension—1 point, 3 of 5 facial features (dolichocephaly, enophthalmos, downslanting palpebral fissures, malar hypoplasia, retrognathia)—1 point, skin striea—1 point, myopia—1 point, mitral valve prolapse—1 point. Genetic testing in the blood for FBN1 and TGFBR1 and 2 mutations are confirmatory but will also identify carriers so that clinical evaluation is essential.

Clinical Findings

The most significant dermatological finding of Marfan syndrome is the presence of hyperextensible skin with striae atrophicae (Fig. 3.43). These lesions represent stretch marks on the skin and tend to form at areas subject to stress, such as the lower back. In patients with Marfan syndrome, striae atrophicae can develop at an early age and do not necessitate weight changes, as is otherwise often the case in individuals without Marfan syndrome.

Imaging Findings

Neuroimaging contributes to establishing the diagnosis and management of Marfan syndrome. Dural ectasia may be observed on spine imaging and manifests as widening of the dural sac, dilatation of the nerve root sleeve, and scalloping of vertebral bodies in the lumbosacral spine on MR and CT images (Fig. 3.44). Radiographs, CT, or MRI can be used to evaluate the extent of scoliosis for surgical planning (Fig. 3.45). Although usually evident on ophthalmological examination, CT and MRI can also demonstrate lens subluxation or dislocation (Fig. 3.46).

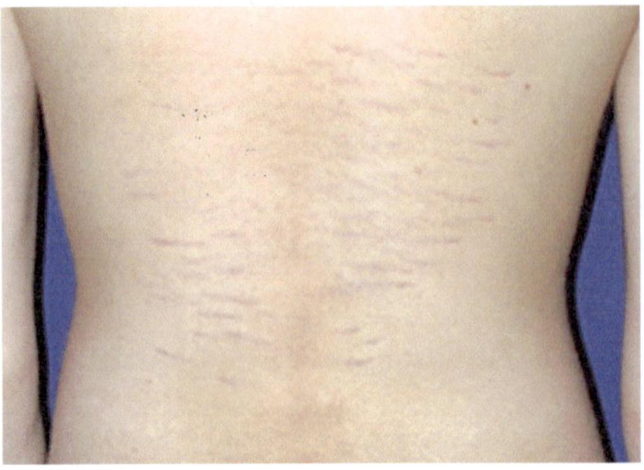

Fig. 3.43 Marfan syndrome. Photograph shows multiple striae atrophicae in the lower back. Courtesy of Min Deng MD and Arlene Ruiz de Luzuriaga MD

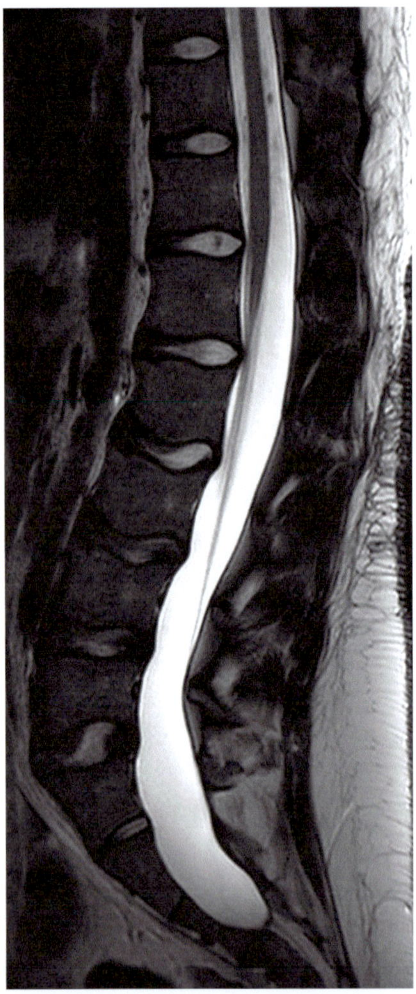

Fig. 3.44 Marfan syndrome. Sagittal T2-weighted MRI shows lumbosacral dural ectasia and multiple malformed vertebral bodies with endplate deformities

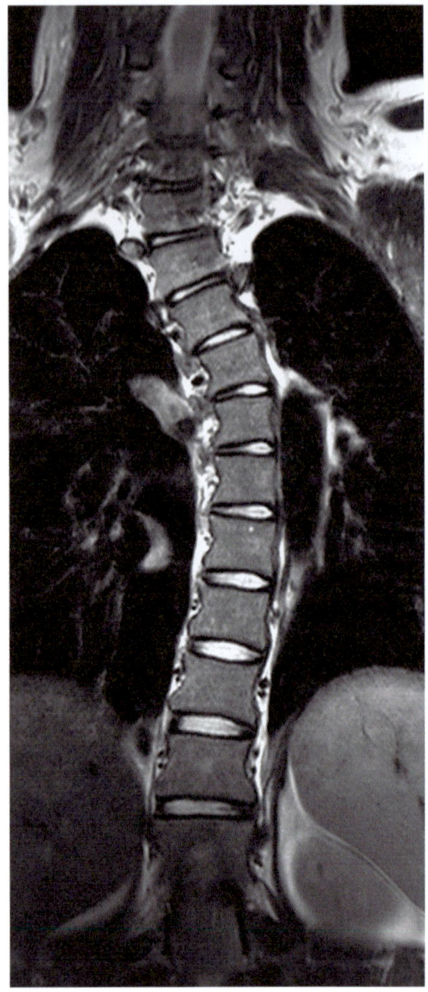

Fig. 3.45 Marfan syndrome. Coronal T2-weighted MRI shows upper thoracic scoliosis

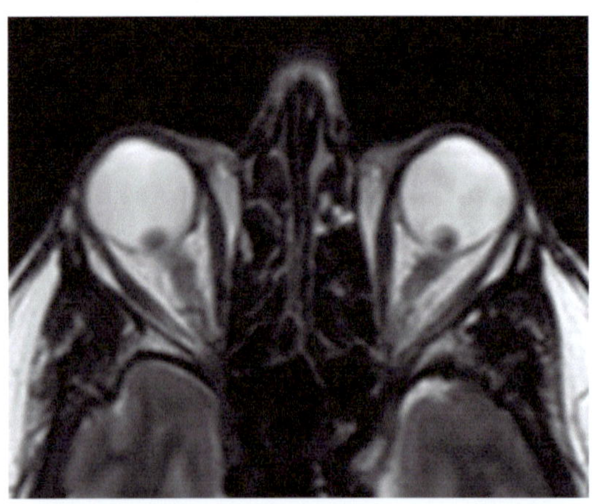

Fig. 3.46 Marfan syndrome. Axial T2-weighted MRI show bilateral posterior lens dislocation

Sjogren-Larsson Syndrome

Overview

Sjogren-Larsson syndrome is an autosomal recessive condition characterized by ichthyosis, mental retardation, spastic paraparesis, macular dystrophy, and leukoencephalopathy. Sjogren-Larsson syndrome has an estimated prevalence of 1 in 250,000 individuals and is caused by a homozygous or compound heterogeneous mutation the fatty aldehyde dehydrogenase (FALDH), a key enzyme in fatty acid oxidation. In individuals with Sjogren-Larsson syndrome, fatty aldehydes are unable to be broken down and accumulate in cells, thereby disrupting cell membranes, resulting in dry, scaly skin. Additionally, the neurological manifestations of Sjogren-Larsson syndrome are believed to be due to disrupted myelin lamellar formation due to excess fat accumulation in cells.

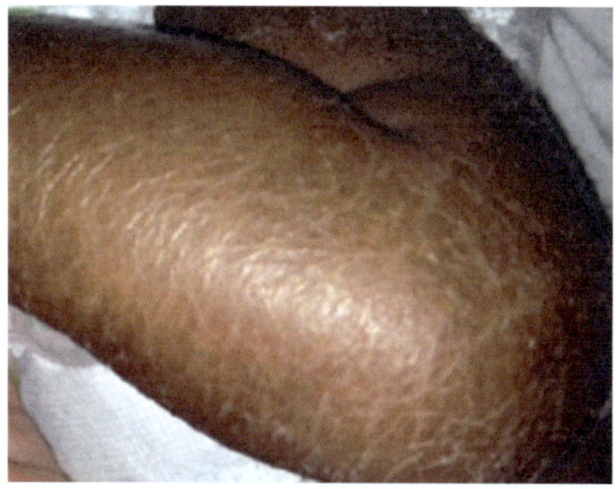

Fig. 3.47 Sjogren-Larson syndrome. Photograph shows scaly lesions involving the extremity, which represents ichthyosis

Diagnosis

The diagnosis is made by genetic testing in the blood for mutations in FALDH.

Clinical Findings

The characteristic dermatologic finding in individuals with Sjogren-Larsson syndrome is ichthyosis, or dry, scaly skin that is often yellowish or brownish in tone (Fig. 3.47). At birth, patients may present with erythematous skin. Ichthyosis develops later in infancy, and these dermatologic findings are usually distributed throughout the body, most notably on the nape of the neck, the trunk, and the extremities. Patients often have global developmental retardation, spasticity, short stature, kyphoscoliosis, visual impairment, and seizures.

Imaging Findings

Individuals affected with Sjogren-Larsson syndrome often present with neurological manifestations thought to be due to leukoencephalopathy. T1-weighted MR images show a paucity of white matter suggestive of severely delayed myelination (Fig. 3.48). Patients may also develop periventricular lesions with high intensity on T2-weighted with associated high lipid and low N-acetyl aspartate peaks on proton MR spectroscopy.

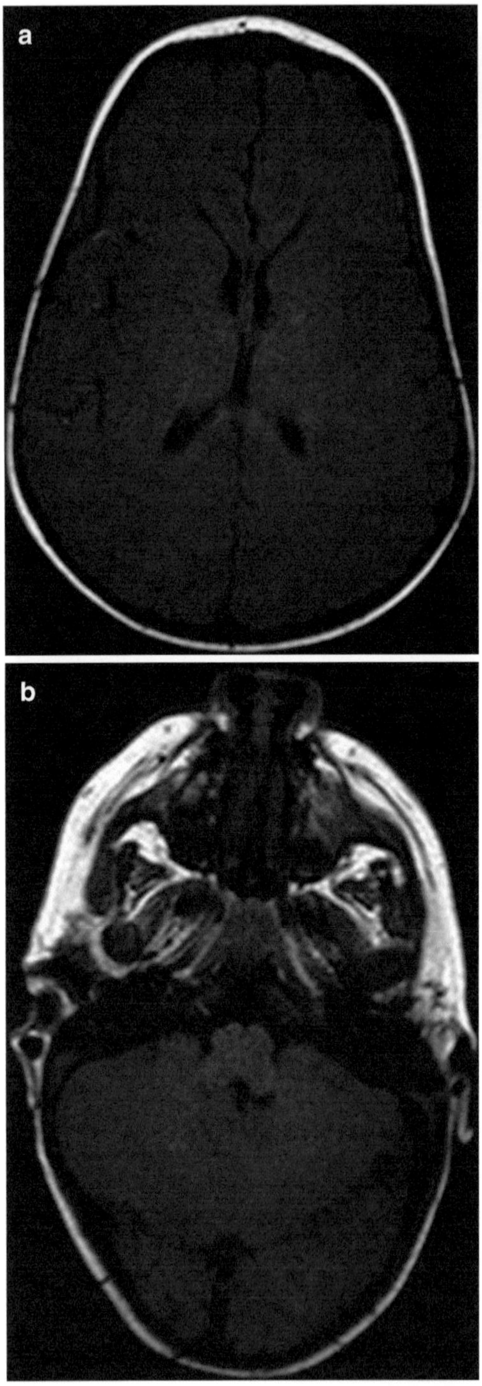

Fig. 3.48 Sjogren-Larsson syndrome. Axial T1-weighted MR images (**a** and **b**) show severely delayed myelination throughout the brain in a 9-month-old infant born at 34 weeks

Waardenburg Syndrome

Overview

Waardenburg syndrome is an autosomal dominant disorder characterized by pigmentary abnormalities of the hair, skin, and eyes, and congenital hearing loss. The disease is divided into four subtypes, with an overall estimated incidence of 1 in 40,000 individuals, and arises from mutations in a group of genes involved in melanocyte formation and development. Unilateral or bilateral congenital hearing loss occurs in 20% of affected individuals. Cleft lip, spina bifida, Hirschsprung disease, dystopia canthorum, or neurological deficits have been described in a subset of patients with WS. Mutations in six genes—PAX3, MITF, EDN3, EDNRB, SOX10, and SNAI2—have been implicated in Waardenburg syndrome.

Diagnosis

The diagnosis is made based on the presence of craniofacial dysmorphisms, pigmentation defects, and severe congenital sensory neural hearing loss. Classification into the different subtypes is based on finding mutations in the blood in one of six genes—PAX3, MITF, EDN3, EDNRB, SOX 10 and SNA12.

Clinical Findings

Waardenburg syndrome often presents with a patchy piebald-like distribution of depigmentation of hair or skin. The most common pigmentation abnormality associated with type I Waardenburg syndrome is the classic white forelock of hair (Fig. 3.49), which can be present from birth or appear later in life. Affected individuals may also have pigmentation anomalies of the irides resulting in heterochromia iridium or bright blue eyes.

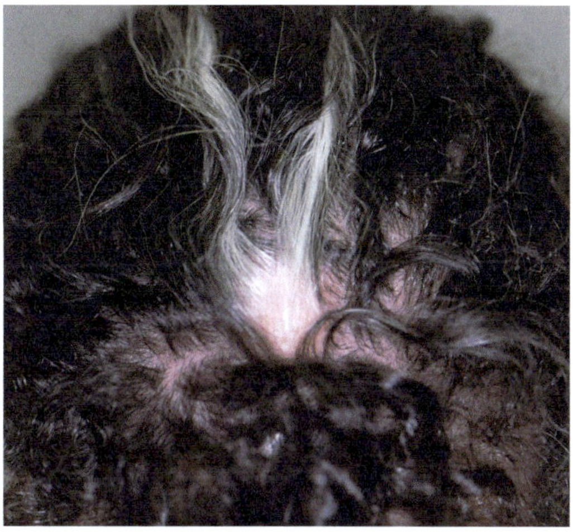

Fig. 3.49 Waardenburg syndrome. Photograph shows an area of hypopigmentation in the scalp and hair, which represents poliosis. Courtesy of Vesna Petronic-Rosic MD

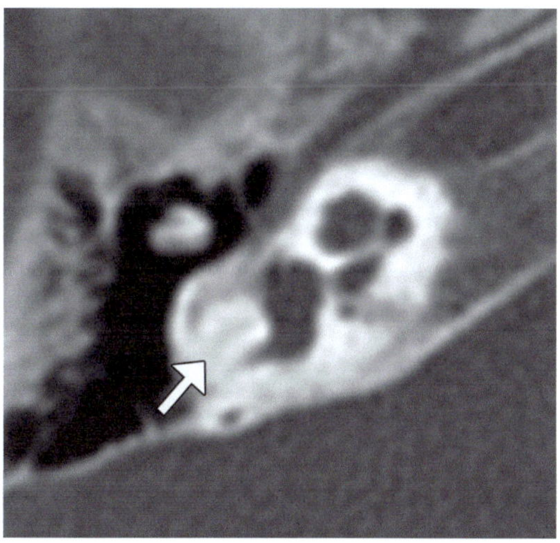

Fig. 3.50 Waardenburg syndrome. Axial CT image shows hypoplasia of the horizontal semicircular canal (*arrow*), a mildly enlarged vestibule, and a mildly dysmorphic cochlea

Imaging Findings

In individuals affected with Waardenburg syndrome due to *SOX10* mutations, MRI or CT of the temporal bones may demonstrate semicircular canal hypoplasia, vestibular enlargement, and a small, dysmorphic cochlea, but with normal partition (Fig. 3.50).

Menkes Disease

Overview
Menkes disease or Menkes kinky hair disease is an X-linked recessive disorder characterized by generalized copper deficiency with an estimated prevalence of 1 in 40,000 to 1 in 298,000 live births. The condition is caused by dysfunction of several copper-dependent enzymes.

Diagnosis

The diagnosis is suggested by the presence of intractale epilepsy and developmental regression and abnormal hair within the first year of life as well as abnormalities in serum copper and ceruloplasmin, and plasma catecholamine. The diagnosis is confirmed by genetic testing in the blood for ATP7A mutations/deletions.

Clinical Findings

The most characteristic cutaneous finding in Menkes disease is sparse, steely, brittle, depigmented hair, which manifests in infancy or early childhood (Fig. 3.51). Patients also have feeding problems, skin laxity and hypopigmentation. The severe copper deficiency in this disease can result in neurodegeneration, including mental retardation, spastic quadriparesis, seizures, and hypothermia. The copper deficiency results in impairment of the following proteins and associated manifestations:

- Tyrosinase: depigmentation
- Lysyl oxidase: defects in elastin and collagen producing arterial intimal defects
- Monoamine oxidase: kinky hair
- Cytochrome c oxidase: hypothermia
- Ascorbase oxidate: skeletal demineralization

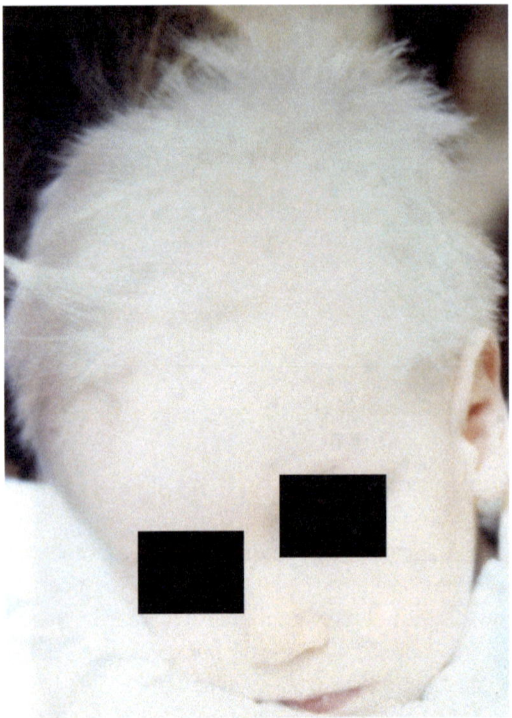

Fig. 3.51 Menkes disease. Photograph shows diffusely depigmented skin and hair

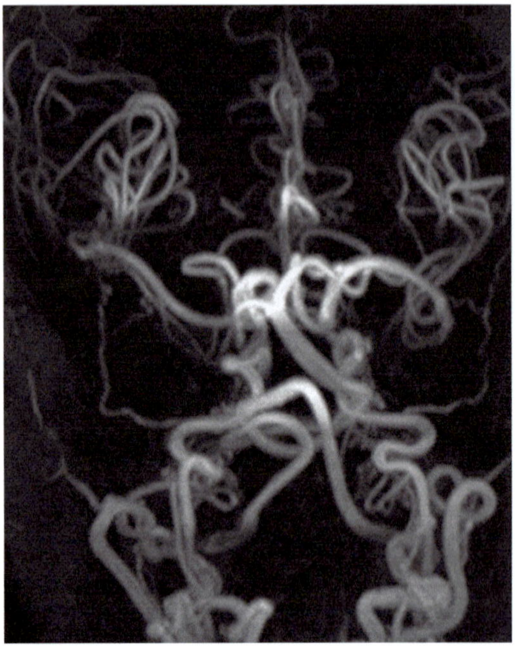

Fig. 3.52 Menkes disease. 3D MRA MIP image shows markedly tortuous head and neck arteries

Imaging Findings

Menkes disease exhibits excessive cerebrovascular tortuosity on angiographic imaging (Fig. 3.52), which is an early and reliable diagnostic biomarker for this condition. Other intracranial abnormalities that can be demonstrated on neuroimaging include cerebral and cerebellar atrophy, delayed myelination, white matter and deep gray-white matter nuclei lesions, and subdural collections.

Ataxia-Telangiectasia

Overview

Ataxia-telangiectasia is an autosomal recessive disorder characterized by cerebellar ataxia, telangiectasias, immunodeficiency, and a predisposition to malignancy. Sensitivity to ionizing radiation and chromosomal breakage are also features of this disorder. The disorder usually becomes apparent during early childhood with progressive ataxia and ocular apraxia. Laboratory studies including alpha-fetoprotein, carcinoembryonic antigen, quantitative immunoglobulin panel, and genetic studies can be performed to confirm diagnosis and elucidate prognosis. There is a strong predilection for cancers including leukemia, medulloblastoma, and gliomas.

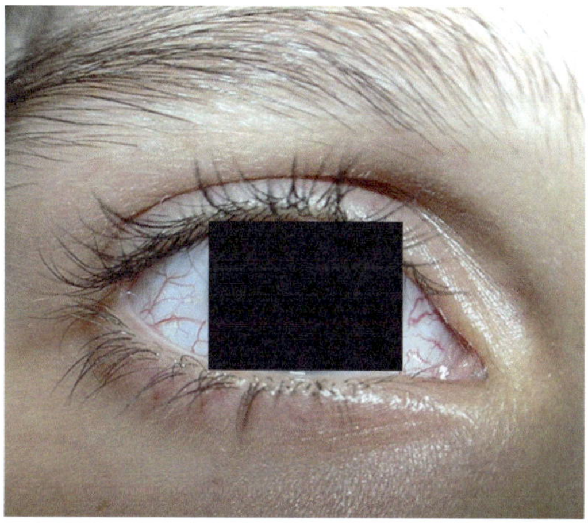

Fig. 3.53 Ataxia-telangiectasia. Photograph shows multiple dilated conjunctival vessels compatible with telangiectasias

Diagnosis

The diagnosis should be suspected in children presenting with ataxia in the first 5 years of life who also have telangiectasias and deficiencies in IgA or IgE and elevated alpha-fetoprotein and CEA. Diagnosis is confirmed by finding a mutation in the ATM gene. It is now known that several diseases associated with abnormal DNA damage response manifest with neurologic symptoms and immunodeficiency.

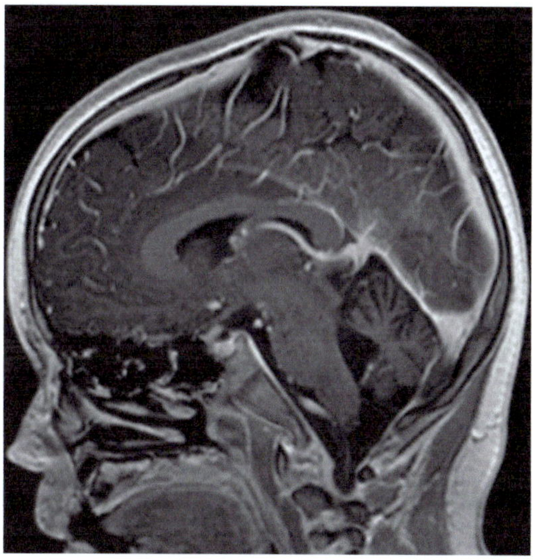

Fig. 3.54 Ataxia-telangiectasia. Sagittal T1-weighted MRI shows diffuse cerebellar atrophy. Courtesy of Jason Johnson MD

Clinical Findings

The clinical hallmark of ataxia-telangiectasia syndrome is the presence of ocular and to a lesser extent cutaneous telangiectases (Fig. 3.53). Other skin anomalies may include café-au-lait macules, hypopigmented macules, melanocytic nevi, facial papulosquamous rash, and hypertrichosis. Neurological manifestations include truncal ataxia and oculomotor apraxia.

Imaging Findings

MRI is the most appropriate neuroimaging modality in patients with ataxia-telangiectasia syndrome; CT should be avoided due to the heightened radiation sensitivity in these patients. Cerebellar atrophy is a characteristic finding in patients with ataxia-telangiectasia (Fig. 3.54). Intracerebral telangiectasias, which appear as punctate foci of susceptibility effect and enhancement on MRI, are also common.

References

Aboukais R, Zairi F, Baroncini M, Bonne NX, Schapira S, Vincent C, Lejeune JP. Intracranial meningiomas and neurofibromatosis type 2. Acta Neurochir. 2013;155(6):997–1001. discussion 1001

Aoki S, Barkovich AJ, Nishimura K, Kjos BO, Machida T, Cogen P, Edwards M, Norman D. Neurofibromatosis types 1 and 2: cranial MR findings. Radiology. 1989;172(2):527–34. PMID: 2501822

Barkovich AJ, Frieden IJ, Williams ML. MR of neurocutaneous melanosis. AJNR Am J Neuroradiol. 1994;15(5):859–67. PMID: 8059652

Benedikt RA, Brown DC, Walker R, Ghaed VN, Mitchell M, Geyer CA. Sturge-Weber syndrome: cranial MR imaging with Gd-DTPA. AJNR Am J Neuroradiol. 1993;14(2):409–15. PMID: 8456721

Bognanno JR, Edwards MK, Lee TA, Dunn DW, Roos KL, Klatte EC. Cranial MR imaging in neurofibromatosis. AJR Am J Roentgenol. 1988;151(2):381–8.

Boyd KP, Korf BR, Theos A. Neurofibromatosis type 1. J Am Acad Dermatol. 2009;61(1):1–14.

Brillante B, Guthrie L, Van Ryzin C. McCune-Albright Syndrome: an overview of clinical features. J Pediatr Nurs. 2015;30(5):815–7. PMID: 26209174

Bronoosh P, Shakibafar AR, Houshyar M, Nafarzade S. Imaging findings in a case of Gorlin-Goltz syndrome: a survey using advanced modalities. Imaging Sci Dent. 2011;41(4):171–5. PMID: 22232727

Cassiman C, Legius E, Spileers W, Casteels I. Ophthalmological assessment of children with neurofibromatosis type 1. Eur J Pediatr. 2013 May.; PMID: 23708214

De Paepe A, Devereux RB, Dietz HC, Hennekam RCM, Pyeritz RE. Revised diagnostic criteria for the Marfan syndrome. Am J Med Genet. 1996;62:417–26.

DeBella K, Szudek J, Friedman JM. Use of the national institutes of health criteria for diagnosis of neurofibromatosis 1 in children. Pediatrics. 2000;105(3):608–14.

Di Rocco C, Tamburrini G. Sturge-Weber syndrome. Childs Nerv Syst. 2006;22(8):909–21. PMID: 16823586

Dietz HC, Cutting GR, Pyeritz RE, Maslen CL, Sakai LY, Corson GM, Puffenberger EG, Hamosh A, Nanthakumar EJ, Curristin SM, et al. Marfan syndrome caused by a recurrent de novo missense mutation in the fibrillin gene. Nature. 1991;352(6333):337–9.

Dirks MS, Butman JA, Kim HJ, Wu T, Morgan K, Tran AP, Lonser RR, Asthagiri AR. Long-term natural history of neurofibromatosis Type 2-associated intracranial tumors. J Neurosurg. 2012;117(1):109–17.

van Domburg PH, Willemsen MA, Rotteveel JJ, de Jong JG, Thijssen HO, Heerschap A, Cruysberg JR, Wanders RJ, Gabreëls FJ, Steijlen PM. Sjögren-Larsson syndrome: clinical and MRI/MRS findings in FALDH-deficient patients. Neurology 1999;52(7):1345–1352.

Dumitrescu CE, Collins MT. McCune-Albright Syndrome. Orphanet J Rare Dis. 2008;3:11. PMID: PMC2459161

Elmaleh-Bergès M, Baumann C, Noël-Pétroff N, Sekkal A, Couloigner V, Devriendt K, Wilson M, Marlin S, Sebag G, Pingault V. Spectrum of temporal bone abnormalities in patients with Waardenburg syndrome and SOX10 mutations. AJNR Am J Neuroradiol. 2013;34(6):1257–63. PMID: 23237859

Evans DGR, Ladusans EJ, Rimmer S, Burnell LD, Thakker N, Farndon PA. Complications of the naevoid basal cell carcinoma syndrome: results of a population based study. J Med Genet. 1993;30:460–4.

Fini G, Belli E, Mici E, Virciglio P, Moricca LM, D'Itri L, Leonardi A, Malavenda MS, Krizzuk D, Merola R, Maturo A, Pasta V. Nevoid basal cell carcinoma syndrome (Gorlin-Goltz syndrome). Case report. G Chir. 2013;34(5–6):176–9. PMID: 23837959

Fortman BJ, Kuszyk BS, Urban BA, Fishman EK. Neurofibromatosis type 1: a diagnostic mimicker at CT. Radiographics. 2001;21(3):601–12. PMID: 11353109

Franz DN, Leonard J, Tudor C, Chuck G, Care M, Sethuraman G, Dinopoulos A, Thomas G, Crone KR. Rapamycin causes regression of astrocytomas in tuberous sclerosis complex. Ann Neurol. 2006;59(3):490–8. PMID: 16453317

Friedrich RE, Stelljes C, Hagel C, Giese M, Scheuer HA. Dysplasia of the orbit and adjacent bone associated with plexiform neurofibroma and ocular disease in 42 NF-1 patients. Anticancer Res. 2010;30(5):1751–64. PMID: 20592374

Greenberger S, Berkun Y, Ben-Zeev B, Levi YB, Barziliai A, Nissenkorn A. Dermatologic manifestations of ataxia-telangiectasia syndrome. J Am Acad Dermatol. 2013;68(6):932–6.

Grønskov K, Ek J, Brondum-Nielsen K. Oculocutaneous albinism. Orphanet J Rare Dis. 2007;2(2):43. PMID: 17980020

Ha HI, Seo JB, Lee SH, Kang JW, Goo HW, Lim TH, Shin MJ. Imaging of Marfan syndrome: multisystemic manifestations. Radiographics. 2007;27(4):989–1004.

Hassell DS, Bancroft LW, Kransdorf MJ, Peterson JJ, Berquist TH, Murphey MD, Fanburg-Smith JC. Imaging appearance of diffuse neurofibroma. AJR Am J Roentgenol. 2008;190(3):582–8.

Jacobs DS, Smith AS, Finelli DA, Lanzieri CF, Wiznitzer M. Menkes kinky hair disease: characteristic MR angiographic findings. AJNR Am J Neuroradiol. 1993;14(5):1160–3.

Jelinek J, Smirniotopoulos JG, Parisi JE, Kanzer M. Lateral ventricular neoplasms of the brain: differential diagnosis based on clinical, CT, and MR findings. AJR Am J Roentgenol. 1990;155(2):365–72. PMID: 2115270

Kalantari BN, Salamon N. Neuroimaging of tuberous sclerosis: spectrum of pathologic findings and frontiers in imaging. AJR Am J Roentgenol. 2008;190(5):W304–9.

Karlsgodt KH, Rosser T, Lutkenhoff ES, Cannon TD, Silva A, Bearden CE. Alterations in white matter microstructure in neurofibromatosis-1. PLoS One. 2012;7(10):e47854. PMID: 23094098

Kim OH, Suh JH. Intracranial and extracranial MR angiography in Menkes disease. Pediatr Radiol. 1997;27(10):782–4.

Lekalakala PT, Khammissa RA, Kramer B, Ayo-Yusuf OA, Lemmer J, Feller L. Oculocutaneous albinism and squamous cell carcinoma of the skin of the head and neck in Sub-Saharan Africa. J Skin Cancer. 2015;2015:167847.

Lin DD, Barker PB, Lederman HM, Crawford TO. Cerebral abnormalities in adults with ataxia-telangiectasia. AJNR Am J Neuroradiol. 2014;35(1):119–23.

Livingstone E, Claviez A, Spengler D, Barth H, Stark AM, Hugo HH, Hauschild A. Neurocutaneous melanosis: a fatal disease in early childhood. J Clin Oncol. 2009;27(13):2290–1. PMID: 19349541

Lo W, Marchuk DA, Ball KL, Juhász C, Jordan LC, Ewen JB, Comi A, Comi A. Updates and future horizons on the understanding, diagnosis, and treatment of Sturge-Weber syndrome brain involvement. Dev Med Child Neurol. 2012;54(3):214–23. PMID: 22191476

Manara R, D'Agata L, Rocco MC, Cusmai R, Freri E, Pinelli L, Darra F, Procopio E, Mardari R, Zanus C, Di Rosa G, Soddu C, Severino M, Ermani M, Longo D, Sartori S; Menkes Working Group in the Italian Neuroimaging Network for Rare Diseases Neuroimaging Changes in Menkes Disease, Part 2. AJNR Am J Neuroradiol 2017a 38 (10) 1858–1865.

Manara R, D'Agata L, Rocco MC, Cusmai R, Freri E, Pinelli L, Darra F, Procopio E, Mardari R, Zanus C, Di Rosa G, Soddu C, Severino M, Ermani M, Longo D, Sartori S, Menkes Working Group in the Italian Neuroimaging Network for Rare Diseases. Neuroimaging Changes in Menkes Disease, Part 1. AJNR Am J Neuroradiol. 2017b;38(10):1850–7.

Mano T, Ono J, Kaminaga T, Imai K, Sakurai K, Harada K, Nagai T, Rizzo WB, Okada S. Proton MR spectroscopy of Sjögren-Larsson's syndrome. AJNR Am J Neuroradiol. 1999;20(9):1671–3.

Mcketton L, Kelly KR, Schneider KA. Abnormal lateral geniculate nucleus and optic chiasm in human albinism. J Comp Neurol. 2014;522(11):2680–7.

McMurdo SK Jr, Moore SG, Brant-Zawadzki M, Berg BO, Koch T, Newton TH, Edwards MS. MR imaging of intracranial tuberous sclerosis. AJR Am J Roentgenol. 1987;148(4):791–6. PMID: 3493666

Meuwissen ME, Mancini GM. Neurological findings in incontinentia pigmenti; a review. Eur J Med Genet. 2012;55(5):323–31.

Nozaki T, Nosaka S, Miyazaki O, Makidono A, Yamamoto A, Niwa T, Tsutsumi Y, Aida N, Masaki H, Saida Y. Syndromes associated with vascular tumors and malformations: a pictorial review. Radiographics. 2013;33(1):175–95. PMID: 23322836

Peleg R, Treister-Goltzman Y. Images in clinical medicine: McCune-Albright syndrome. J Clin Endocrinol Metab. 2014;99(4):1105–6. PMID: 24476078

Perrini P, Caniglia M, Pieroni M, Castagna M, Parenti GF. Malignant transformation of intramedullary melanocytoma: case report. Neurosurgery. 2010;67(3):E867–9. PMID: 20657325

Pingault V, Ente D, Dastot-Le Moal F, Goossens M, Marlin S, Bondurand N. Review and update of mutations causing Waardenburg syndrome. Hum Mutat. 2010;31(4):391–406. PMID: 20127975

Plotkin SR, O'Donnell CC, Curry WT, Bove CM, MacCollin M, Nunes FP. Spinal ependymomas in neurofibromatosis Type 2: a retrospective analysis of 55 patients. J Neurosurg Spine. 2011;14(4):543–7.

Poziomczyk CS, Recuero JK, Bringhenti L, Maria FD, Campos CW, Travi GM, Freitas AM, Maahs MA, Zen PR, Fiegenbaum M, Almeida ST, Bonamigo RR, Bau AE. Incontinentia pigmenti. An Bras Dermatol. 2014;89(1):26–36. PMID: 24626645

Ramaswamy V, Delaney H, Haque S, Marghoob A, Khakoo Y. Spectrum of central nervous system abnormalities in neurocutaneous melanocytosis. Dev Med Child Neurol. 2012;54(6):563–8. PMID: 22469364

Rea D, Brandsema JF, Armstrong D, Parkin PC, deVeber G, MacGregor D, Logan WJ, Askalan R. Cerebral arteriopathy in children with neurofibromatosis type 1. Pediatrics. 2009;124(3):e476–83.

Rehefeldt-Erne S, Nägeli MC, Winterton N, Felderer L, Weibel L, Hafner J, Dummer R. Nevoid basal cell carcinoma syndrome: report from the Zurich Nevoid Basal Cell Carcinoma Syndrome Cohort. Dermatology. 2016;232(3):285–92.

Sahama I, Sinclair K, Pannek K, Lavin M, Rose S. Radiological imaging in ataxia telangiectasia: a review. Cerebellum. 2014;13(4):521–30.

Sartip K, Kaplan A, Obeid G, Kadom N. Neuroimaging of nevoid basal cell carcinoma syndrome (NBCCS) in children. Pediatr Radiol. 2013;43(5):620–7. PMID: 23151728

Schroeder RD, Angelo LS, Kurzrock R. NF2/Merlin in hereditary neurofibromatosis 2 versus cancer: biologic mechanisms and clinical associations. Oncotarget. 2013. [Epub ahead of print). PMID: 24393766.

Sevick RJ, Barkovich AJ, Edwards MS, Koch T, Berg B, Lempert T. Evolution of white matter lesions in neurofibromatosis type 1: MR findings. AJR Am J Roentgenol. 1992;159(1):171–5. PMID: 1609692

Slattery WH. Neurofibromatosis type 2. Otolaryngol Clin N Am. 2015;48(3):443–60.

Spritz RA. Piebaldism, Waardenburg syndrome, and related disorders of melanocyte development. Semin Cutan Med Surg. 1997;16(1):15–23. PMID: 9125761

Tavani F, Zimmerman RA, Berry GT, Sullivan K, Gatti R, Bingham P. Ataxia-telangiectasia: the pattern of cerebellar atrophy on MRI. Neuroradiology. 2003;45(5):315–9.

Umeoka S, Koyama T, Miki Y, Akai M, Tsutsui K, Togashi K. Pictorial review of tuberous sclerosis in various organs. Radiographics. 2008;28(7):e32. PMID: 18772274

Van Mieghem F, Van Goethem JW, Parizel PM, van den Hauwe L, Cras P, De Meirleire J, De Schepper AM. MR of the brain in Sjögren-Larsson syndrome. AJNR Am J Neuroradiol. 1997;18(8):1561–3.

Wasenko JJ, Rosenbloom SA, Duchesneau PM, Lanzieri CF, Weinstein MA. The Sturge-Weber syndrome: comparison of MR and CT characteristics. AJNR Am J Neuroradiol. 1990;11(1):131–4. PMID: 2105594

Willemsen MA, Van Der Graaf M, Van Der Knaap MS, Heerschap A, Van Domburg PH, Gabreëls FJ, Rotteveel JJ. MR imaging and proton MR spectroscopic studies in Sjögren-Larsson syndrome: characterization of the leukoencephalopathy. AJNR Am J Neuroradiol. 2004;25(4):649–57.

Zafeiriou DI, Vargiami E, Hatzidimitriou V, Kyriazi M. Incontinentia pigmenti: a skin, brain, and eye matter. J Pediatr. 2013;163(5):1520. PMID: 23896188

4 Neuroimaging of Infectious, Inflammatory, and Autoimmune Skin and Subcutaneous Lesions

Daniel Thomas Ginat, Nicole Cipriani, and Jason Michael Johnson

Contents

D. T. Ginat (✉)
Department of Radiology, University of Chicago, Pritzker School of Medicine, Chicago, IL, USA
e-mail: dtg1@uchicago.edu

N. Cipriani
Department of Pathology, University of Chicago, Chicago, IL, USA

J. M. Johnson
Department of Diagnostic Radiology, The University of Texas MD Anderson Cancer Center, Houston, TX, USA

D. T. Ginat (ed.), *Neuroradiological Imaging of Skin Diseases and Related Conditions*,
https://doi.org/10.1007/978-3-319-90931-8_4

Abstract

Many infections, inflammatory conditions, and immune disorders can involve the skin and subcutaneous tissues. Diagnostic imaging often plays an important role in evaluating these conditions, including both local and distant manifestations. The clinicopathologic and neuroimaging features of the following topics are reviewed in this chapter: bacterial, viral, and fungal infections, histiocytic disorders, rheumatoid arthritis, sarcoidosis, systemic lupus erythematosus, Sjogren syndrome, scleroderma, immunoglobin G4-related disease, Kimura disease, benign osteoma cutis, and Parry Romberg syndrome.

Bacterial Skin Infections

Overview

There is a broad spectrum of bacterial skin infections that can have neuroimaging findings, including the following main categories:

- Pyogenic skin infections, which have the propensity to form pus and are most commonly caused by Staphylococcus aureus and group A streptococcus.
- Necrotizing infections, which may be caused by *Clostridium*, *Proteus*, *Escherichia coli*, *Bacteroides*, and *Enterobacteriaceae*.
- Acne, associated with Propionibacterium acnes, an anaerobic, Gram-positive rod present in pores and follicles tends to be a chronic condition associated with increased sebum secretion.
- Mycobacterial skin and soft tissue infections include nontuberculous mycobacterial diseases, tuberculosis, and leprosy. There are over 130 identified species of nontuberculous mycobacteria, including most notably *Mycobacterium fortuitum*, *abscessus*, *chelonae*, *avium* complex, *marinum*, and *kansasii*.
- Tick-borne infections can lead to local skin rashes and systemic disease. This is epitomized by Lyme disease, which is a multisystemic disease caused by the spirochete *Borrelia burgdorferi* that is transmitted by ixodid ticks.

Clinicopathologic Findings

Pyogenic Infections: cellulitis, erysipelas, erythrasma, folliculitis, and skin abscesses, including furuncles and carbuncles, hidradenitis suppurativa, impetigo, and ecthyma, and scalded skin syndrome. Bacteria can enter and infect the skin through hair follicles and associated glands, or open wounds. Alternatively, an infection can spread to the skin via underlying sinusitis, dental disease, or from systemic infections. In general, the clinical presentation of pyogenic bacterial skin infections ranges from areas of skin discoloration from erythema and cellulitis (Fig. 4.1) to abscess formation, with or without drainage (Fig. 4.2). Acute infections contain neutrophilic infiltrates, while chronic infections are characterized by lymphoplasmacytic inflammation, and there may be associated fibrosis with abscess formation (Fig. 4.3). The specific types of infections include the following:

- Impetigo is a superficial infection can manifest as yellow, crusting lesions that may be itchy or bullous impetigo or as bullae that rupture to form a brown crust.
- Erysipelas involves the upper dermis and superficial lymphatics and can manifest as well-demarcated areas of raised erythema.

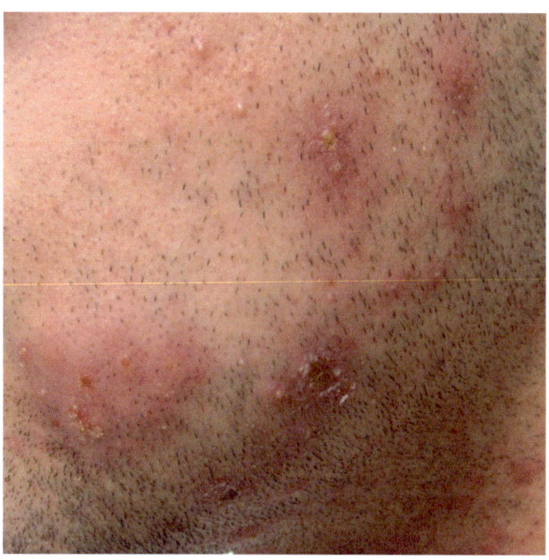

Fig. 4.1 Cellulitis. Photograph shows mildly raised areas of erythema associated with impetigo. Courtesy of Vesna Petronic-Rosic, MD, MSc

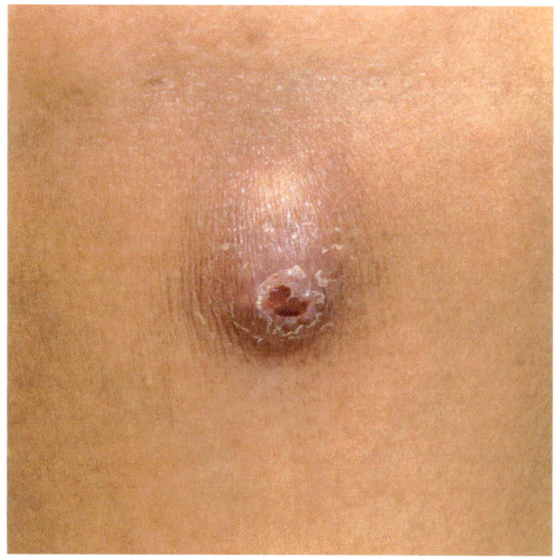

Fig. 4.2 Abscess. Photograph shows a nodular lesion with erythema and an opening in the skin. Courtesy of Vesna Petronic-Rosic, MD, MSc

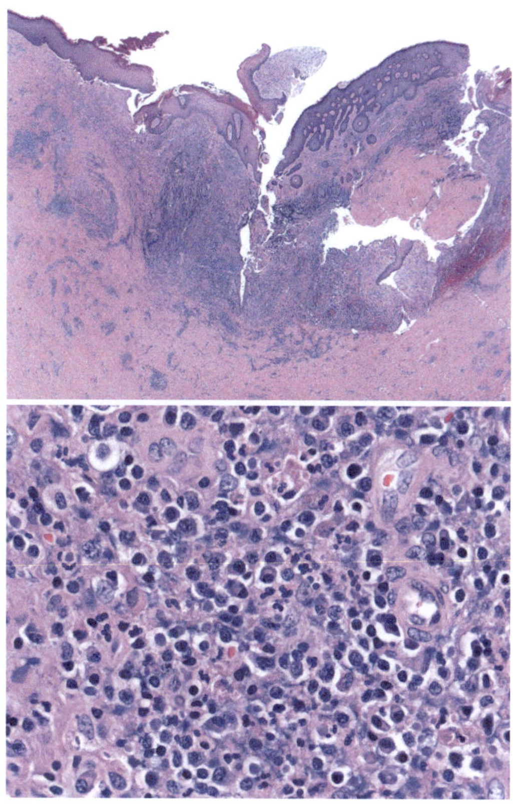

Fig. 4.3 Cellulitis and abscess. Low and high power hematoxylin and eosin stained photomicrographs show dense acute neutrophilic and chronic lymphoplasmacytic inflammation involving dermis with associated fibrosis

- Cellulitis involves the deep dermis and subcutaneous tissue and can present as diffuse erythema and swelling.
- Furuncles (boils) and carbuncles are associated with hair follicle infection (folliculitis) and extend into subcutaneous tissues in the form of purulent fluid collections. The lesions are tender and painful, fluctuant, and erythematous nodules, frequently surmounted by a pustule and surrounded by a rim of erythematous swelling.
- External hordeolum arises from obstruction and infection of Zeiss or Moll sebaceous glands, while internal hordeolum represents a secondary infection of meibomian glands in the tarsal plate of the eyelid.
- Hidradenitis suppurativa (acne inversa) is characterized by recurrent nodules or abscesses and chronic suppurative lesions, which often present as painful, extensive, and deep-seated nodules accompanied by sinus tracts and hypertrophic scars. A histopathological examination may reveal dermal lymphoplasmacytic inflammation and giant cells and deep epithelial-lined sinuses (Fig. 4.4).

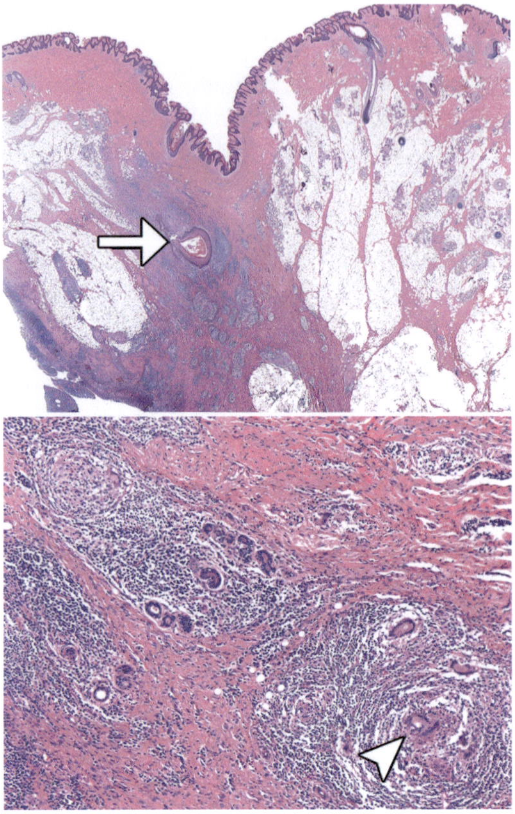

Fig. 4.4 Hidradenitis. Low and high power hematoxylin and eosin stained photomicrographs show dense lymphoplasmacytic inflammation and giant cells (arrowhead) involving dermis/subcutis, including surrounding skin adnexal glands and deep epithelial-lined sinuses (arrow)

Necrotizing Infections: Necrotizing fasciitis can be a rapidly progressive and life-threatening condition that requires emergent treatment. Necrotizing fasciitis can present with crepitus, edema, and even hemorrhage in the setting of sepsis due to gas-forming bacteria. Histological examination can reveal edematous and necrotic tissues with mixed inflammatory cell infiltrates and early fibroblastic proliferation (Fig. 4.5). Inflammation and edema are caused by vasculitis with microthromboses at the margins of the infection.

Acne Vulgaris: Skin findings associated with acne include comedones, papules, pustules, and nodules primarily located on the face, chest, and back. The main component of acne is the comedo, which represents an enlarged and plugged hair follicle. A comedo that remains beneath the skin is a closed comedo or whitehead. On the other hand, a comedo that extends through the skin surface is an open comedo or blackhead. The black discoloration is due to oxidation of the sebum exposed to air. There can also be scarring and an associated acneiform rash that consists of papules and pustules (Fig. 4.6).

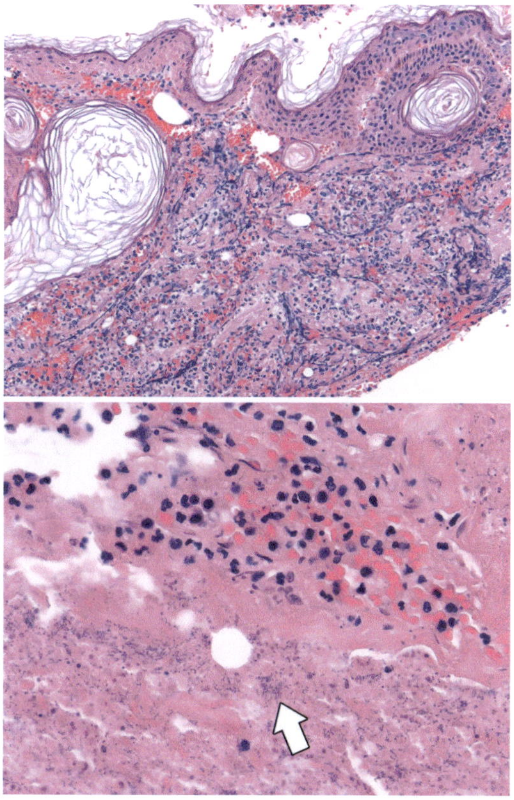

Fig. 4.5 Necrotizing fasciitis. Low (top) and high (bottom) power hematoxylin and eosin stained photomicrographs show skin with dermal involvement by a dense neutrophilic infiltrate and bacterial colonies (arrow)

Mycobacterial Infections: The characteristic feature that the many types of mycobacteria have in common is that they are acid-fast (Fig. 4.7). However, the acid-fast bacillus stain does not differentiate between mycobacterial species and histopathology is nonspecific. Mycobacterial cultures are needed for primary species identification and drug susceptibility testing. Skin lesions can occur as one isolated lesion or as multiple lesions at multiple sites. The disseminated

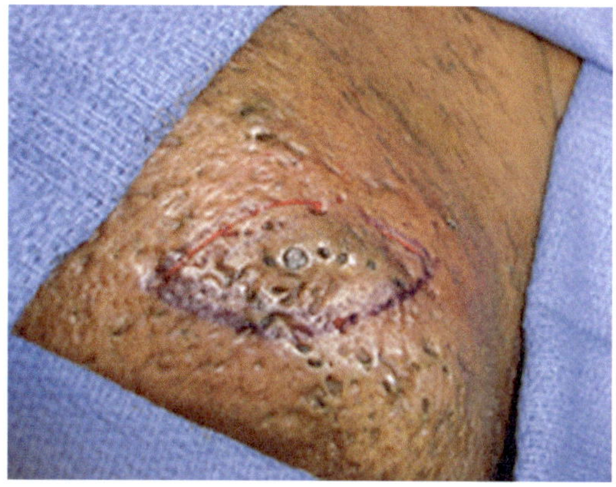

Fig. 4.6 Acne vulgaris. Photograph shows blackheads and irregular scarring

disease tends to affect immunocompromised individuals.

There are three main categories of cutaneous tuberculosis, including lesions containing the bacilli, such as chancre, cutis verrucosa, lupus vulgaris, acute miliary, gumma, orificial tuberculosis, and scrofuloderma, tuberculids, such as papulonecrotic tuberculid and lichen scrofulosorum, and lesions without bacilli, such as erythema induratum.

The skin lesions associated with nontuberculous mycobacterial infections are also quite varied, including erythematous papules and nodules, ulcers with drainage, and scarring. These may be accompanied by abscesses and cervical lymphadenitis. Nontuberculous mycobacterial infections can be rapidly growing and present within days of exposure or slow growing. Despite aggressive medical treatment and surgical intervention, results may be suboptimal.

The skin lesions associated with leprosy have decreased or loss of sensation may be single or multiple, hypopigmented, and associated with skin thickening and hair loss.

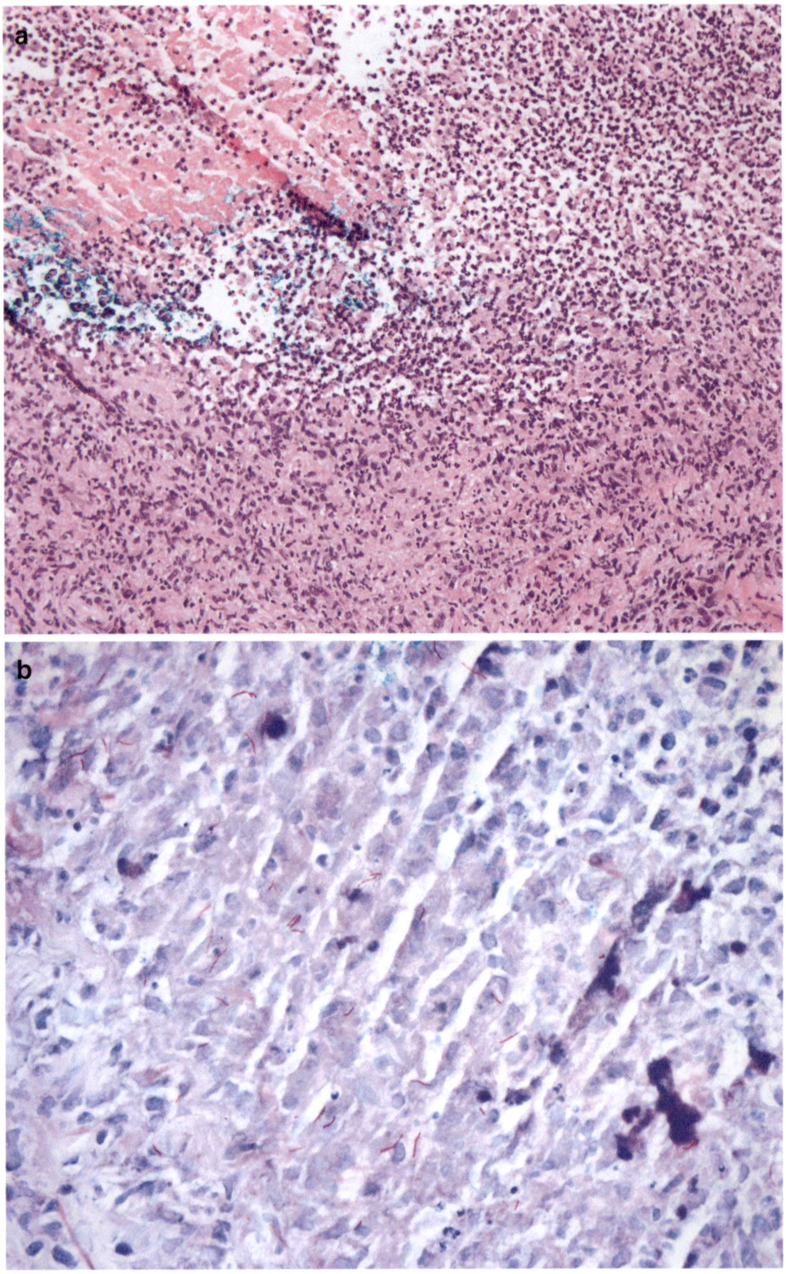

Fig. 4.7 Mycobacterial infection. Hematoxylin and eosin stained photomicrographs demonstrate neutrophilic granulomatous dermatitis and necrosis (**a**). AFB staining shows scattered acid-fast organisms (**b**). Courtesy of Lohini Sundharkrishnan, MD

Tick-borne Disease: There are three rather distinct clinical stages of Lyme disease:

- Stage 1: an expanding skin lesion with a "bulls-eye appearance" (erythema chronicum migrans) around the site of the tick bite, which may be accompanied by flu-like symptoms 2–30 days after the tick bite.
- Stage 2: cardiac and neurologic symptoms 1–4 months after infection. The triad of

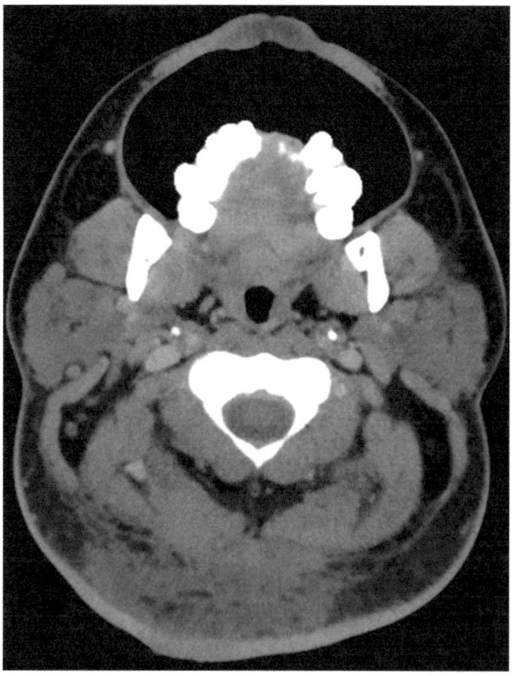

Fig. 4.8 Cellulitis. Axial CT image shows posterior enck skin thickening and extensive subcutanaeous fat stranding with extension to the underlying muscles in a dibeteric patient

neurologic manifestations of Lyme disease includes meningitis, cranial neuritis, particularly facial palsy, and radiculoneuritis is characteristic.

- Stage 3: arthritic and chronic neurologic symptoms that occur up to several years later.

Imaging Findings

In general, the role of imaging is to determine the type and extent of infection for treatment planning and monitoring of the treatment response. In general, ultrasound may be useful for detecting superficial fluid collections, while CT and MRI are well-suited for identifying superficial and deep manifestations of infection in the head and neck.

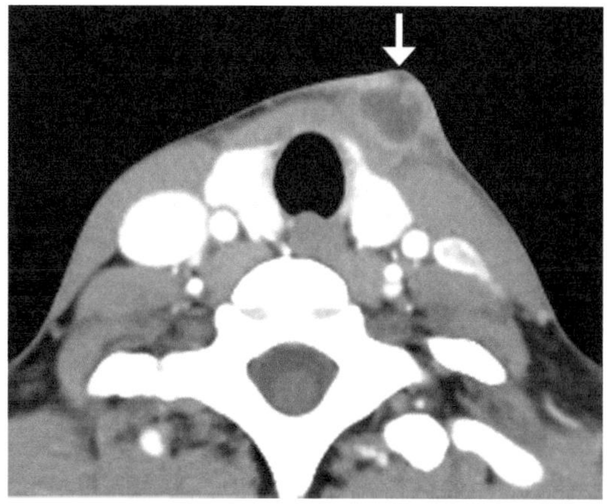

Fig. 4.9 Abscess. Axial CT image shows a rim-enhancing fluid collection (arrow) in the anterior neck with stranding of the surrounding subcutaneous tissues and thickening of the overlying skin

Pyogenic Infections: On routine diagnostic imaging, the primary forms of pyogenic skin infection that can be discerned include cellulitis and abscess. Cellulitis appears as stranding and swelling of the subcutaneous fat, along with what may sometimes be visible skin thickening (Fig. 4.8), while abscess appears as a rim-enhancing fluid collection (Fig. 4.9), but is often associated with cellulitis. In the orbital region, diagnostic imaging is often obtained to determine if there is postseptal extension or abscess, since this is pertinent to clinical management. In addition, diagnostic imaging can sometimes help identify the underlying cause of the skin infection, such as dacryocystitis or dental disease. In particular, cutaneous sinus tracts can result from chronically draining deep head and neck infections, such as those of odontogenic origin with periapical abscess and associated osteomyelitis, which can be evaluated via CT (Fig. 4.10). Furthermore, bacteria can enter the bloodstream via open skin wounds, catheters, and intravenous drug use, for example. This can lead to complications such as septic brain emboli, discitis-osteomyelitis, and septic arthritis, which are best depicted on MRI. In particular, septic emboli in the brain typically appear ring-enhancing lesions

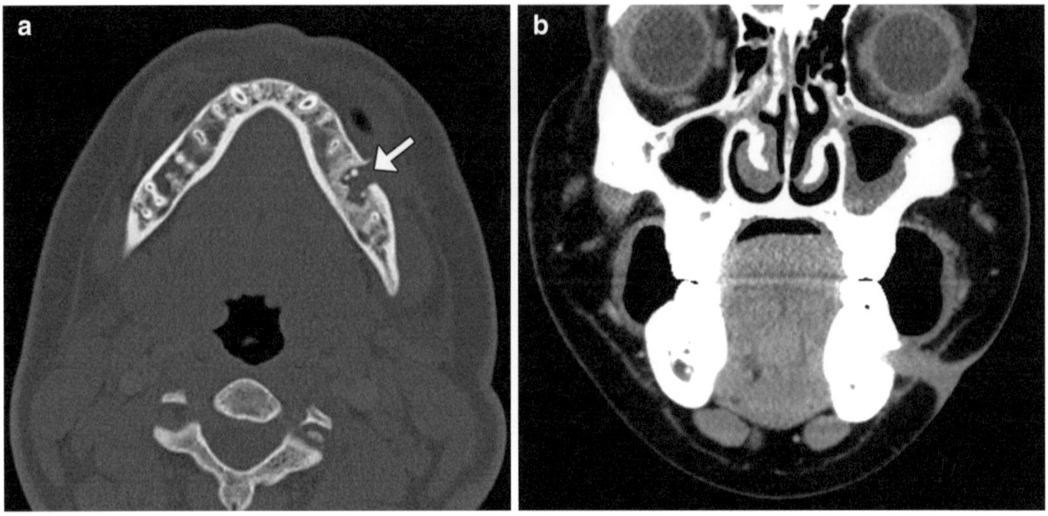

Fig. 4.10 Sinus tract. Coronal CT image (**a**) shows a left lower face cutaneous sinus tract that extends from the mandible to the overlying skin. Axial CT image (**b**) shows underlying periodontal disease with cortical dehiscence (arrow) and surrounding sclerosis from chronic osteomyelitis

with restricted diffusion and surrounding vasogenic edema (Fig. 4.11). Discitis-osteomyelitis and septic arthritis usually appear as a disc or joint space enhancement, adjacent bone marrow enhancement, and often surrounding soft tissue inflammation with or without fluid collections from abscess formation (Fig. 4.12). There can also be osteolysis that eventually becomes apparent on CT.

Necrotizing Infections: The presence of soft tissue emphysema, which may be accompanied by subfascial fluid collections and fat stranding, is characteristic of necrotizing fasciitis (Fig. 4.13), but the diagnosis is not excluded when it is absent. Alternatively, recent traumatic injury and surgery can have similar imaging features. Treatment of clinically suspected necrotizing fasciitis should not be delayed to obtain imaging.

Acne Vulgaris: Stigmata of acne can be encountered on cross-sectional imaging as skin nodularity, which may be associated with subcutaneous fat stranding, depending on the severity of the disease (Fig. 4.14). Acne can also appear hypermetabolic on ^{18}FDG-PET due to the inflammation and can appear similar to other hypermetabolic lesions such as neoplasms and metastases.

Mycobacterial Infections: Tuberculous meningitis and tuberculoma are the two most salient manifestations of Mycobacterium tuberculosis infection of the central nervous system. Intracranial tuberculomas can be solitary or multiple and can mimic neoplasms. Tuberculomas can appear as peripherally enhancing masses without restricted diffusion (Fig. 4.15). The presence of a lipid peak at 1.3 ppm on MR spectroscopy can be helpful in differentiating tuberculomas from neoplasms. In addition, the granulomatous disease may be suspected if calcifications are identified on CT. Basal meningitis is also a typical manifestation of tuberculosis, which can be associated with vasculopathy and cerebral infarction (Fig. 4.16). Tuberculous cervical lymphadenitis, or scrofula, usually presents as necrotic/cystic lymphadenopathy, often in the posterior triangle of the neck, although the imaging features may not be specific. Otherwise, nontuberculous Mycobacterial infections of the head and neck typically present as asymmetric cervical

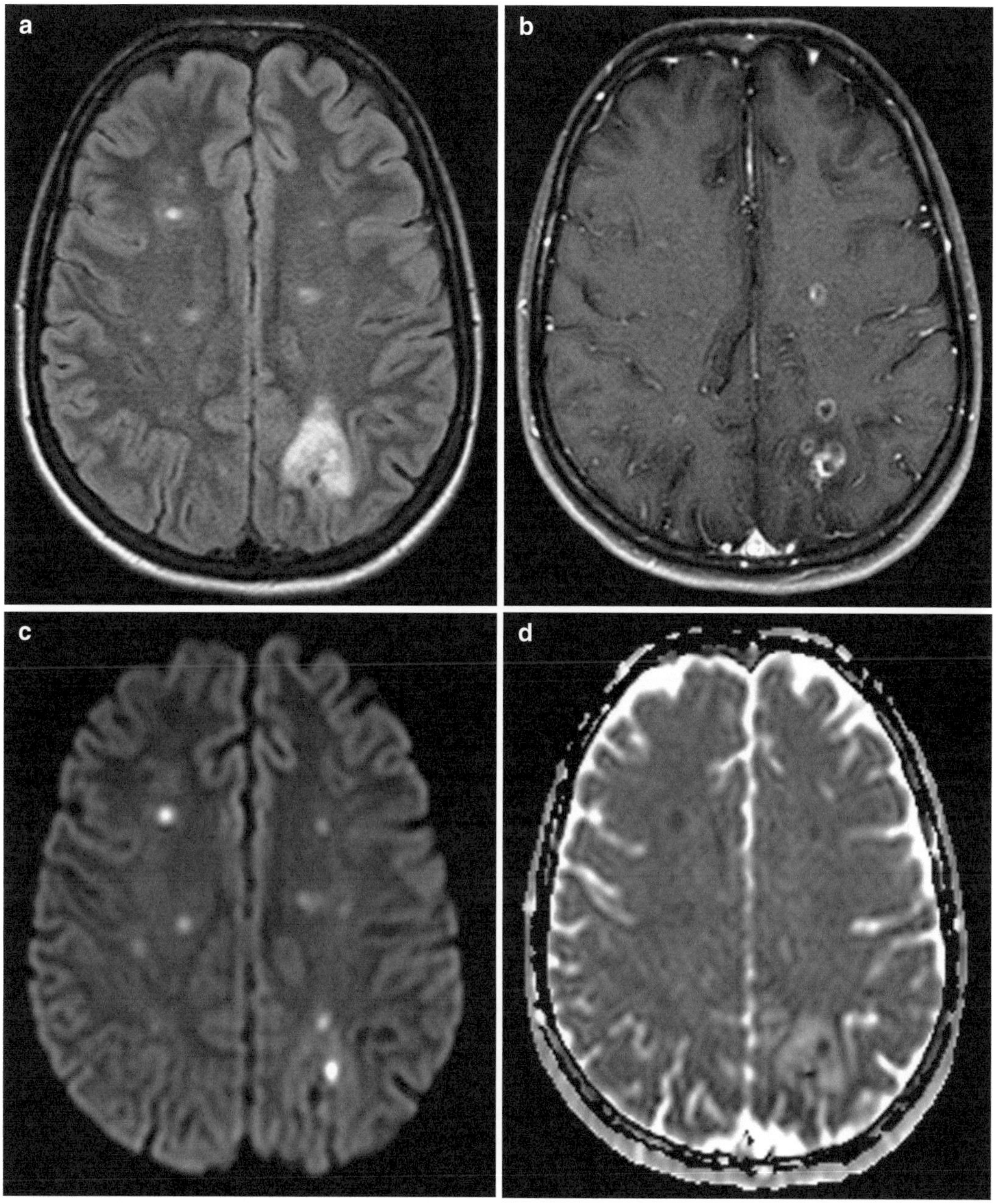

Fig. 4.11 Septic emboli. Axial T2-weighted FLAIR (**a**), post-contrast T1-weighted MRI (**b**), DWI (**c**), and ADC map (**d**) show multiple ring-enhancing lesions with central restricted diffusion and surrounding vasogenic edema in the bilateral cerebral hemispheres

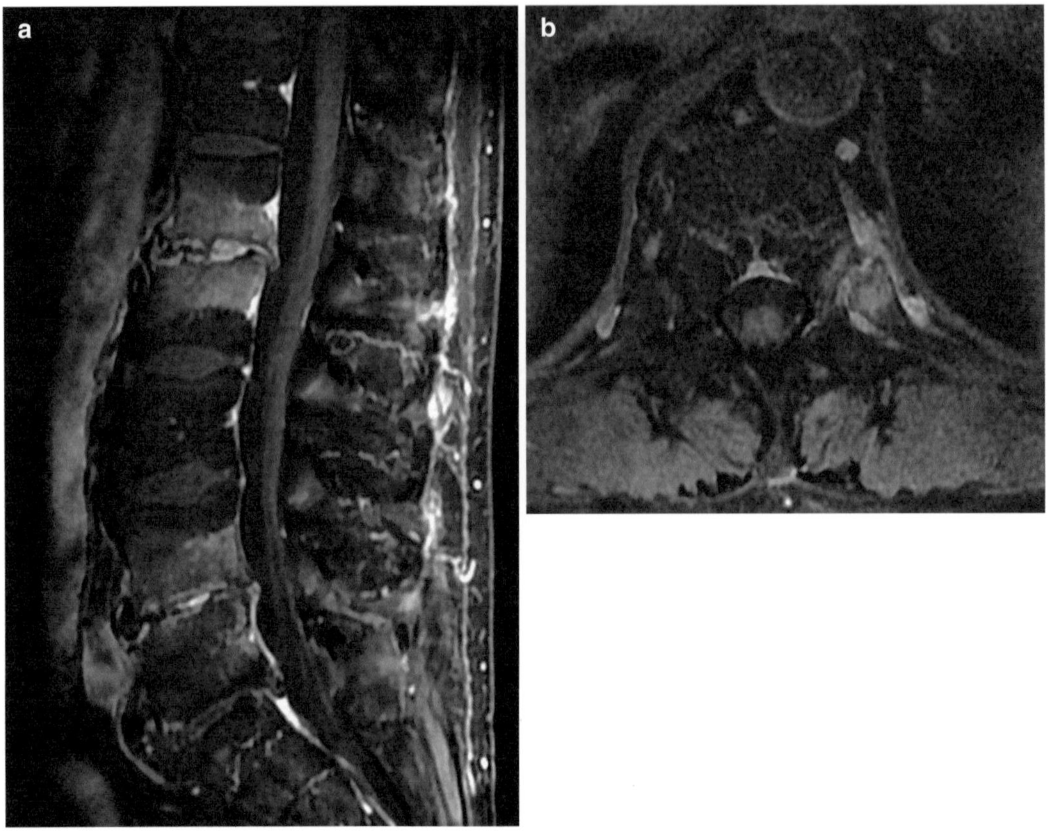

Fig. 4.12 Discitis-osteomyelitis and septic arthritis. The patient has a history of intravenous drug use. Sagittal fat-suppressed post-contrast T1-weighted MRI (**a**) shows disc space and adjacent vertebral bone marrow enhancement L1–2 and L4–5. Axial fat-suppressed post-contrast T1-weighted MRI (**b**) shows enhancement in the bone marrow and soft tissues surrounding a left costovertebral joint

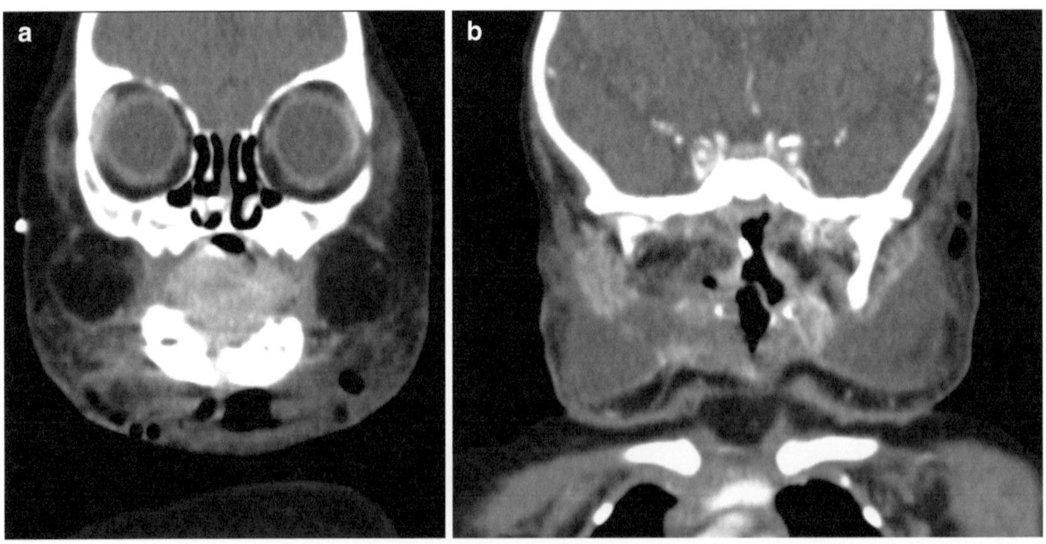

Fig. 4.13 Necrotizing fasciitis. Coronal CT images (**a**, **b**) show diffuse stranding of the subcutaneous fat, fluid collections, and foci of gas in the face

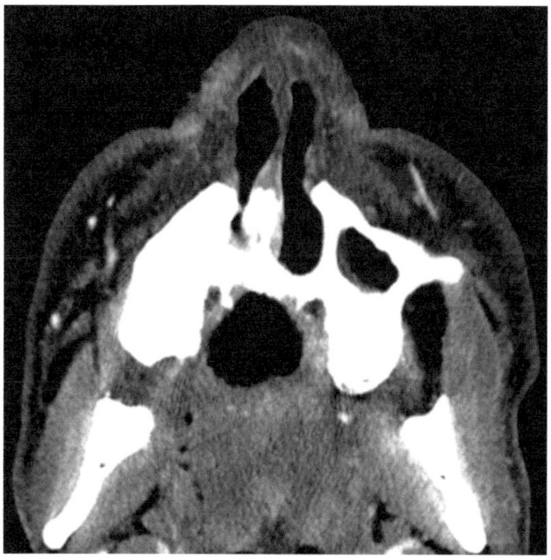

Fig. 4.14 Acne vulgaris. Axial CT shows skin thickening and areas of hyperattenuation along the nasal ala bilaterally

lymphadenopathy, often in the submandibular and preauricular regions, with low-attenuation areas and granuloma formation in the subcutaneous fat and skin (Fig. 4.17). However, there is usually negligible inflammatory stranding of the surrounding subcutaneous fat.

Tick-borne Disease: MRI is the modality of choice for imaging suspected neuroborreliosis. However, positive neuroimaging is evident in less than half of patients with Lyme disease, for example. Among those with positive neuroimaging findings, leptomeningeal and nerve-root enhancement, mainly involving the facial nerves, are relatively common findings associated with Lyme disease that may be encountered on MRI (Fig. 4.18). Besides, white matter lesions manifesting as T2 hyperintensities on MRI may also be present, but are nonspecific (Fig. 4.19).

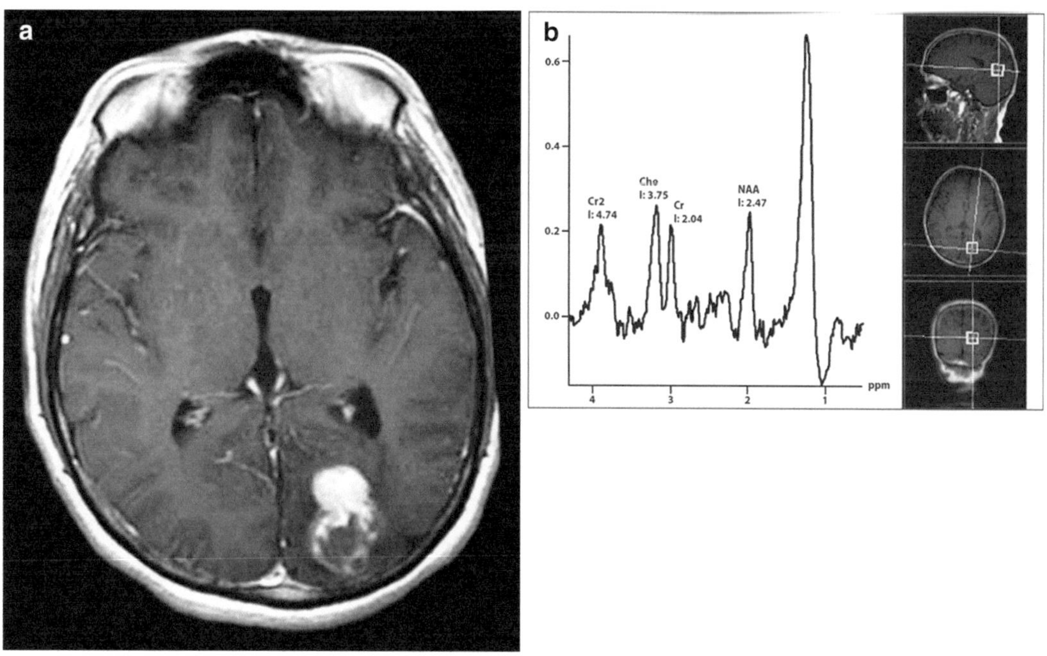

Fig. 4.15 Tuberculoma. The patient from Nepal presented with visual field deficits. Axial contrast-enhanced T1-weighted MRI (**a**) shows a left occipital lobe mass with irregular peripheral enhancement. MR spectroscopy of the lesion (**b**) shows prominent lipid peak at 1.3 ppm

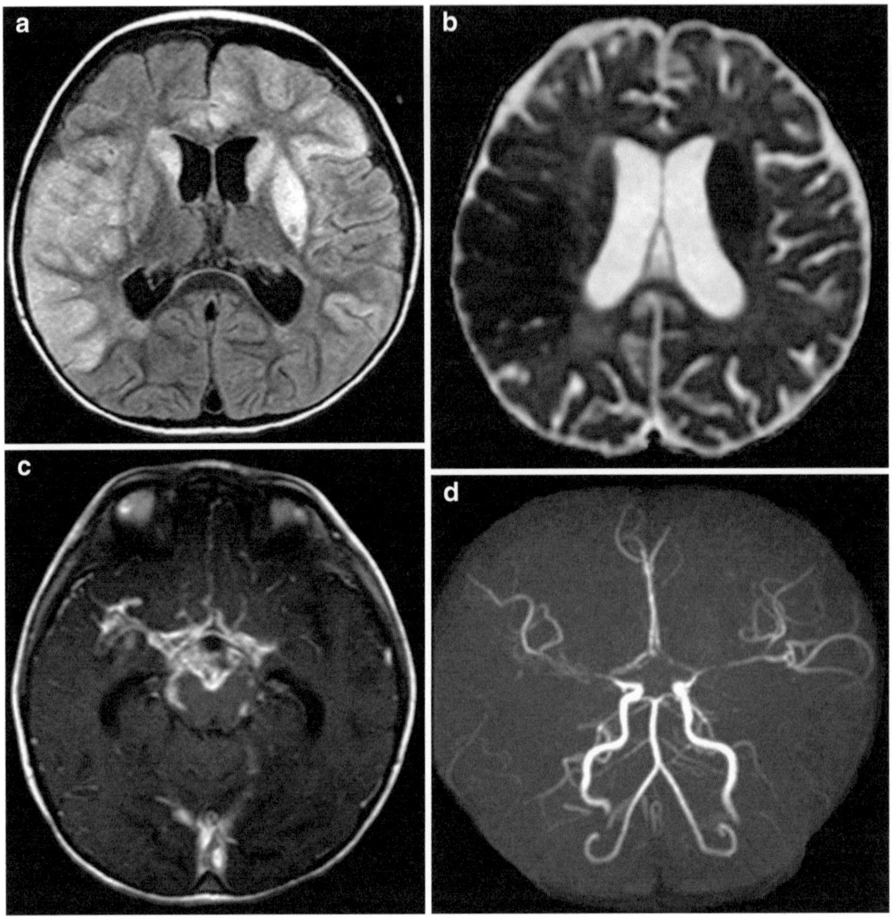

Fig. 4.16 Tuberculous meningitis and vasculitis. Axial T2-weighted FLAIR MRI (**a**), ADC map (**b**), and post-contrast T1-weighted (**c**) MRI show bilateral middle cerebral artery territory infarcts and basilar predominant leptomeningeal enhancement. MRA MIP image (**d**) shows bilateral middle cerebral artery stenoses due to vasculitis

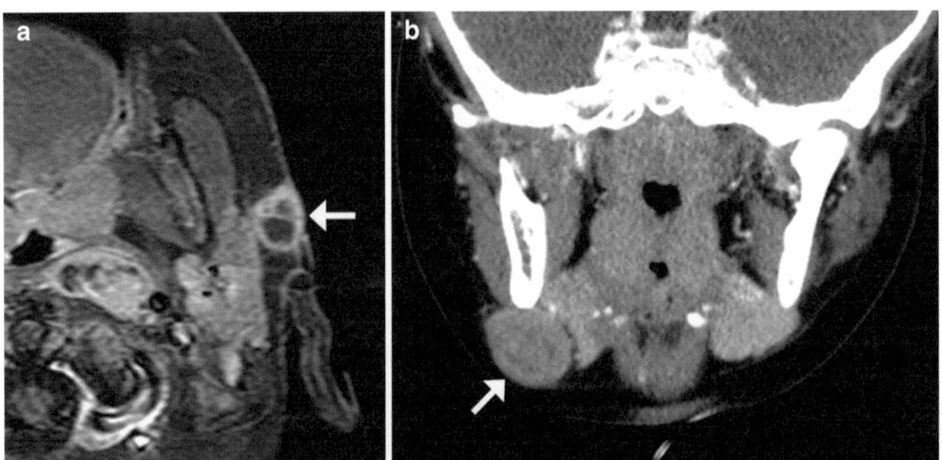

Fig. 4.17 Nontuberculous Mycobacterial infection. Axial fat-suppressed post-contrast T1-weighted MRI (**a**) shows ring-enhancing lesion in the preauricular subcutaneous tissues that extends to the skin surface (arrow). Coronal CT image (**b**) in a different patient shows an enlarged right submandibular lymph node with areas of hypoattenuation, but no surrounding inflammation (arrow)

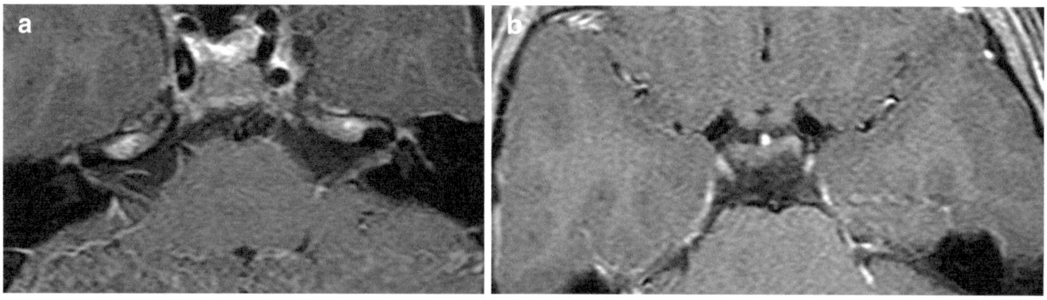

Fig. 4.18 Lyme disease. Axial post-contrast T1-weighted MR images (**a**, **b**) show enhancement of the bilateral facial and oculomotor nerves

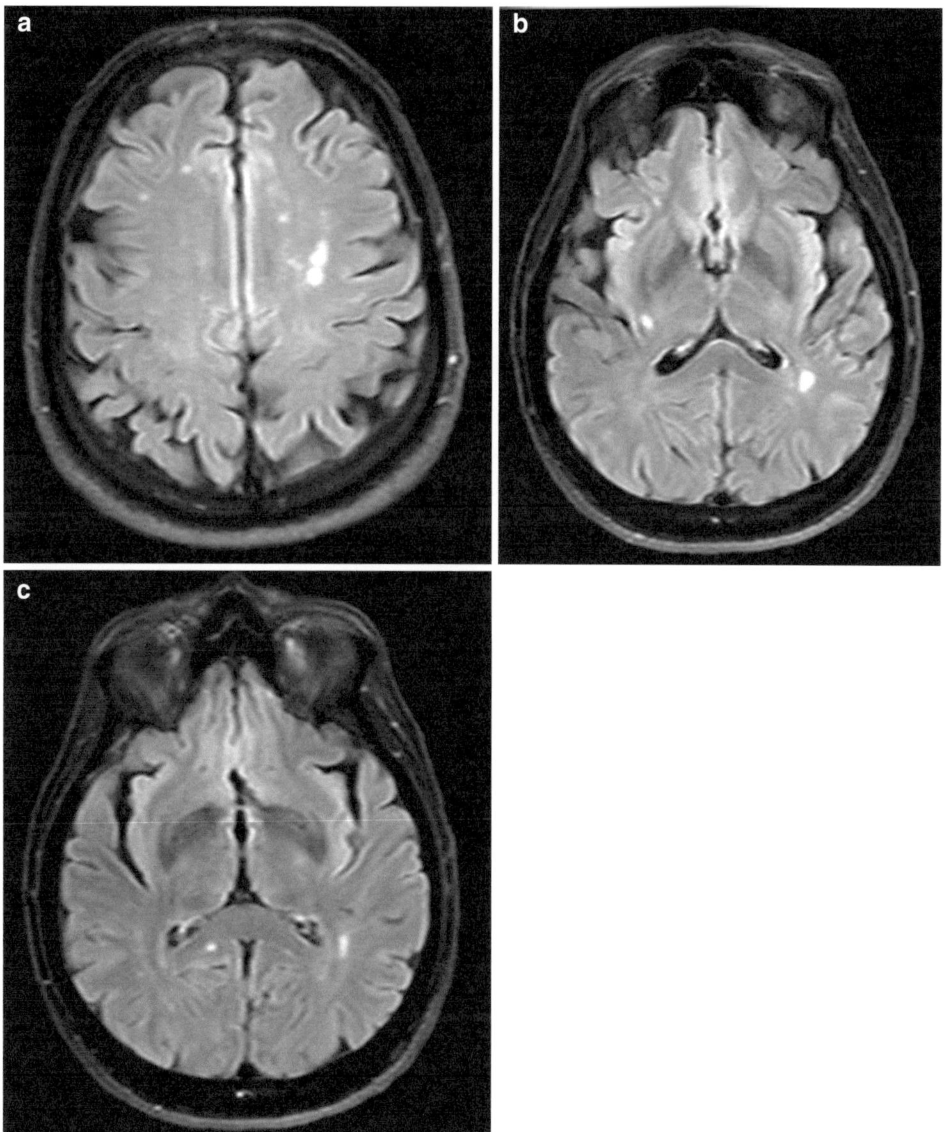

Fig. 4.19 Lyme disease. Axial T2-weighted FLAIR MR images (**a–c**) show multiple cerebral white matter lesions

Viral Skin Diseases

Overview

Viral infections often present with an exanthem, which is a skin rash. Viral exanthems can be caused by many viruses, including enteroviruses, adenovirus, chickenpox, measles, rubella, mononucleosis, and certain types of herpes, and can occur during the primary infection or reactivation of the disease. Furthermore, skin lesions can have a delayed appearance, such as with trigeminal trophic syndrome related to herpes zoster, in which chronic injury to the trigeminal nerve is associated with skin ulceration in the distribution of the nerve.

Viruses can attain the central nervous system by infecting and migrating along peripheral nerves. For example, herpes simplex virus initially infects keratinocytes and then migrates to peripheral sensory neurons. Alternatively, viruses can reach the central nervous system via olfactory nerves or hematogenously through a variety of mechanisms. Viruses that remain within cells of the meninges or ventricular lining tend to induce meningitis or ventriculitis, while those that infect the central nervous system parenchyma result in meningoencephalitis, encephalitis, or myelitis. Ultimately, the particular distribution of viruses and the ensuing immune response determine how the infection will manifest clinically. In particular, Guillain-Barré syndrome, which comprises acute inflammatory immune-mediated polyradiculoneuropathy, Miller Fisher syndrome, which affects the oculomotor nerves and the brainstem, and Bickerstaff's brainstem encephalitis, result from myelin or axonal damage by immunoglobulins that share antigenic epitopes with some viral antigens.

Clinicopathologic Findings

Viral exanthems can have a wide variety of clinical presentations, including vesicular, maculopapular, morbilliform, urticarial, and scarlatiniform rashes. The lesions may or may not be pruritic. Although viral exanthems are often nonspecific, some have characteristic features. For example, herpes zoster, which remains dormant in the dorsal root ganglia of peripheral nerves and becomes reactivated, resulting in a painful, hyperesthetic, and pruritic vesicular rash in the dermatomal distribution of the nerve and are known as shingles (Fig. 4.20). In particular, Ramsay Hunt syndrome, or herpes zoster oticus is a form of shingles that affects the ears with associated facial nerve paralysis and hearing loss. Trigeminal trophic syndrome is another potential sequela of herpes zoster. The clinical triad of trigeminal trophic syndrome includes anesthesia, paresthesia, and skin ulceration of the trigeminal dermatome.

Many viruses are transmitted via mosquito bites. There is often mild, transient inflammation in the skin at the site of the bite. However, in rare cases, there can be associated hypersensitivity characterized by intense local skin reactions, including bullae and necrosis, along with general

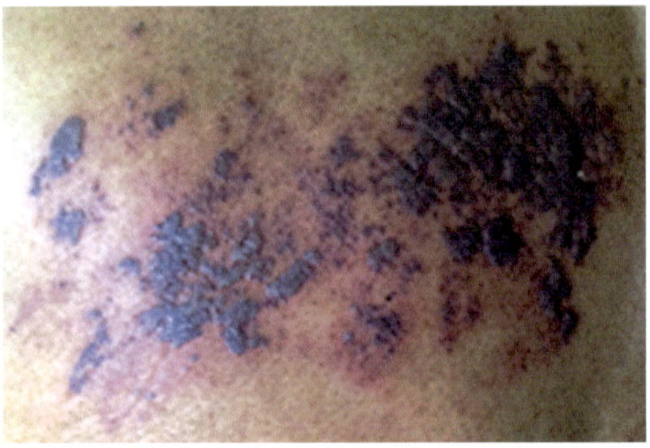

Fig. 4.20 Viral infection. Photograph shows crusting erythematous patches on the neck that represent shingles from Herpes Zoster. Courtesy of Min Deng MD and Arlene Ruiz de Luzuriaga MD

symptoms, such as fever and regional lymphadenopathy. On histology, such skin lesions demonstrate features of vasculitis. Following a mosquito bite, there can be viral replication and seeding of the reticuloendothelial system, viremia, neurotropic spread, as well as the effects of the elicited immune response that can involve the central nervous system. Some of the clinical manifestations related central nervous system involvement by viral infections include the following:

- *Aseptic meningitis*: typically presents with a headache, fever, photophobia, and meningeal signs, and may be accompanied by myalgias and rash.
- *Meningoencephalitis*: typically presents with altered mental status, fever, and headache, often accompanied by seizures and variable neurological deficits depending on what areas of the brain are affected. The presence of an altered level of consciousness or focal neurologic findings distinguishes encephalitis from meningitis. Otherwise, alteration of healthy immune function in the setting of a previous viral infection can lead to acute disseminated encephalomyelitis (ADEM) and antibody-associated encephalitides, such as *N*-methyl-D-aspartate receptor antibody.
- *Guillain-Barré syndrome and transverse myelitis*: likely results from aberrant immune response triggered by a recent infection or vaccination and characteristically presents as progressive ascending symmetric weakness, mild sensory loss, and hypo- or areflexia. Patients may also experience autonomic dysfunction, which consists of sinus tachycardia or sometimes bradycardia, labile blood pressure, orthostatic hypotension, arrhythmias, neurogenic pulmonary edema, and bowel and bladder problems. Electrophysiologic testing shows a pattern of multifocal demyelination, and there is cerebrospinal fluid protein elevation.

Ultimately, the diagnosis of viral central nervous system infections is typically based on cerebrospinal fluid analysis to identify antibodies of the remnants of viral DNA or RNA through polymerase chain reaction (PCR) assays that indicate the presence of a particular virus or group of viral pathogens.

Imaging Findings

A high-resolution internal auditory canal MRI protocol can reveal enhancement along cranial nerves 7 and 8 associated with acute herpes zoster oticus (Fig. 4.21). Similarly, high-resolution T2-weighted cisternographic MRI sequences can demonstrate atrophy of the trigeminal nerve in cases of the trigeminal trophic syndrome (Fig. 4.22).

Neuroimaging can also be used to delineate the extent of the inflammatory changes in the brain and spine from viral infections, but the findings are usually not specific enough to suggest a single entity. Nevertheless, specific imaging features are suggestive of viral infections in the differential diagnosis. For example, herpes simplex viral encephalitis typically appears as high T2 signal involving the cortex and underlying white matter with a predilection for the temporal and inferior frontal lobes, as well as the insula, and cingulate gyri. Early stages of disease are unilateral but may progress to bilateral involvement, which can be asymmetric. Associated diffusion restriction due to cytotoxic injury is often present (Fig. 4.23).

The consequence of autoimmune responses to various viral antigens on the central nervous system, such as acute disseminated encephalomyelitis and acute inflammatory immune-mediated polyradiculoneuropathy, also often have characteristic findings that are otherwise not specific to a particular antigen. For example, acute inflammatory immune-mediated polyradiculoneuropathy can be demonstrated on MRI as diffuse cauda equina enhancement with preferential involvement of the anterior nerve roots (Fig. 4.24).

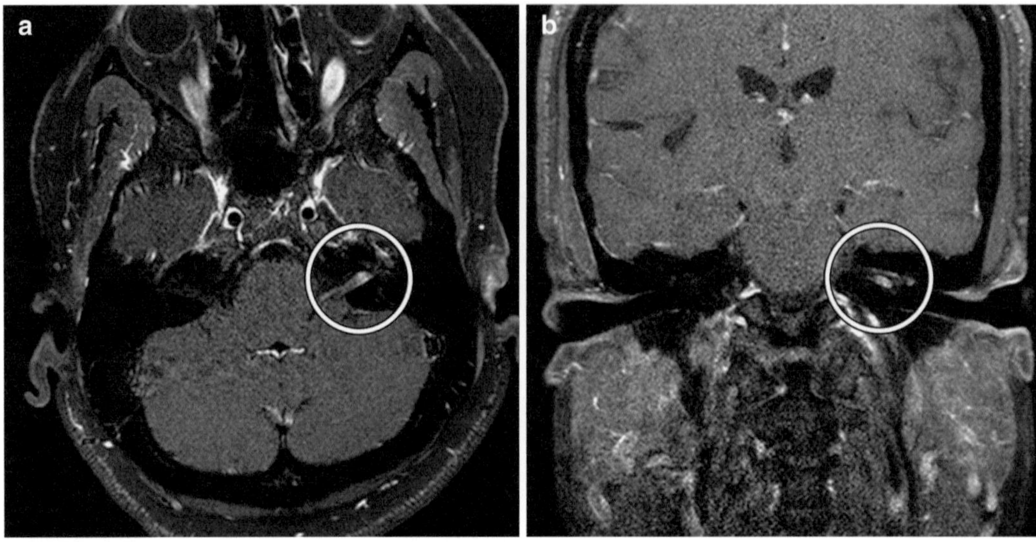

Fig. 4.21 Ramsay Hunt syndrome. Axial post-contrast T1-weighted MRI shows enhancement of the left facial and vestibulocochlear nerves (encircled). There is also a suggestion of left auricular and external auditory canal cutaneous enhancement

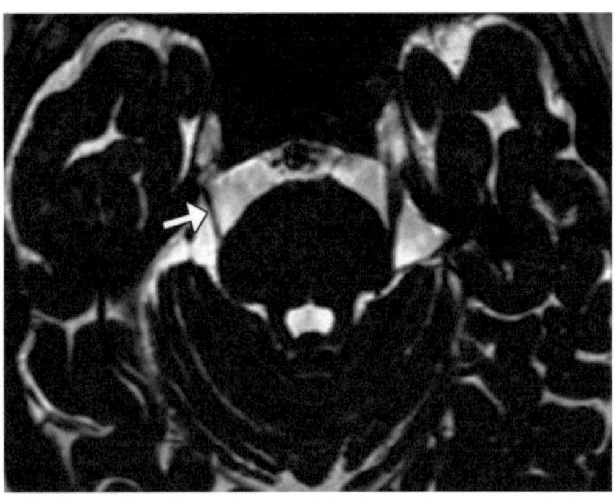

Fig. 4.22 Trigeminal trophic syndrome. Axial T2-weighted MRI shows an atrophic right trigeminal nerve (arrow)

Fungal Skin Infections

Overview

Fungal skin infections can be caused by a wide variety of yeasts, molds, and dimorphic fungi and tend to occur in immunocompromised individuals. Cutaneous manifestations of fungal infections can be primary or secondary. Primary lesions contain the fungal organisms, which can be identified in cultures or histopathology and can result from skin injury, such as near intravenous access catheter sites, at sites of traumatic injection, and in areas associated with dressings, burns, or surgery. Secondary cutaneous lesions result either from contiguous extension to the skin from infected underlying structures or widespread blood-borne seeding of the skin. These include erythema nodosum, erythema multiforme, acute generalized exanthema, reactive interstitial granulomatous dermatitis, and Sweet syndrome. Mucormycosis and aspergillosis, in particular, tend to be angioinvasive and are associated with high morbidity and mortality.

Clinicopathologic Findings

Fungal skin lesions may result from direct implantation, such as with tinea capitis, invasion from adjacent tissues, such as from sinonasal infection, or disseminated disease from hematogenous spread. Skin lesions associated with

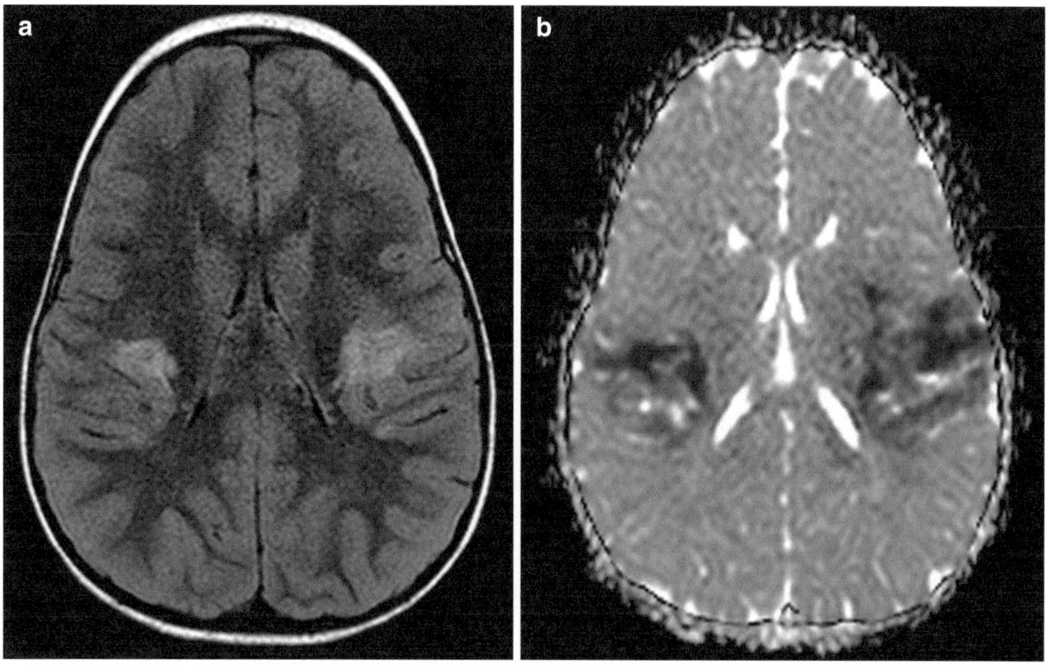

Fig. 4.23 Viral encephalitis. Axial T2-weighted FLAIR MRI (**a**) and ADC map (**b**) show cytotoxic edema in the bilateral peri-Sylvian regions. The patient tested positive for herpes simplex virus

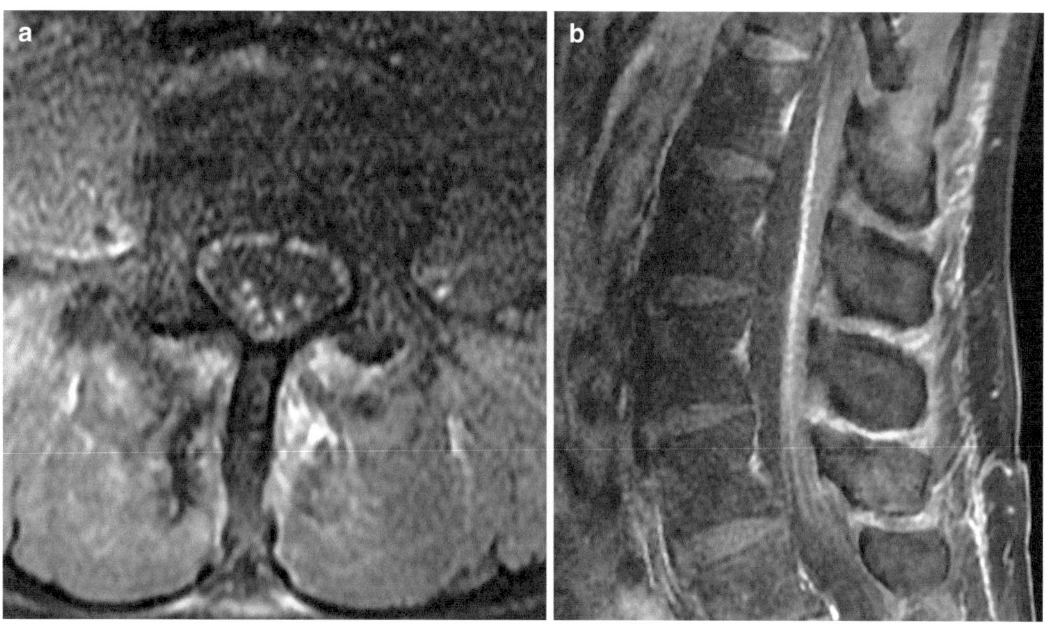

Fig. 4.24 Viral acute inflammatory immune-mediated polyradiculoneuropathy. The patient contracted West Nile virus after being stung in the back of the neck by an insect described as an "unusual mosquito" that led to a rash at the site of the sting. Axial (**a**) and sagittal (**b**) fat-suppressed post-contrast T1-weighted MR images obtained about 1 week after the insect bite show diffuse enhancement of multiple cauda equina nerve roots

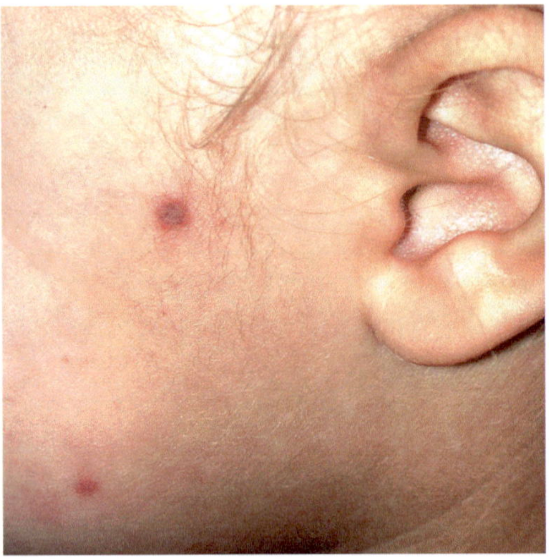

Fig. 4.25 Fungal infection. The patient has a history of relapsed AML. Photograph shows erythematous papules and plaques with central ulceration scattered across the face, which proved to be caused by Fusarium species. Courtesy of Sarah Stein MD

disseminated fungal infections may present as macules, papules, pustules, or subcutaneous nodules. For example, multiple red or gray macules with central ulceration or black eschar are characteristic of Fusarium skin infection (Fig. 4.25).

Most of the systemic fungal pathogens are associated with potential central nervous system involvement. In order to achieve favorable outcomes, prompt diagnosis and treatment are essential. CNS fungal infections may present with various clinical syndromes which may be specific for particular fungi. Among these, common syndromes are basal meningitis, hydrocephalus, space occupying lesions, such as cerebral abscesses, granulomas, stroke syndromes, particularly with aspergillosis, zygomycosis, and spinal infections. Identifying the etiological agent as fungal and not bacterial is vital since antibacterial therapy is not effective against fungi and CNS mycoses lead to high morbidity and mortality. Histopathologic examination of tissues detects fungal invasion of tissues and vessels, as well as the host reaction to the fungus (Fig. 4.26). There are only rare instances in which the morphologic characteristics of fungi are specific, and in general, speciation is best performed on tissue culture in the microbiology lab

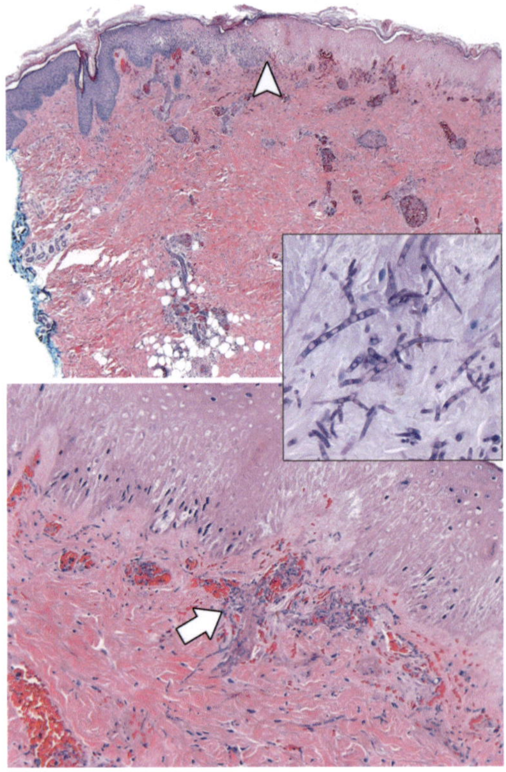

Fig. 4.26 Fungal infection. Low power hematoxylin and eosin stained photomicrograph (**top**) shows viable skin (left of arrowhead) and necrotic epidermis (right of arrowhead). High power hematoxylin and eosin stained photomicrograph (**bottom**) shows necrotic epidermis and an underlying dermal vessel infiltrated by fungal hyphae (*arrow*). PAS stain (inset) shows branching fungal hyphae. Fungal typing is best performed on culture rather than tissue morphology

or PCR from fresh or Formalin-fixed, Paraffin-embedded tissue. Histologic examination remains a valuable tool to define the diagnostic significance of positive culture isolates or results of PCR testing.

Imaging Findings

Fungal skin lesions from disseminated disease may be identified on imaging as scattered punctate foci of enhancement (Fig. 4.27). Fungal infection can also extend to the skin and subcutaneous tissues from underlying cervical lymphadenopathy, particularly following inter-

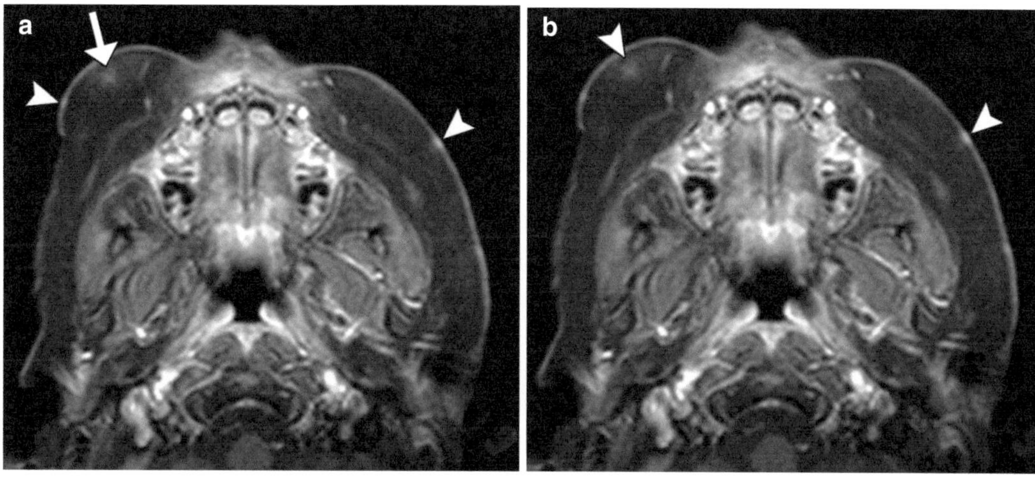

Fig. 4.27 Fungal infection. Axial post-contrast T1-weighted MR images (**a**, **b**) in the same patient as in Fig. 4.25 show multiple small enhancing lesions in the skin (*arrowheads*) and subcutaneous tissues (*arrow*)

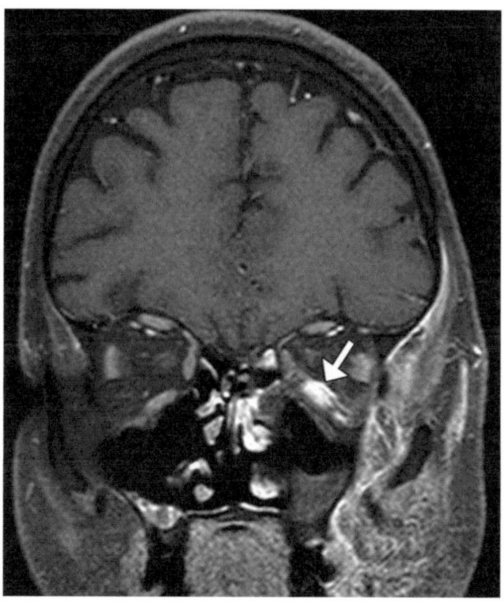

Fig. 4.28 Fungal infection. Coronal fat-suppressed post-contrast T1-weighted MR image shows left maxillary sinus mucosal inflammation, as well as an inflamed left inferior rectus muscle (arrow) and left facial soft tissues, extending to the skin in a patient with invasive Mucor infection

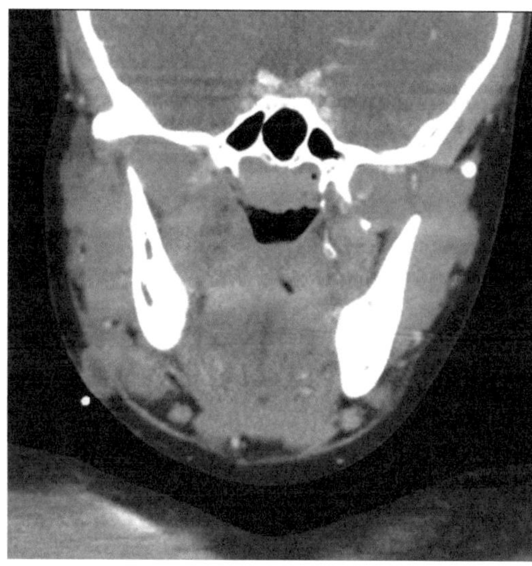

Fig. 4.29 Fungal infection. Coronal CT image (**a**) at initial presentation shows a heterogeneous bulky right submandibular lymphadenopathy. Follow-up coronal CT image (**b**) after antibiotics and biopsy shows decrease in size of the adenopathy, but a new fluid collection in the overlying skin and subcutaneous tissues

ventions (Fig. 4.28). Otherwise, diffuse enhancement of the subcutaneous tissues of the face may be a sign of invasive fungal rhinosinusitis, along with other imaging findings, including bone dehiscence, orbital invasion, septal ulceration, and pterygopalatine fossa involvement (Fig. 4.29). Associated necrosis may appear as areas of non-enhancement on imaging, as exemplified by the "black turbinate sign" on sinonasal imaging.

The main categories of fungal infection of the central nervous system include the following:

- Extra-axial, such as meningitis. Fungal meningitis is best depicted on MRI and can appear as diffuse or nodular leptomeningeal enhancement, which can be complicated by communicating hydrocephalus (Fig. 4.30).
- Parenchymal, such as cerebritis, granuloma, or abscess formation. For example, granulomas can appear nonspecific, but may contain foci of susceptibility effect and may enhance (Fig. 4.31). Otherwise, cerebritis appears as areas of high T2 signal on MRI with variable enhancement and restricted diffusion.
- Vascular, such as vasculitis and mycotic aneurysms. For example, there is a predilection of medium-sized vessels around the circle of Willis with fungal cerebral arteritis (Fig. 4.32), which may be complicated by cerebral infarction.

In general, fungal morphology correlates with the imaging manifestations with large, hyphal species having a predilection for brain parenchymal involvement, while small, unicellular organisms typically result in meningitis.

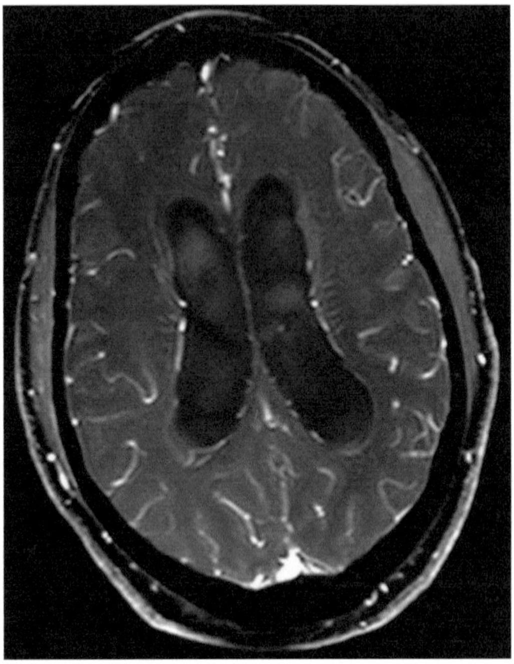

Fig. 4.30 Fungal infection. Axial post-contrast T1-weighted MRI shows diffuse leptomeningeal enhancement and ventriculomegaly

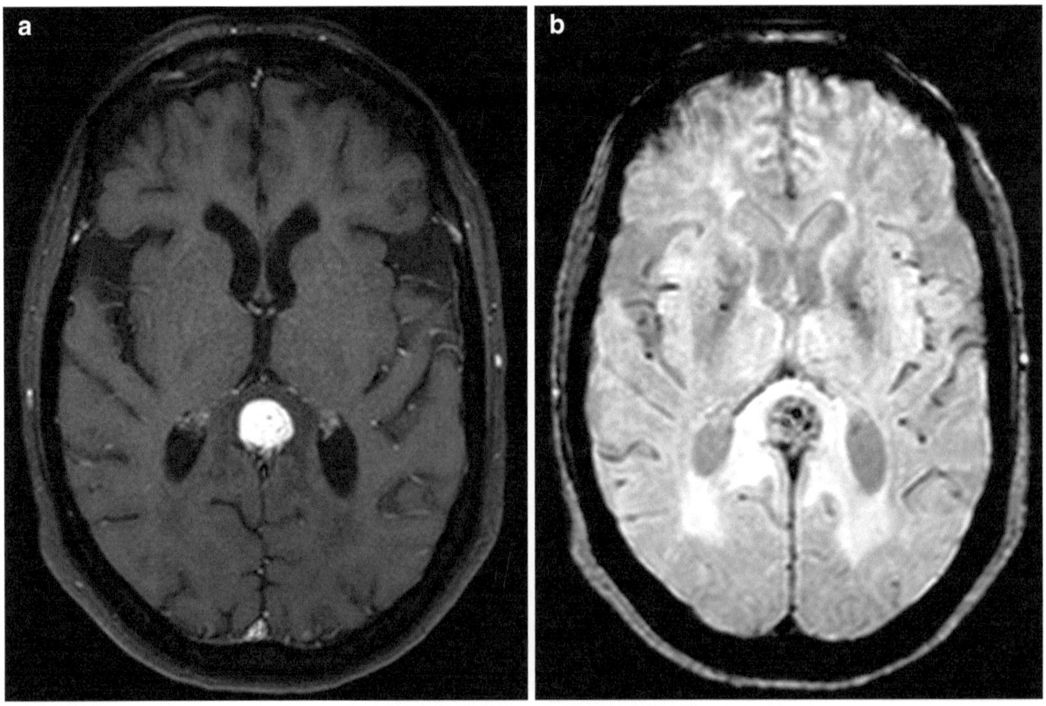

Fig. 4.31 Fungal infection. The patient has a history of disseminated Nocardia, including skin lesions. Axial post-contrast T1-weighted (**a**) and SWI (**b**) MR images show an enhancing mass in the posterior corpus callosum with associated susceptibility effect

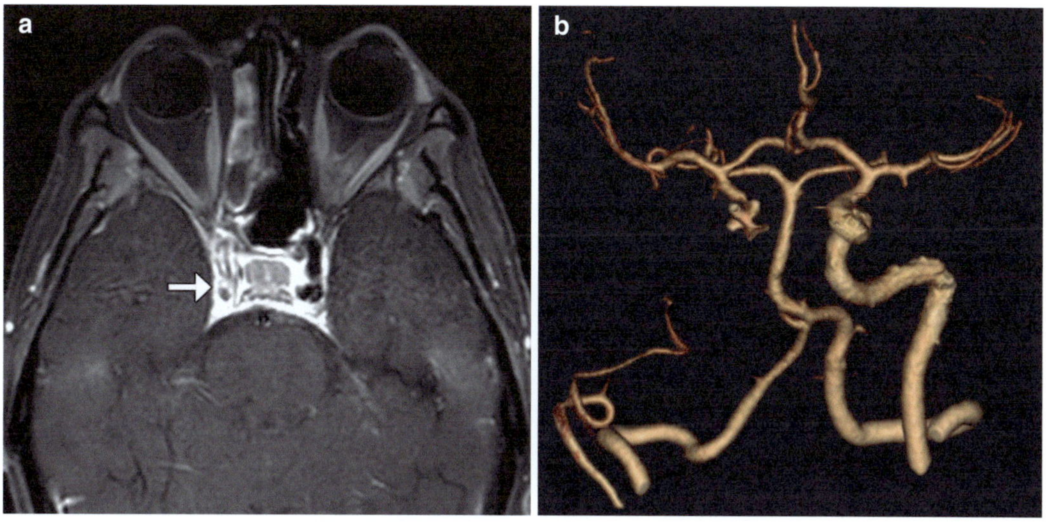

Fig. 4.32 Fungal infection. Axial fat-suppressed post-contrast T1-weighted MRI (**a**) shows right sphenoid and ethmoid sinusitis and an abnormal right cavernous carotid artery flow void (arrow). The corresponding 3D CTA image (b) shows significant steno-occlusive disease involving the right internal carotid artery due to vasculitis

Dendritic Cell Histiocytic Disorders

Overview

Dendritic cells are antigen-presenting cells located in the skin, mucosa, and lymphoid tissues. Histiocytic disorders of dendritic cell proliferation include Langerhans cell histiocytosis, juvenile xanthogranuloma, and Erdheim-Chester disease. Langerhans cell histiocytosis is the most common of these diseases and can be unifocal, multifocal unisystem, or multifocal multisystem, mainly occurring in the pediatric population. Juvenile xanthogranuloma may represent a granulomatous histiocytic reaction that most commonly affects infants and is typically confined to the skin. Erdheim-Chester disease tends to be a systemic disorder that mainly occurs in adults and is likely attributable to systemic immune Th-1 disruption and can be associated with mutations in the BRAF proto-oncogene.

Clinicopathologic Findings

Langerhans cell histiocytosis. Depending on the extent of the disease, patients may present with palpable craniofacial bone masses that are often associated with exophthalmos, disorders of the hypothalamic-pituitary system primarily with diabetes insipidus, progressive neurological deterioration with mainly cerebellar-pontine symptoms and abnormal brainstem evoked potentials. The skin rash associated with Langerhans cell histiocytosis is often present in the form of papulosquamous granulomatous lesions, which are frequently found on the face and scalp (Fig. 4.33). Other clinical manifestations of Langerhans cell histiocytosis in the head and neck include uveitis and lymphadenopathy. In the spine, vertebra plana can present with pain and even neurological deficits if there is spinal canal compromise. While previously thought to be a reactive process, the presence of *BRAF* V600E mutation in >50% likely indicates that Langerhans cell histiocytosis is actually a neoplastic proliferation. Affected tissues are infiltrated by monotonous

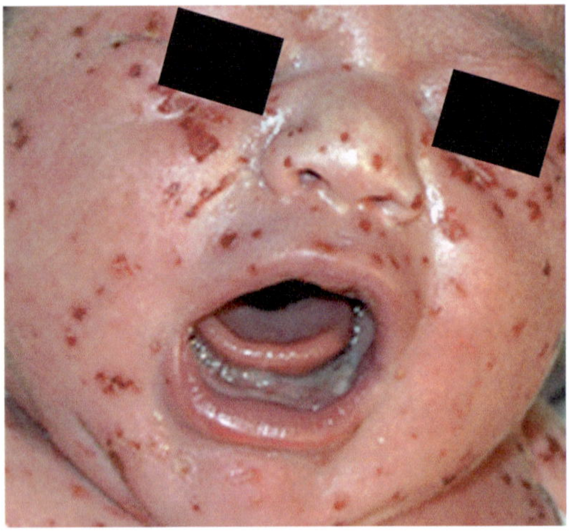

Fig. 4.33 Langerhans cell histiocytosis. Photograph shows extensive facial papulosquamous rashes. Courtesy of Min Deng MD and Arlene Ruiz de Luzuriaga MD

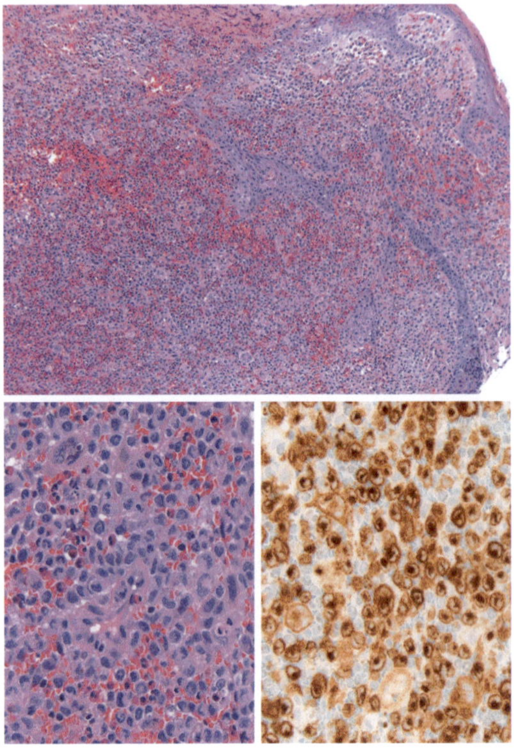

Fig. 4.34 Langerhans cell histiocytosis. Hematoxylin and eosin stained photomicrographs show sheets of cells expanding dermis with adjacent reactive epithelium (top), with Langerhans cells that have kidney-bean, horse-shoe, or grooved nuclei (bottom left). Scattered eosinophils are also present. Langerin immunostain is positive with perinuclear dot-like accentuation (bottom right)

cells with kidney-bean, horse-shoe, or grooved nuclei that stain positively for S100, Langerin, and CD1a (Fig. 4.34). Associated giant cells or eosinophils may be prominent.

Juvenile Xanthogranuloma. The skin lesions typically appear as yellow, red, or brown papules or nodules (Fig. 4.35). Several extracutaneous sites have been reported in the head and neck region, including the tympanic membrane, nasal cavity, tongue, orbit, subglottic region, intracranial compartment, and muscles, for example. On histology, juvenile xanthogranulomas display proliferations of foamy histiocytes (Fig. 4.36), and many contain multinucleated Touton cells, as well as lymphocytes and eosinophils. The lesional cells stain positively for histiocyte marker CD68, but not for Langerhans markers (S100, Langerin, CD1a). Juvenile xanthogranulomas often regress spontaneously.

Erdheim-Chester Disease. Cutaneous involvement in Erdheim-Chester disease manifest as xanthelasmas and papulonodular skin lesions (Fig. 4.37). Otherwise, the most common clinical presentation of Erdheim-Chester disease is bone pain, mainly affecting the lower extremities. Central nervous system involvement can present as cerebellar and pyramidal syndromes, headaches, seizures, cognitive impairment, cranial nerve palsies, and sensory disturbances. Furthermore, pituitary gland infiltration can lead

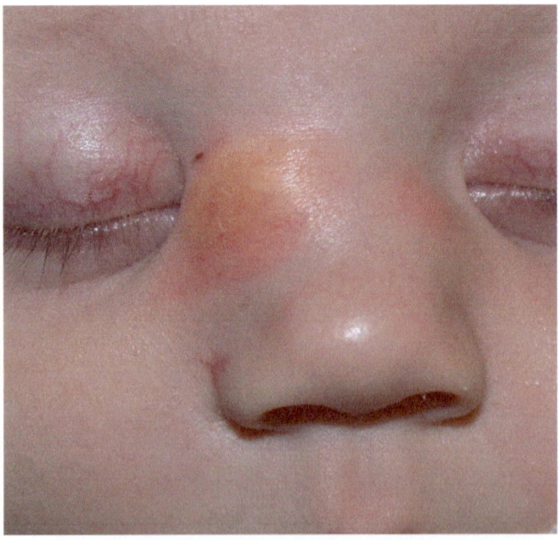

Fig. 4.35 Juvenile xanthogranuloma. Photograph shows a smooth lump along the right aspect of the glabella with associated yellowish discoloration of the skin. Courtesy of Mark Volk MD

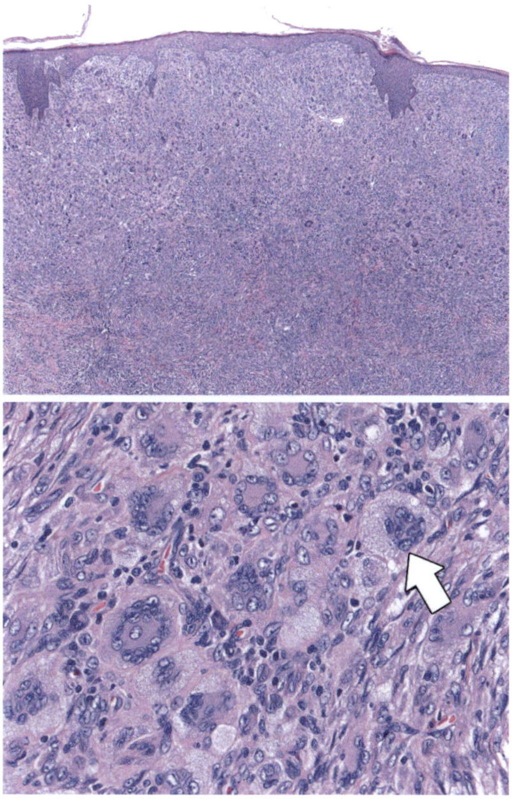

Fig. 4.36 Juvenile xanthogranuloma. Low (top) and high (bottom) power hematoxylin and eosin stained photomicrographs show dermis filled with sheets of histiocytoid cells with associated giant cells with foamy (xanthomatous) cytoplasm (arrow)

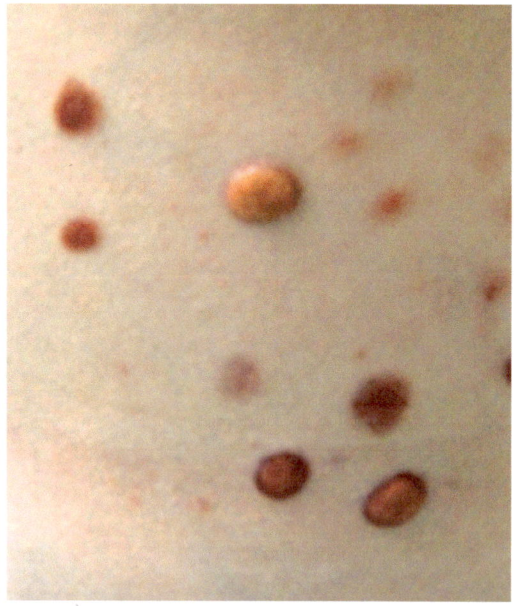

Fig. 4.37 Erdheim-Chester disease. Photograph shows multiple yellow-red pigmented papulonodular skin lesions. Courtesy of Min Deng MD and Arlene Ruiz de Luzuriaga MD

to diabetes insipidus and rarely hyperprolactinemia and gonadotropin insufficiency. Involvement of the orbits can lead to exophthalmos, papilledema. Constitutional symptoms include fever, weakness, and weight loss. On histology, cases that involve the reticular dermis tend to form xanthogranulomatous or xanthomatous infiltration with Touton cells and infiltrating foamy histiocytes that are CD68-positive and CD1a/S100-negative. Also, *BRAF* V600E mutation is frequently present in patients with cutaneous involvement.

Imaging Findings

Langerhans cell histiocytosis. Diagnostic imaging can reveal lytic lesions in the skull in patients with Langerhans cell histiocytosis, which classically have beveled edges and an avidly enhancing soft tissue component (Fig. 4.38). Vertebra plana is another classic skeletal lesion of Langerhans cell histiocytosis, which consists of marked flattening of the affected vertebral bodies (Fig. 4.39). MRI in patients with diabetes insipidus may demonstrate thickening of the pituitary stalk and absence of the posterior pituitary bright spot (Fig. 4.40). In the neurodegenerative form of Langerhans cell histiocytosis, symmetrical T2 hyperintensity in the cerebellar white matter and the surrounding pontine tegmentum white matter can be observed on MRI (Fig. 4.41). There can also be T1 hyperintensity the basal ganglia, but these lesions do not enhance or have mass effect.

Juvenile xanthogranuloma. In the head and neck region, juvenile xanthogranuloma usually appears as smooth, well-defined subcutaneous masses. When these involve the subgaleal space or dura, they tend to have a dome-shaped configuration. Furthermore, pachymeningeal juvenile xanthogranuloma lesions can display a dural tail and mimic meningiomas.

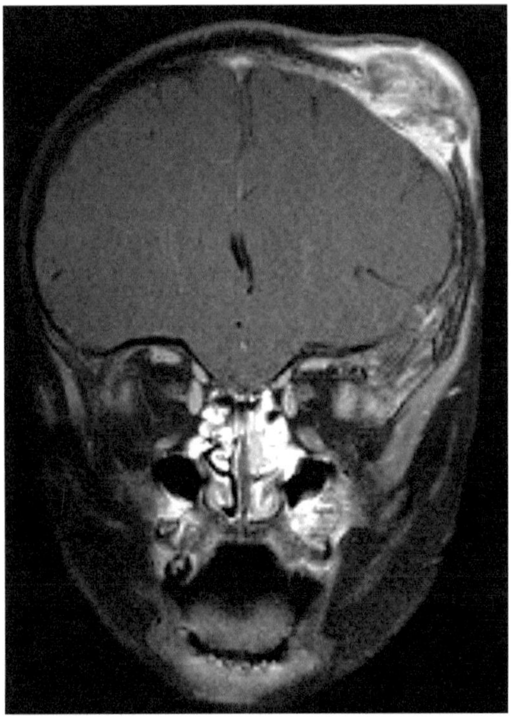

Fig. 4.38 Langerhans cell histiocytosis. Coronal fat-suppressed post-contrast T1-weighted MRI shows an enhancing skull mass with beveled edges that extends into the scalp

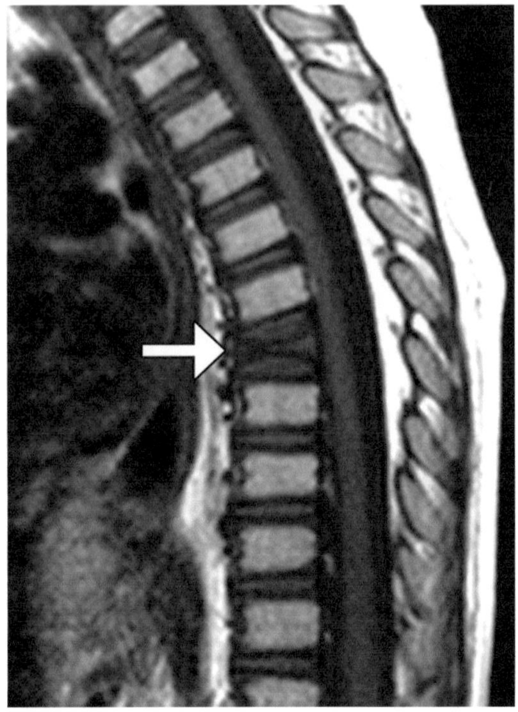

Fig. 4.39 Langerhans cell histiocytosis. Sagittal T1-weighted MRI shows thoracic vertebra plana (arrow)

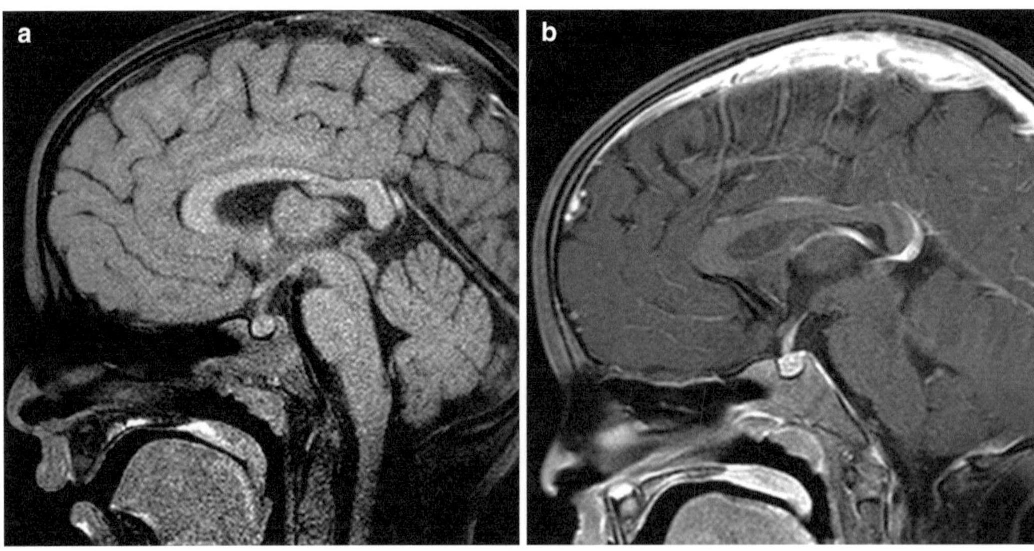

Fig. 4.40 Langerhans cell histiocytosis. Sagittal T1-weighted (**a**) and post-contrast T1-weighted (**b**) MR images show an absence of the posterior pituitary bright spot and thickening of the pituitary stalk in a patient with diabetes insipidus

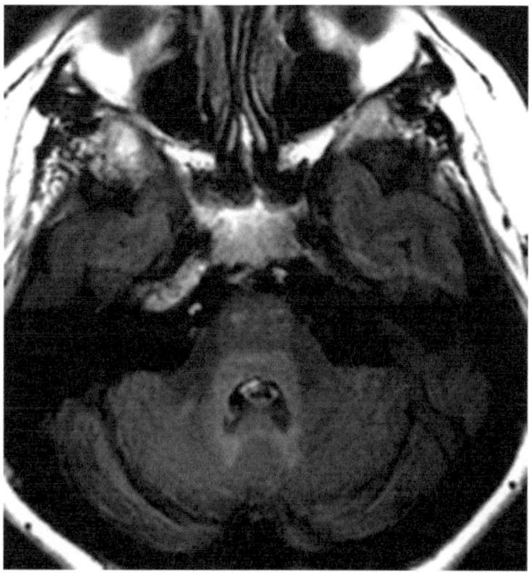

Fig. 4.41 Langerhans cell histiocytosis. Axial T2-weighted FLAIR MRI shows abnormal high signal surrounding the fourth ventricle

Occasionally, the lesions can appear more infiltrative and aggressive. On CT, the lesions appear as soft tissue attenuation and enhance diffusely. On MRI, the lesions often display low to intermediate signal on T2-weighted sequences and intermediate to high signal on T1-weighted sequences and typically enhance avidly and homogeneously (Fig. 4.42). On diffusion-weighted imaging, juvenile xanthogranuloma can display low diffusivity, which is likely attributable to the highly cellular nature of these lesions.

Erdheim-Chester disease: Lesions of the brain, meninges, bones, and orbits are often observed on MR and CT, even if these patients are asymptomatic. In particular, neuroimaging findings may include nodular masses of the pituitary stalk, meningeal lesions, bilateral

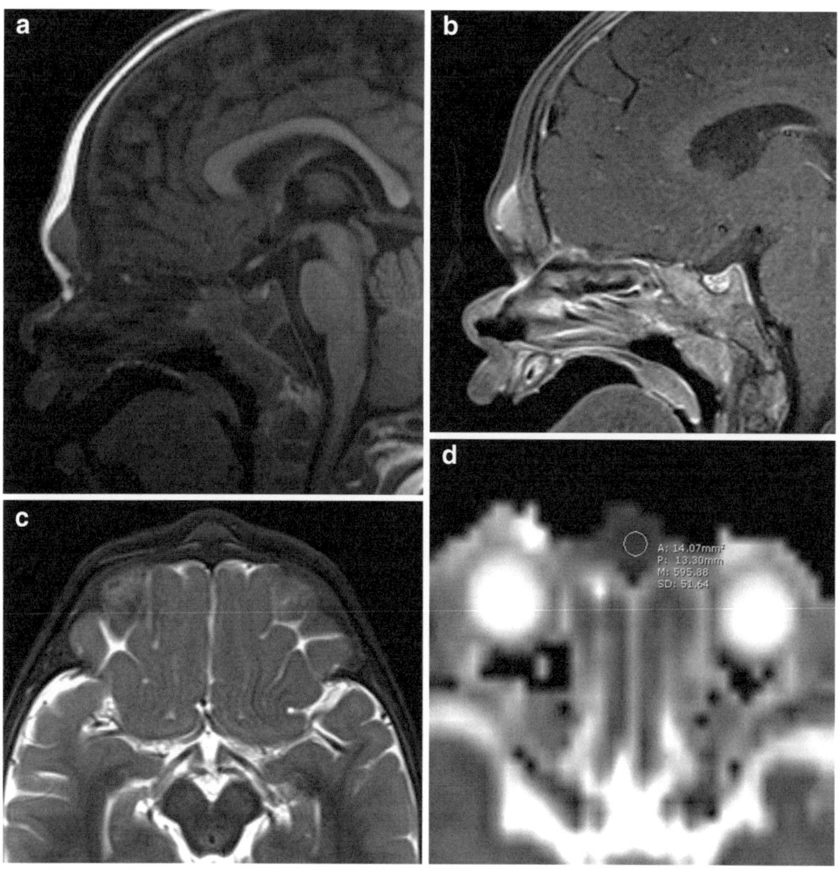

Fig. 4.42 Juvenile xanthogranuloma. Sagittal T1-weighted (**a**) and fat-suppressed post-contrast T1-weighted (**b**), axial fat-suppressed T2-weighted (**c**) MR images, and ADC map (**d**) show a well-defined, T2 hypointense, enhancing mass with low diffusivity in the midline frontal scalp that appears to arise from the periosteum of the underlying skull

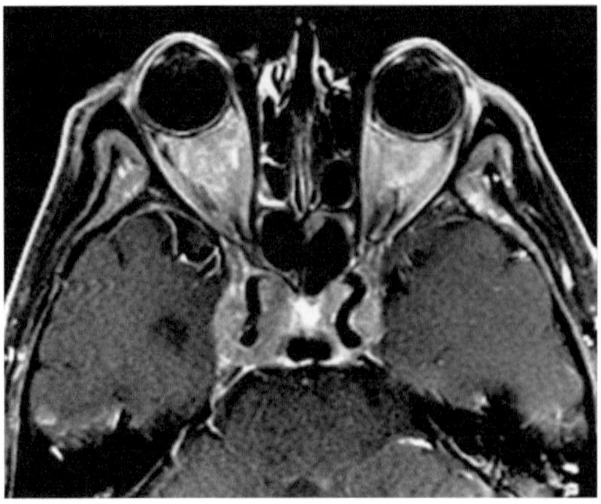

Fig. 4.43 Erdheim-Chester disease. Axial fat-suppressed post-contrast T1-weighted MRI shows bilateral retrobulbar enhancing masses and involvement of the bilateral cavernous sinuses

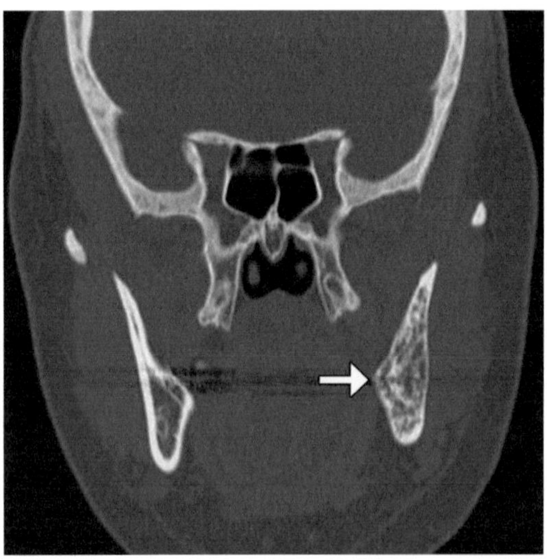

Fig. 4.44 Erdheim-Chester disease. Coronal CT image shows permeative sclerosis in the left mandibular body (arrow). Courtesy of Gul Moonis MD

symmetric T2 high signal intensity in the dentate nucleus areas, and enhancing nodules in the brain. Orbital involvement can appear as infiltrative low T1 and T2 signal intensity masses with avid enhancement (Fig. 4.43). Bone lesions associated with Erdheim-Chester disease are typically sclerotic, as depicted on CT (Fig. 4.44).

Rheumatoid Arthritis

Overview

Rheumatoid arthritis is an autoimmune inflammatory condition that primarily targets the synovium of the diarthrodial joints; however, many nonarticular tissues can also be involved. For example, patients with rheumatoid arthritis may incur neurological symptoms as a result of atlantoaxial subluxation, peripheral neuropathy; rheumatoid nodules in central and peripheral nervous system, and rheumatoid vasculitis, which can result in stroke and/or neuropathy. Likewise, rheumatoid nodules can form in the subcutaneous tissues and associated skin manifestations may include Raynaud phenomenon, urticarial vasculitis, pyoderma gangrenosum, and Sweet syndrome. Furthermore, there is a higher incidence of skin malignancies in patients with rheumatoid arthritis, particularly those treated with immunosuppressive agents.

Clinicopathologic Findings

The tradition diagnostic criteria for rheumatoid arthritis include the following:

- Morning joint stiffness
- Periarticular soft tissue swelling
- Symmetric articular swelling
- Subcutaneous rheumatoid nodules
- Positive rheumatoid factor
- Supportive imaging findings

Rheumatoid nodules are the main dermatological finding in rheumatoid arthritis and are usually painless, well-demarcated, flesh-colored, subcutaneous lumps (Fig. 4.45). The nodules are typically painless, but may occasionally become inflamed or ulcerated. Histologically, the nodules are composed of a fibrous shell with inner necrosis (Fig. 4.46). Other potential dermatological

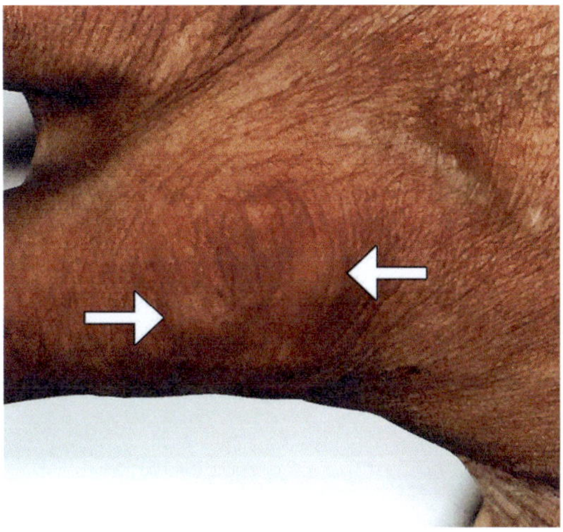

Fig. 4.45 Rheumatoid arthritis. Photograph shows periarticular rheumatoid nodules on the dorsum of the hand (arrows). Courtesy of Anisha Dua, MD, MPH

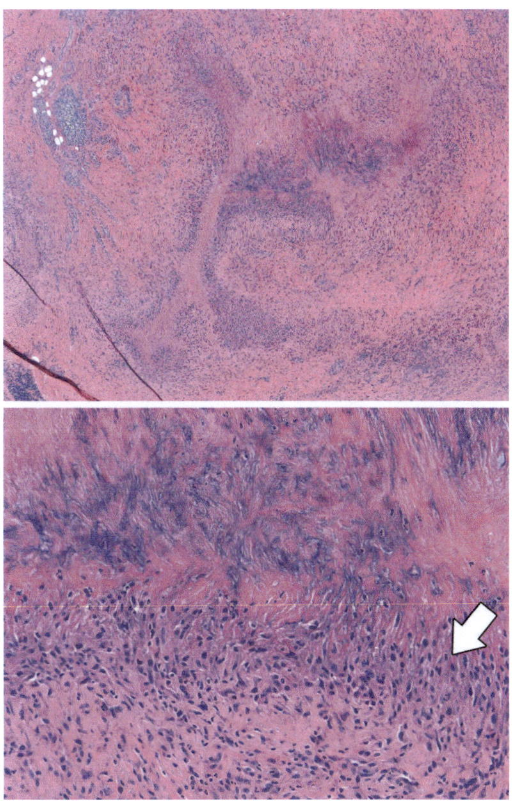

Fig. 4.46 Rheumatoid nodule. Low (top) and high (bottom) power hematoxylin and eosin stained photomicrographs show a nodule composed of epithelioid histiocytes (arrow) surrounding paucicellular "necrobiotic" collagen

findings in patients with rheumatoid arthritis include skin atrophy, hyperpigmentation, petechiae, purpura, ulcers, and gangrene.

Involvement of the cervical spine in rheumatoid arthritis can result in atlantoaxial instability, with cervical pain and neurological deficits, as well as sudden death due to impingement of the medulla by an eroded, vertically subluxed dens. Other potential neurologic manifestations of rheumatoid arthritis include meningitis from mononuclear cell infiltration and ischemic neuropathies from necrotizing arteritis of the vasa vasorum.

Imaging Findings

The most common site affected by rheumatoid arthritis is the atlantoaxial joint, potentially resulting in atlantoaxial instability, with cervical pain and neurological deficits. Another common site of involvement is the subaxial cervical spine, in which there can be multilevel vertebral subluxation that can in nerve root or spinal cord compression. Plain radiographs obtained in flexion and extension views can be performed to evaluate cervical instabilities associated with rheumatoid arthritis (Fig. 4.47). Otherwise, CT is useful for evaluating the presence of erosions, ankyloses, and pseudarthrosis (Fig. 4.48), while MRI is useful for evaluating potential spinal cord compromise related to subluxation and inflammatory tissues (Fig. 4.49). Finally, hypertrophic pachymeningitis associated with rheumatoid arthritis is best depicted via MRI as dural thickening and enhancement that is usually focal, but can be diffuse (Fig. 4.50). The lesions also often display low signal on T2-weighted MRI sequences.

Sarcoidosis

Sarcoidosis is a multifactorial inflammatory disorder that results from a complex interplay of multiple genetic loci and an exaggerated T-cell antigen response. The disease is characterized

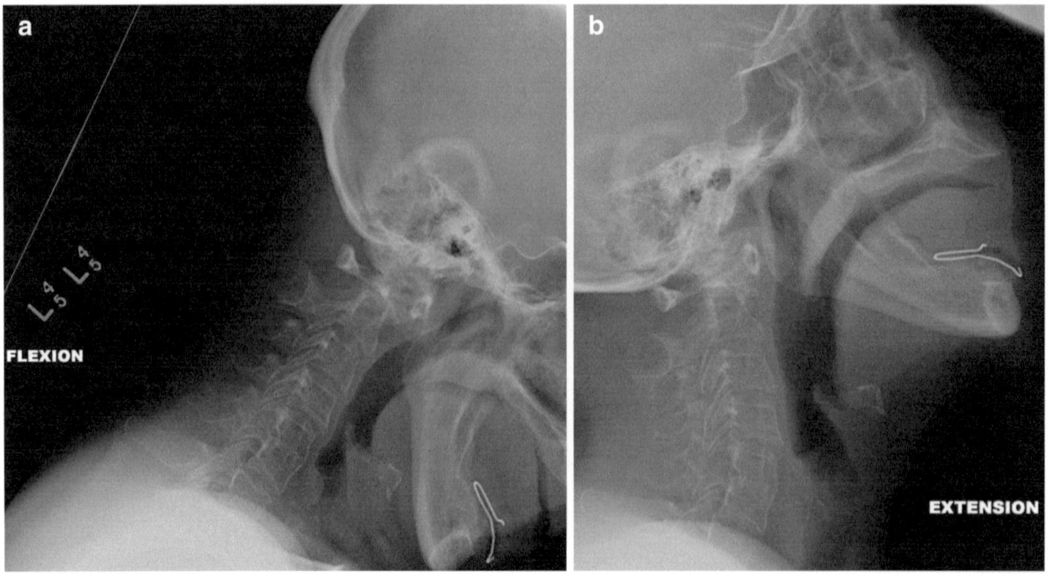

Fig. 4.47 Rheumatoid arthritis. Lateral radiographs of the cervical spine in flexion (**a**) and extension (**b**) reveal anterior subluxation of C1 on C2

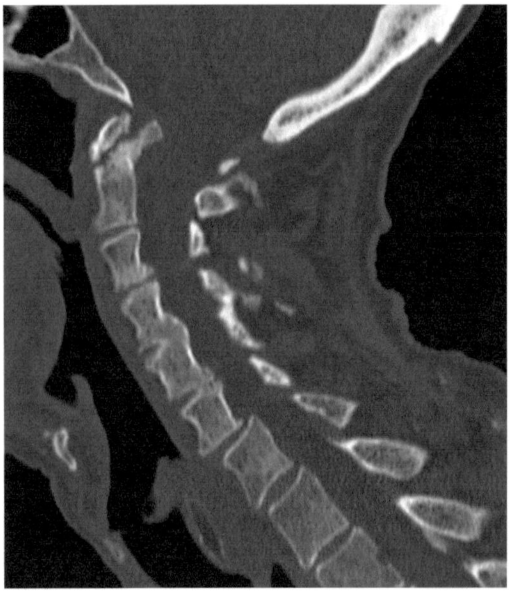

Fig. 4.48 Rheumatoid arthritis. Sagittal CT image shows deformity and erosions of the dens and multilevel stepwise anterolisthesis, as well as anklosis between C4 and C5

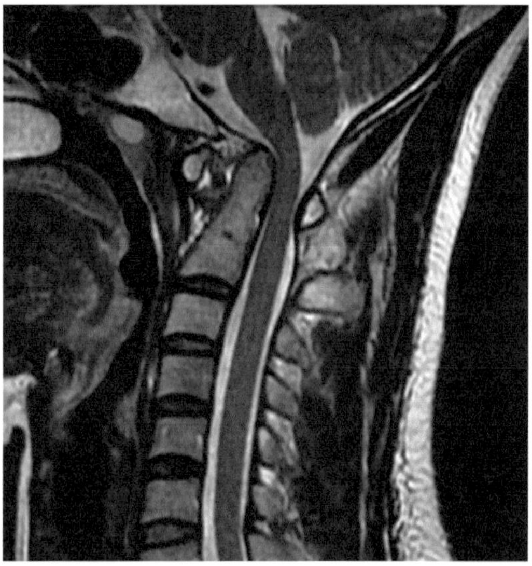

Fig. 4.49 Rheumatoid arthritis. Sagittal T2-weighted MRI shows impingement of the medulla due to basilar invagination

by noncaseating granulomas that can affect multiple organ systems, particularly the lungs, heart, skin, central nervous system, and salivary glands.

Clinicopathologic Findings

Cutaneous manifestations of sarcoidosis include macules, plaques, papules, nodules, and ulcerative lesions. In particular, lupus pernio is characteristic of sarcoidosis and appears as a chronic

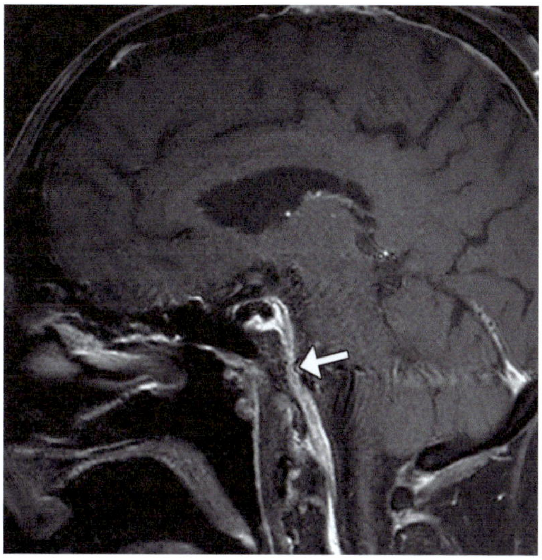

Fig. 4.50 Rheumatoid arthritis. Sagittal fat-suppressed post-contrast T1-weighted MRI shows thickened dura along the clivus (arrow), which represents hypertrophic pachymeningitis

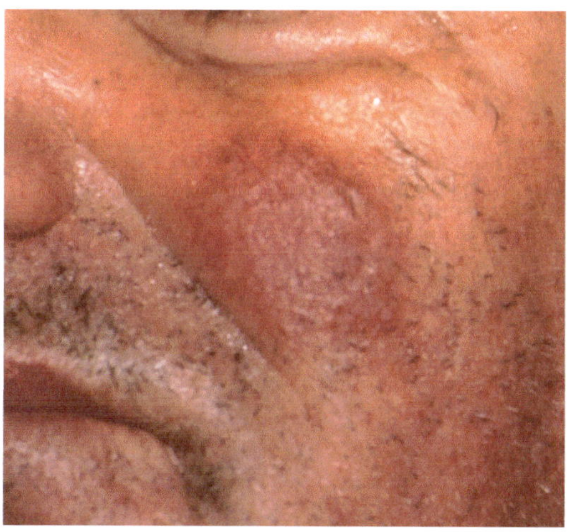

Fig. 4.51 Sarcoidosis. Photograph shows lupus pernio in the cheek manifesting as a raised violaceous lesion. Courtesy of Vesna Petronic-Rosic, MD, MSc

raised, purplish, indurated skin lesion that is often present in the face (Fig. 4.51).

Neurologic manifestations occur in approximately 5% of patients with sarcoidosis. Neurosarcoidosis can have a plethora of manifestations, including cranial neuropathy, aseptic meningitis, mass lesions, encephalopathy, vasculopathy, seizures, hypothalamic-pituitary disorders, hydrocephalus, myelopathy, peripheral neuropathy, and myopathy. The diagnosis of neurosarcoidosis is usually based on the identification of neurologic findings in an individual with proven systemic sarcoidosis as established by clinical, imaging, or histologic findings.

On histology, sarcoidosis is characterized by noncaseating granulomas. Granulomas typically consist of a central area of epithelioid histiocytes and multinucleated giant cells, as well as scattered lymphocytes within and around the granuloma (Fig. 4.52). Schaumann's bodies, asteroid bodies, birefringent crystals, and Hamazaki-Wesenberg bodies may be present, but are nonspecific. Lymphocytes within granulomas tend to be CD4+ T helper cells, while those around the periphery are predominantly CD8+ T cells, as well as B cells. There is minimal to no necrosis within sarcoid granulomas.

Imaging Findings

MRI can be used to evaluate clinically suspected of neurosarcoidosis and the response of pathologic lesions to treatment. There is a broad spectrum of potential manifestations of sarcoidosis on neuroimaging, as exemplified by the following:

- Leptomeningeal involvement: one of the most common neuroimaging findings of neurosarcoidosis, which can appear as diffuse or nodular enhancement, particularly in the basilar region (Fig. 4.53).
- Dural involvement: dural-based lesions in sarcoidosis can appear as low T2 signal enhancing tumors that can resemble hypertrophic pachymeningitis in rheumatoid arthritis or even meningiomas (Fig. 4.54).
- Intraparenchymal lesions: the appearance ranges from nonenhancing periventricular white matter lesions with high signal intensity on T2-weighted sequences, similar to multiple sclerosis, to nodular enhancing lesions along perivascular spaces, resembling lymphoma or other neoplasms, but there can be accompanying ischemia due to vasculopathy (Fig. 4.55).

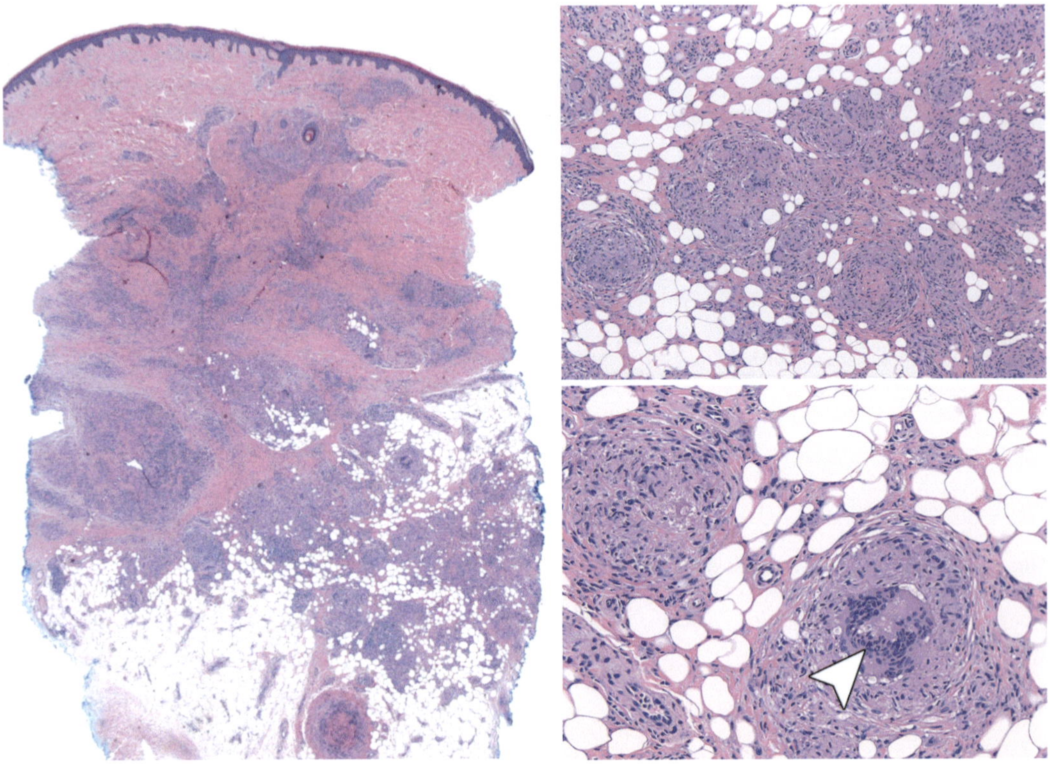

Fig. 4.52 Sarcoidosis. Low power hematoxylin and eosin stained photomicrograph (left) shows skin and subcutis diffusely involved by a nodular infiltrate. Higher power photomicromicrograph shows small non-necrotizing granulomas (top right), some of which also contain multinucleated giant cells (bottom right, arrowhead)

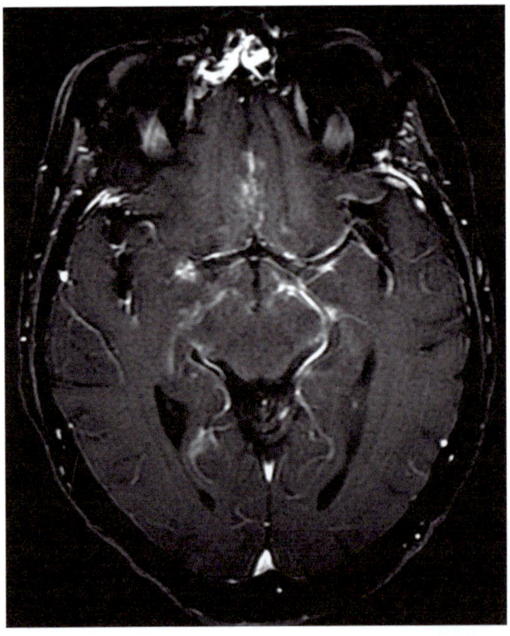

Fig. 4.53 Sarcoidosis. Axial post-contrast T1-weighted MRI shows diffuse basilar region leptomeningeal enhancement

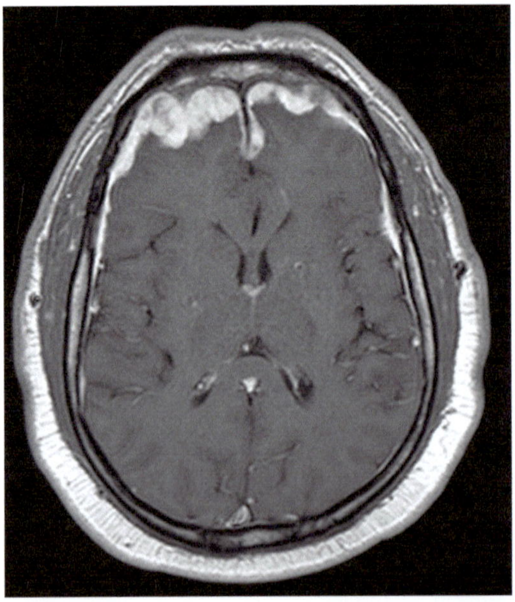

Fig. 4.54 Sarcoidosis. Axial post-contrast T1-weighted MRI shows bilateral cerebral convexity dural-based enhancing lesions

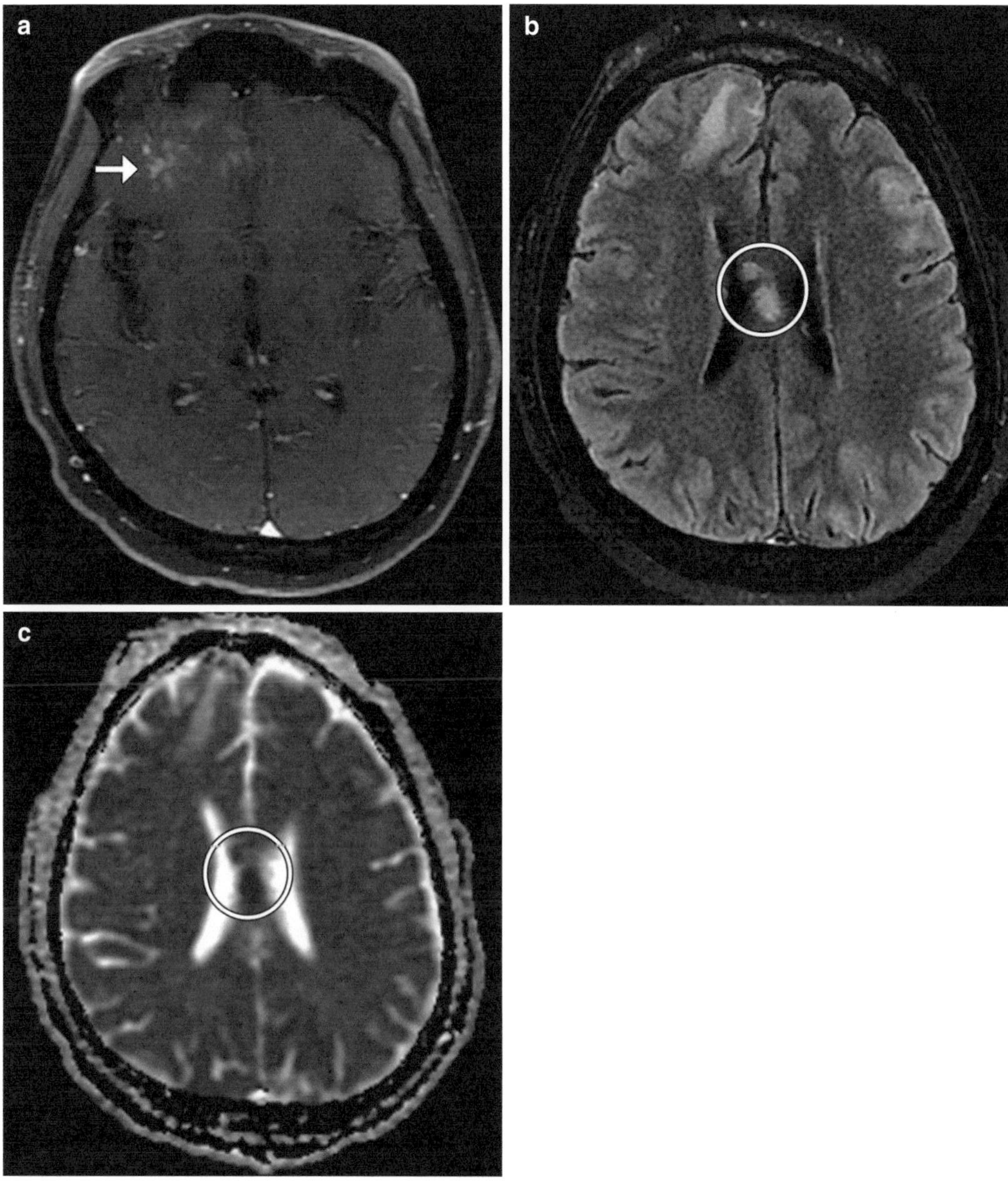

Fig. 4.55 Sarcoidosis. Axial post-contrast T1-weighted (a), T2-weighted FLAIR (**b**), and ADC map (**c**) MRI show punctate foci of enhancement in the right frontal lobe (arrow), as well as scattered areas of vasogenic edema and acute ischemia (encircled)

- Cranial nerve involvement: the facial and optic nerves are most often affected in sarcoidosis, whereby imaging may demonstrate swelling and enhancement (Fig. 4.56).
- Hypothalamus-pituitary axis involvement: thickening and enhancement of the pituitary stalk is a characteristic feature on imaging (Fig. 4.57). This can be associated diabetes insipidus and resemble Langerhans cell histiocytosis.
- Orbital involvement: sarcoidosis can involve virtually any part of the eye and adnexal tissues, especially the lacrimal glands, which

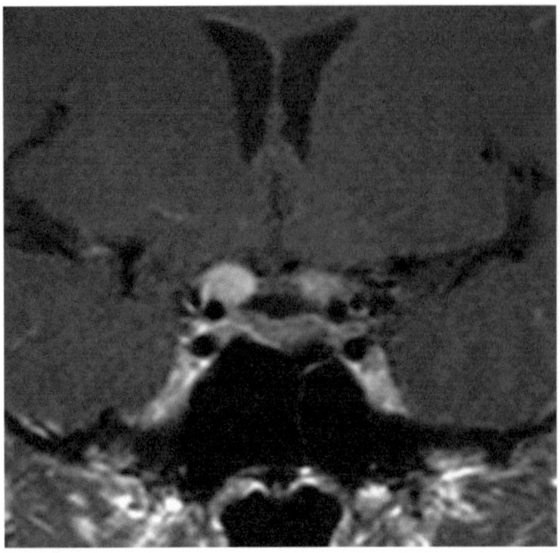

Fig. 4.56 Sarcoidosis. Coronal post-contrast T1-weighted MRI shows swelling and enhancement of the bilateral optic nerves

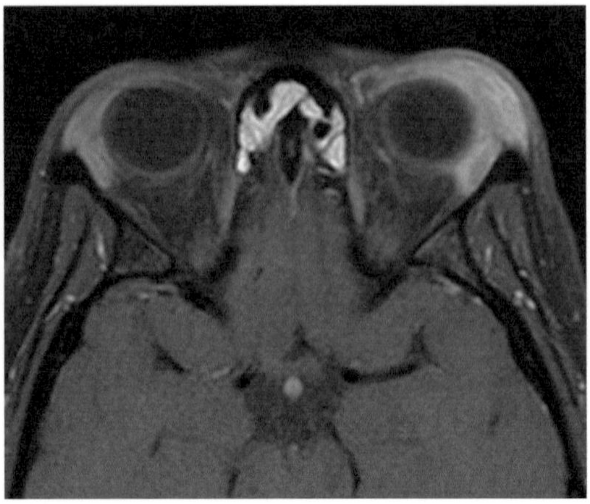

Fig. 4.58 Sarcoidosis. Axial fat-suppressed post-contrast T1-weighted MRI shows enlargement and hyperenhancement of the left lacrimal gland

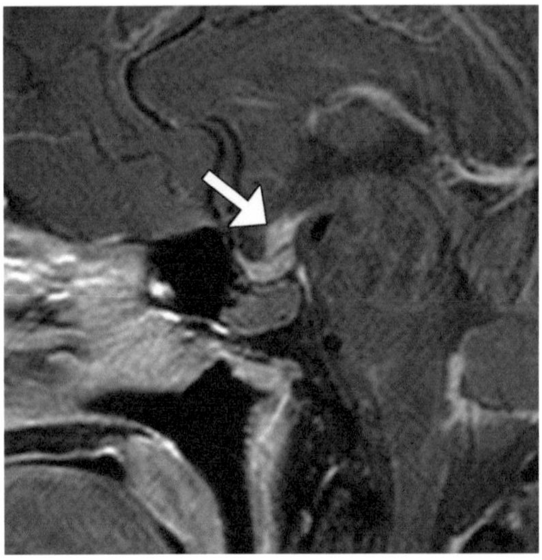

Fig. 4.57 Sarcoidosis. Sagittal post-contrast T1-weighted MRI shows diffuse enlargement and enhancement of the pituitary infundibulum (arrow), which later resolved with steroids

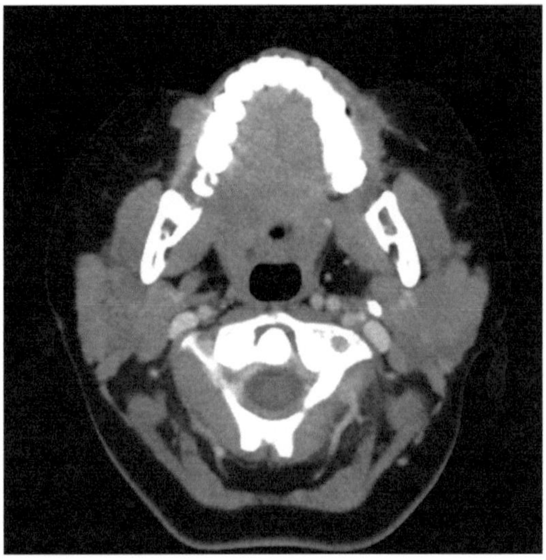

Fig. 4.59 Sarcoidosis. Axial CT image shows diffuse enlargement of the bilateral parotid glands. The patient also had systemic lupus erythematosus

can manifest as swelling and enhancement on imaging (Fig. 4.58).

- Parotid gland involvement: imaging typically demonstrates unilateral or bilateral parotid enlargement (Fig. 4.59). When bilateral and accompanied by lacrimal gland involvement, the appearance is known as the "panda sign" on ^{67}Ga-citrate scintigraphy and ^{18}FDG PET.
- Laryngotracheal involvement: sarcoid granulomas appear as soft tissue nodules on imaging, most often along the epiglottis and aryepiglottic folds (Fig. 4.60).

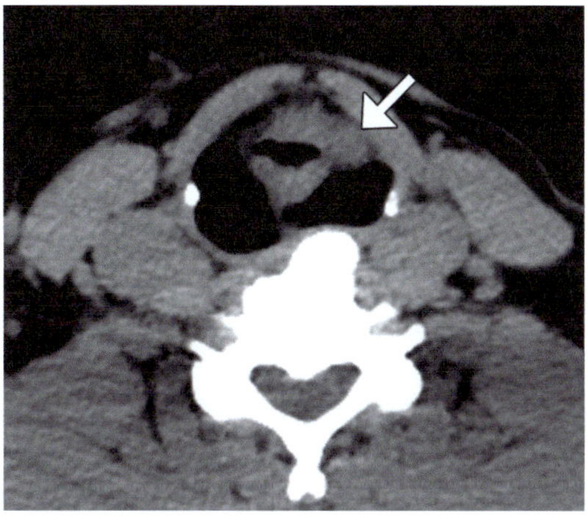

Fig. 4.60 Sarcoidosis. Axial CT image shows nodular soft tissue thickening in the left pre-epiglottic space (arrow)

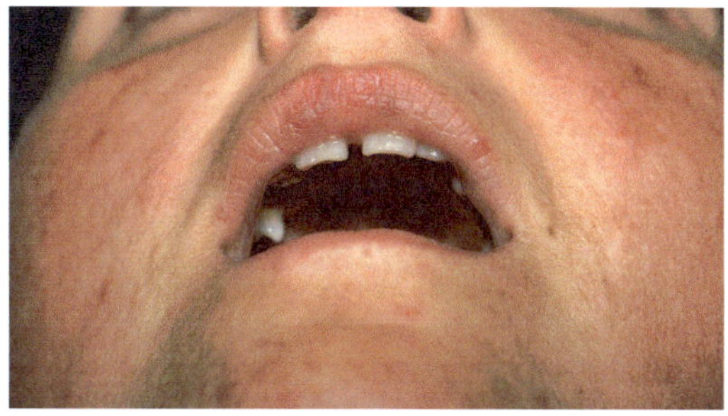

Fig. 4.61 Systemic lupus erythematosus. Photograph shows a malar rash. Courtesy of Vesna Petronic-Rosic, MD, MSc

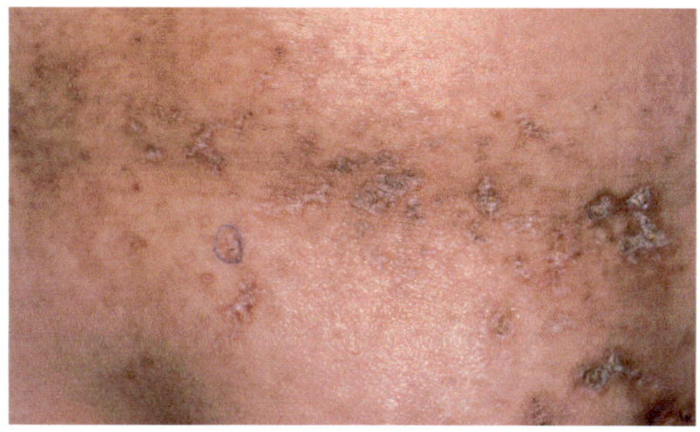

Fig. 4.62 Systemic lupus erythematosus. Photograph show a discoid rash. Courtesy of Vesna Petronic-Rosic, MD, MSc

Systemic Lupus Erythematosus

Overview

Systemic lupus erythematosus is a chronic inflammatory autoimmune disease that can affect virtually any organ, particularly the skin, heart, lungs, kidneys, and nervous system. Vasculitis is also an important feature of systemic lupus erythematosus, in which vessels ranging from small to large can be affected.

Clinicopathologic Findings

A characteristic skin finding of systemic lupus erythematosus is the malar rash (Fig. 4.61), which appears as erythema in a butterfly shape over the nose and cheeks with sun exposure. Photosensitivity is common, and a macular and papular rash can appear in sun-exposed areas of the skin. Other cutaneous findings include inflammatory discoid lesions, painless oral/nasal ulcers, and alopecia. Discoid lupus frequently occurs in the skin of the face and head and consists of thick erythematous (Fig. 4.62), discoid lesions with inflammation that eventually results in a scar. Calcinosis may also occur, resulting in painful nodular lesions from a buildup of calcium deposits. Ultimately, the diagnosis of systemic lupus erythematosus relies on characteristic clinical manifestations, serology, cerebrospinal fluid findings, neuroimaging findings, and exclusion of alternative etiologies. In particular, anti-Smith and anti-double-stranded DNA antibodies are specific, but not very specific for systemic lupus erythematosus.

Imaging Findings

Subcortical and periventricular white matter and spinal cord lesions due to vasculitis are

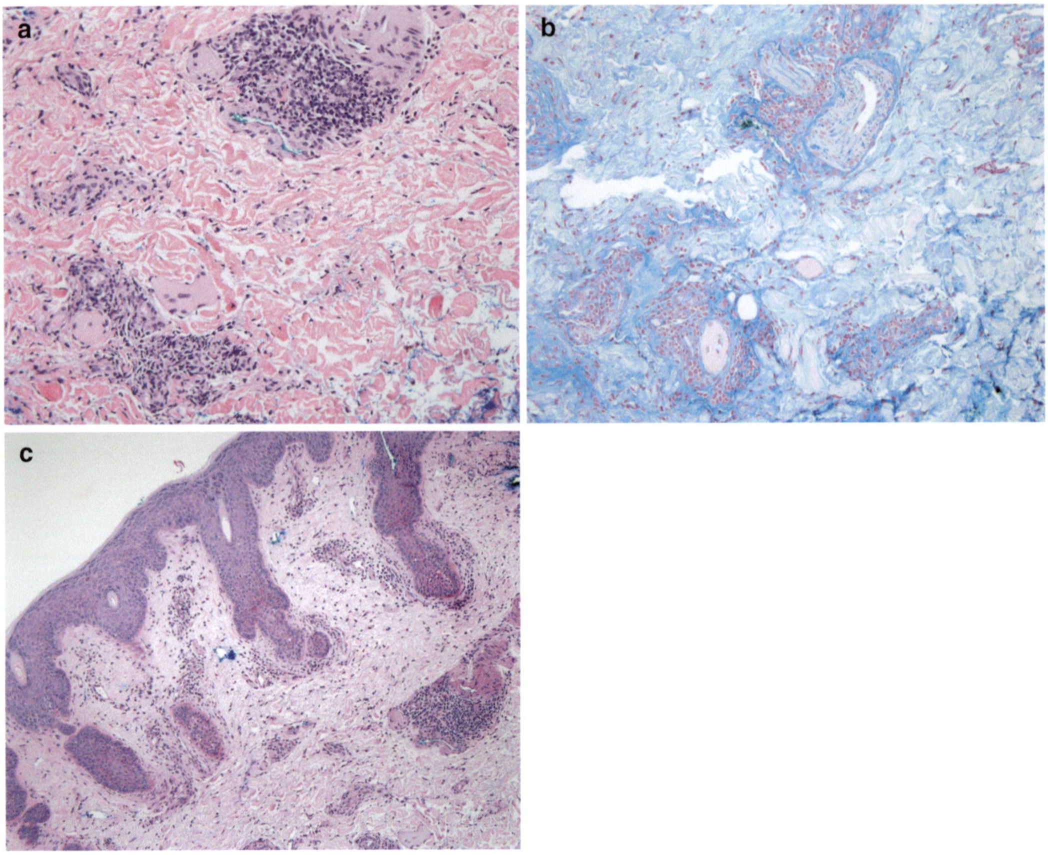

Fig. 4.63 Systemic lupus erythematosus. Hematoxylin and eosin (**a**) and colloidal iron (**b**) stained photomicrographs show skin demonstrate a perivascular and periadnexal lymphocytic infiltrate with increased dermal mucin, highlighted by PAS (**c**). Courtesy of Lohini Sundharkrishnan, MD

frequently apparent on neuroimaging in patients with systemic lupus erythematosus. MRI is most useful for depicting acute infarcts from the vasculitis and angiographic studies may demonstrate steno-occlusive of the cerebral arteries (Fig. 4.64). The vasculitis can be accompanied by hemorrhage, which can be in parenchymal, subarachnoid, or subdural locations, and can lead to cerebral atrophy. Another less common potential neuroimaging finding associated with systemic lupus erythematosus is periorbital dermatitis. The imaging features are rather nonspecific, but typically include bilateral skin thickening, subcutaneous fat stranding, and enhancement (Fig. 4.65).

Sjogren Syndrome

Overview

Sjogren syndrome is a chronic autoimmune inflammatory disease that mainly involves exocrine glands, including the lacrimal and salivary gland, resulting in dry eyes and dry mouth. Other manifestations of Sjogren disease include arthritis, pulmonary fibrosis, interstitial nephritis, and various skin lesions. Certain skin lesions encountered with Sjogren syndrome herald an increased risk for serious extraglandular complications. Sjogren syndrome can also occur in the setting of other rheumatological diseases, in which case it is considered secondary.

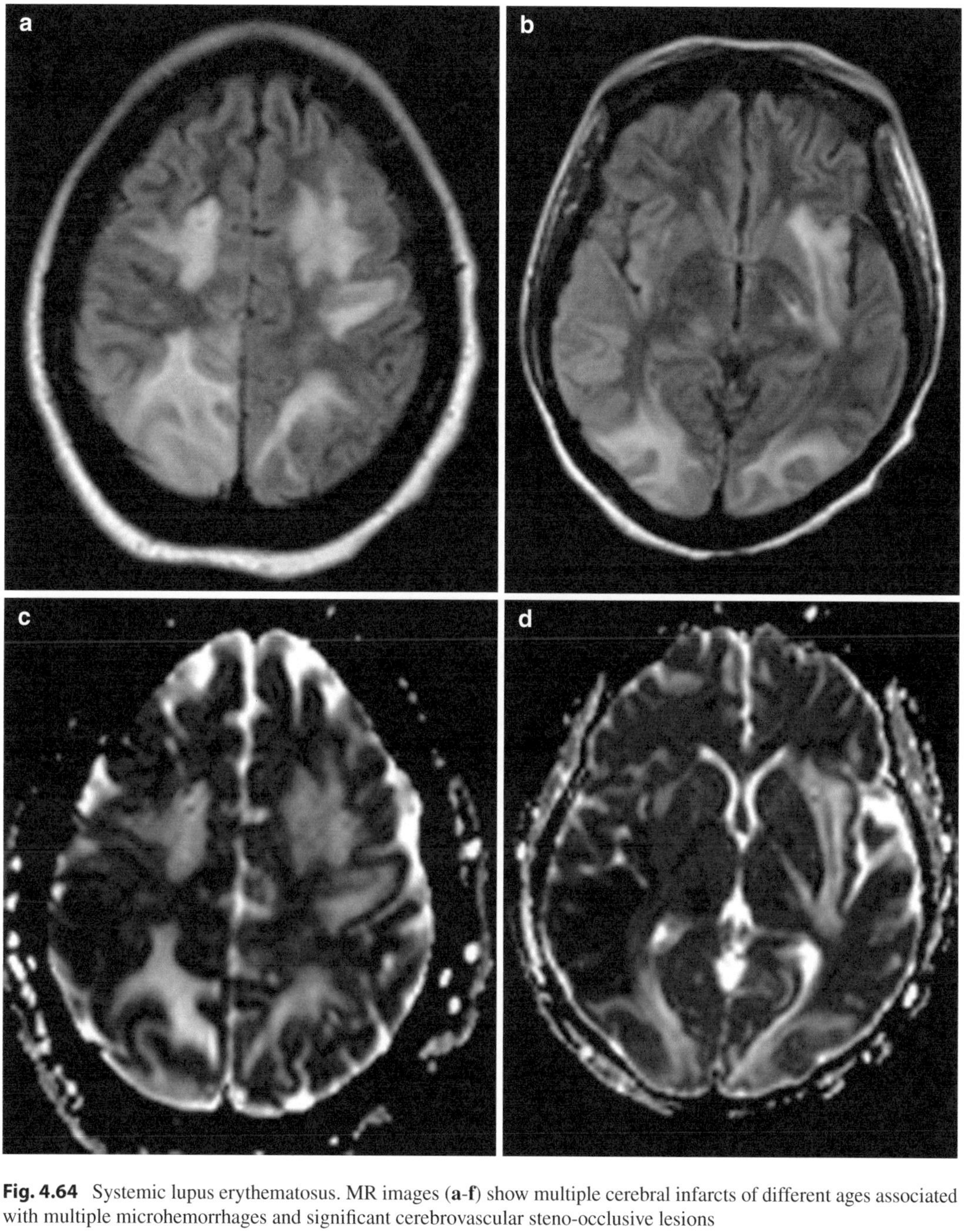

Fig. 4.64 Systemic lupus erythematosus. MR images (**a**-**f**) show multiple cerebral infarcts of different ages associated with multiple microhemorrhages and significant cerebrovascular steno-occlusive lesions

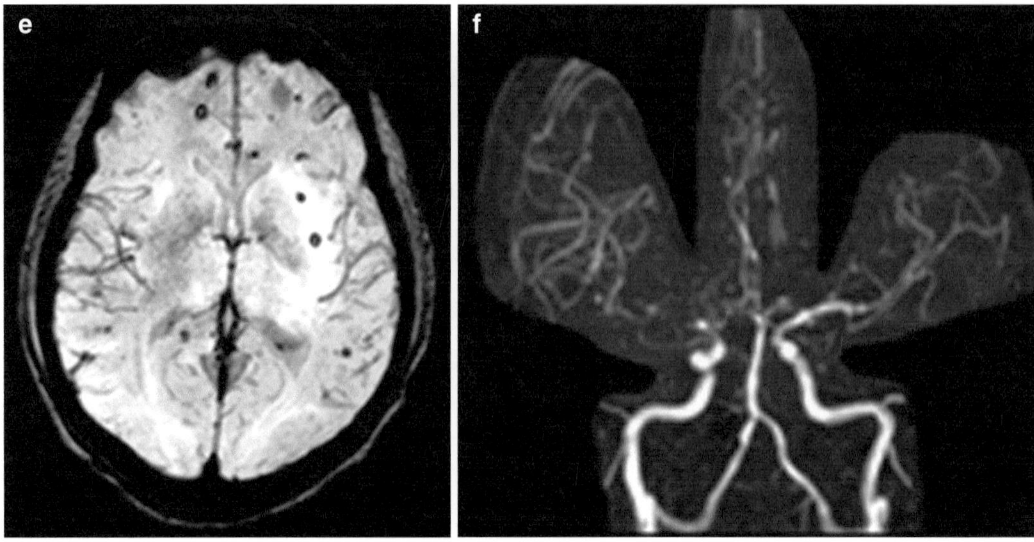

Fig. 4.64 (continued)

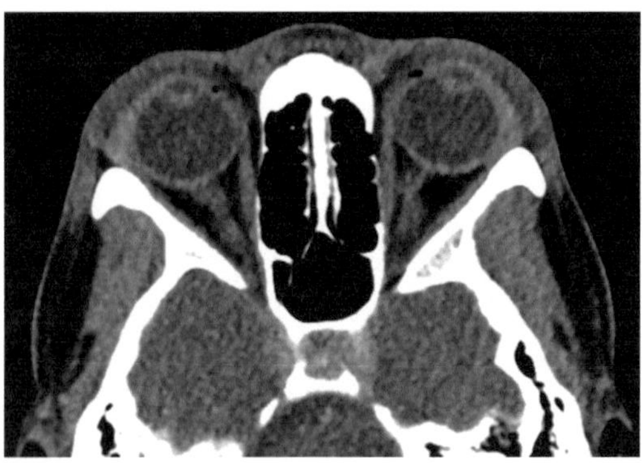

Fig. 4.65 Systemic lupus erythematosus. Axial CT image shows bilateral diffuse periorbital swelling that corresponds to lupus dermatitis

Clinicopathologic Findings

Sjogren syndrome is associated with seropositivity for anti-Ro and anti-La and is characterized histopathologically by the presence of focal lymphocytic infiltrates of the salivary glands, followed by interstitial fibrosis and acinar atrophy. Cutaneous manifestations are present in nearly 50% of patients with Sjogren syndrome and may include dry skin, purpura, urticaria-like lesions, and Raynaud phenomenon. In particular, Raynaud phenomenon occurs in 13–20% of patients with Sjogren syndrome and is a vascular disorder that consists of episodes of reversible digital ischemia in response to cold or stress. The phases of Raynaud phenomenon include pallor followed by cyanosis and subsequently rubor with blood return (Fig. 4.66). Arthritis, vasculitis, and pulmonary fibrosis are more common in Sjogren syndrome when these patients are also afflicted by Raynaud phenomenon.

Imaging Findings

The imaging findings of Sjogren syndrome vary through the course of the disease. The salivary gland may appear normal at first, but the swollen acinar structures can be discerned on imaging as military nodules in enlarged glands (Fig. 4.67). Overtime, the acinar cavities become dilated, forming cystic structures in the glands (Fig. 4.68). With chronic disease, fatty atrophy occurs and punctate calcifications appear within the parotid glands, which are best depicted on CT (Fig. 4.69). In addition, chronic fibrosis results in strictures and dilatation of the salivary ducts caused by chronic fibrosis can be depicted via sialography (Fig. 4.70). The presence of enlarging and ^{18}FDG-PET avid lymph nodes raises the possibility of superimposed lymphoma (Fig. 4.71).

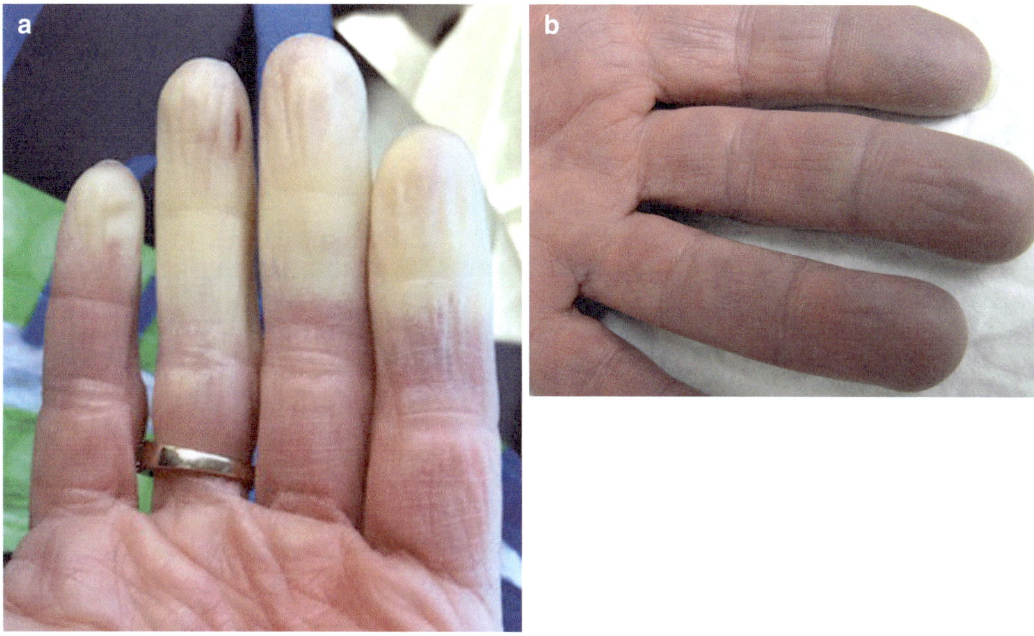

Fig. 4.66 Raynaud phenomenon. Photographs show the pallor phase (**a**) and cyanotic phase (**b**). Courtesy of Fredrick Wigley MD

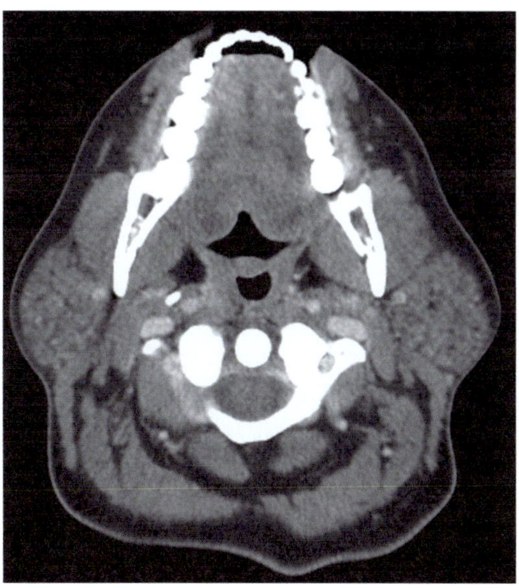

Fig. 4.67 Sjogren syndrome. Axial CT image shows a military pattern of small nodules in the bilateral swollen parotid glands

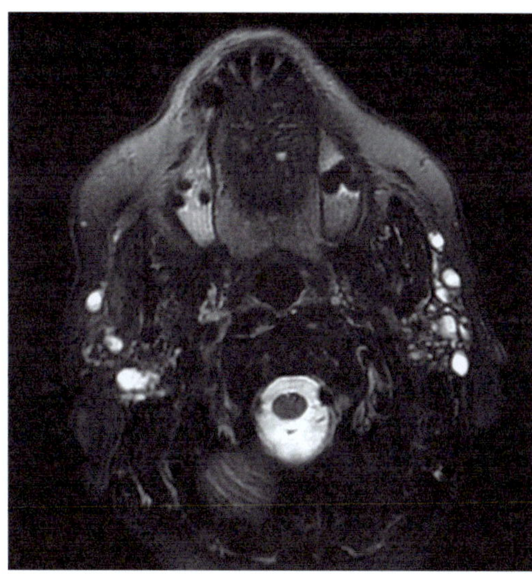

Fig. 4.68 Sjogren syndrome. Axial fat-suppressed T2-weighted MRI shows multiple cystic lesions in the bilateral parotid glands

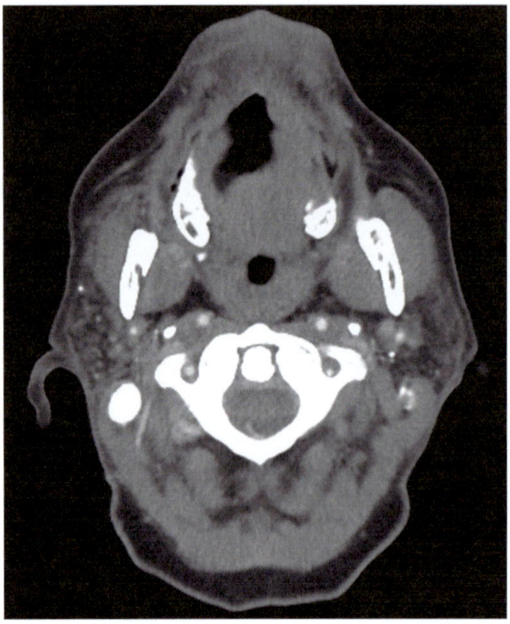

Fig. 4.69 Sjogren syndrome. Axial CT image shows fatty atrophy and punctate calculi in the bilateral parotid glands in a patient with chronic disease

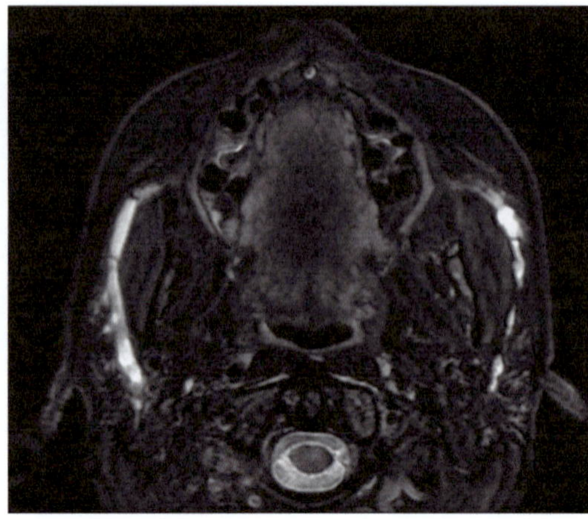

Fig. 4.70 Sjogren syndrome. Axial STIR MRI shows alternating areas of narrowing and dilatation of the parotid ducts bilaterally

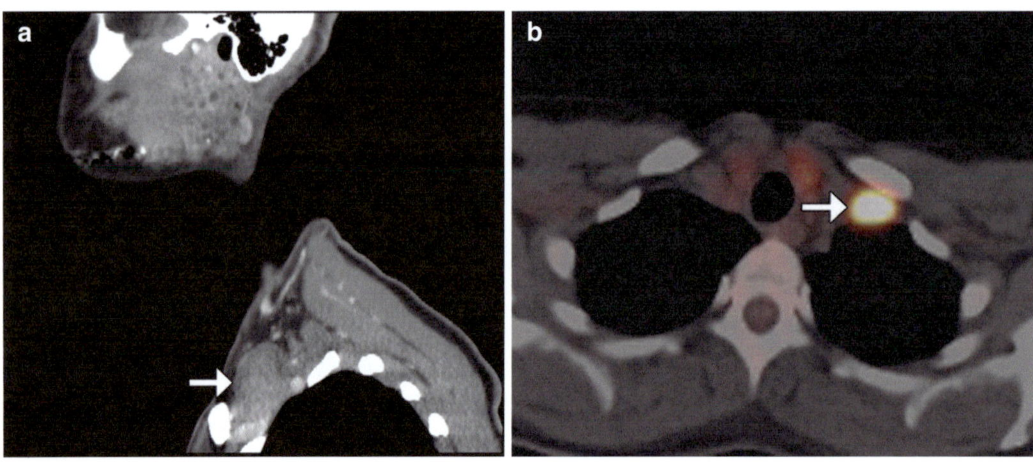

Fig. 4.71 Sjogren syndrome. Sagittal CT image shows multiple small cystic lesions in the parotid gland and supraclavicular lymphadenopathy (arrow). There is corresponding hypermetabolism in the left supraclavicular lymph node (arrow), which proved to be non-Hodgkin lymphoma

Scleroderma

Overview

Scleroderma or systemic sclerosis is an immune-mediated rheumatic disease that is characterized by fibrosis of the skin and internal organs and vasculopathy, manifestations of the disease, such as renal disease, pulmonary arterial hypertension, digital ulceration, and gastroesophageal reflux. CREST syndrome is a variant of systemic sclerosis that consists of calcinosis, Raynaud's phenomenon, esophageal dysmotility, sclerodactyly, and telangiectasia.

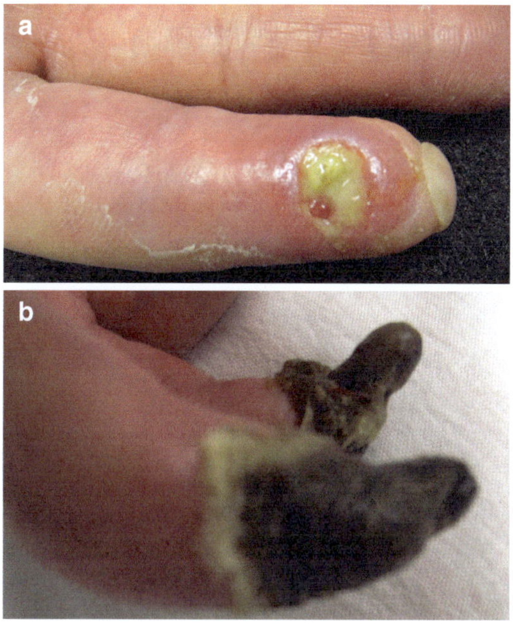

Fig. 4.72 Scleroderma. Photograph (a) shows a digital ulcer in patient with CREST syndrome Photograph (b) shows deep digital infarcts. Courtesy of Fredrick Wigley MD

Clinicopathologic Findings

There is a wide variety of skin manifestations associated with scleroderma/CREST syndrome including the following:

- Fibrosis: the diffuse excess deposition and accumulation of extracellular matrix, mainly type I collagen, in the dermis and leads to a tight, smooth, and shiny appearance of the skin.
- Raynaud phenomenon: often an initial manifestation of scleroderma. The general features of this condition are otherwise described in the preceding section.
- Digital ulcers: occur in about 30–50% of patients with scleroderma and result from ischemia, which if severe can result in skin necrosis (Fig. 4.72).
- Telangiectasias: these macroscopically dilated skin vessels that are mainly present on the hands and face in most patients with scleroderma. The telangiectasias may be a marker of more widespread abnormal microvascular disease in scleroderma.

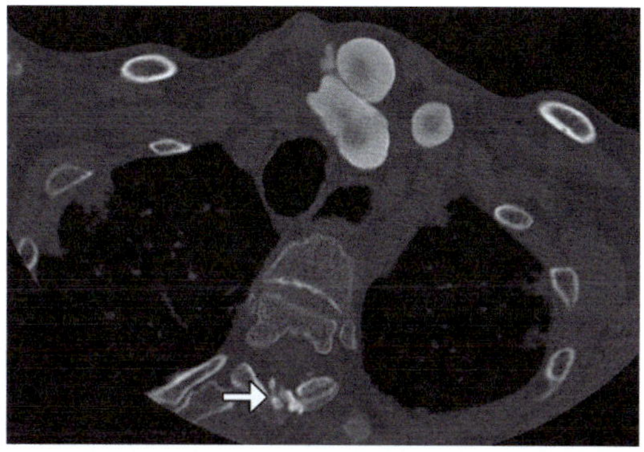

Fig. 4.73 Scleroderma. Axial CT image shows tumoral calcinosis in the anterior neck and spinal canal (arrow). In addition, the esophagus is dilated and there are interstitial lung opacities

- Calcinosis: the abnormal deposition of calcium in soft tissues is a common finding in systemic sclerosis and can be painful.

Imaging Findings

CT is useful for depicting tumoral calcinosis, which can appear as amorphous calcified masses, often with lobulated appearance, in the tissues around large joints, including the spine (Fig. 4.73). Other findings related to scleroderma that may be encountered on neuroimaging include esophageal dilatation with accompanying abnormal motility, which can be best assessed via esophagograms, as well as osteolysis, particularly involving the mandible.

Immunoglobin G4-Related Disease

Overview

Immunoglobin G4 (IgG4)-related disease is a systemic condition characterized by inflammatory lymphoplasmacytic infiltrates with the following diagnostic criteria:

- Serum IgG4 concentration >135 mg/dL
- >40% of IgG+ plasma cells being IgG4+

The head and neck is commonly involved, particularly the salivary glands, lacrimal glands, orbits, thyroid gland, lymph nodes, sinonasal cavities, pituitary gland, and larynx.

Clinicopathologic Findings

IgG4-related skin disease is defined as IgG4(+) plasma-cell-infiltrating skin lesions that form plaques, nodules, or tumors that are often multicentric (Fig. 4.74). Otherwise, head and neck manifestations may include sclerosing sialadenitis, various forms of orbital pseudotumor. Characteristic features of IgG4-related disease on histology include storiform-type fibrosis and obliterative phlebitis (Fig. 4.75). The lesions typically respond to immunosuppressive therapy.

Imaging Findings

Cross-sectional imaging is nonspecific and shows bilateral symmetric swelling of the involved glands. During the active phase, IgG4 lesions often demonstrate infiltrative margins on imaging, particularly in the orbit with lacrimal gland and extraoacular involvement (Fig. 4.76). There can also be associated perineural disease in the periorbital region, with marked enlargement of the involved cranial nerve branches, which can mimic malignant neoplasms (Fig. 4.77). Active

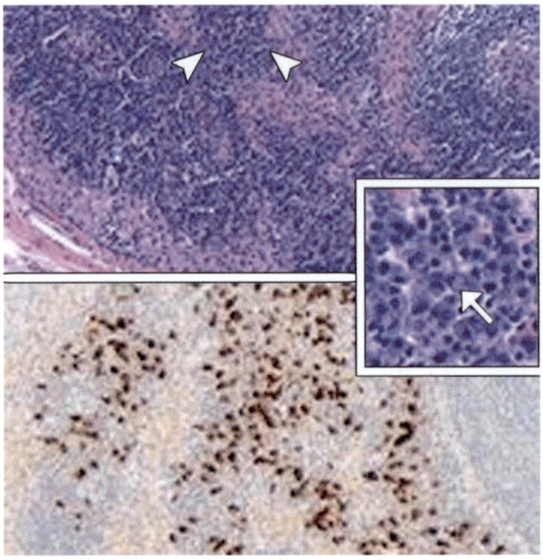

Fig. 4.75 IgG4-related disease. A lymph node containing increased plasma cells (arrowheads, top) that stain positively for IgG4 immunostain (bottom). Plasma cells (inset) show characteristic eccentrically placed nuclei with "clock-face" chromatin and perinuclear eosinophilic hoff (arrow) containing the Golgi apparatus

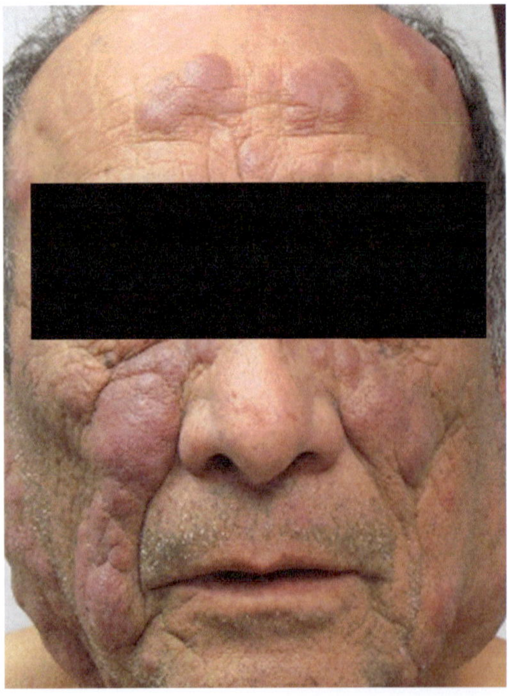

Fig. 4.74 IgG4-related disease. Photograph shows multiple well-circumscribed violaceous plaques and nodules on the scalp and face

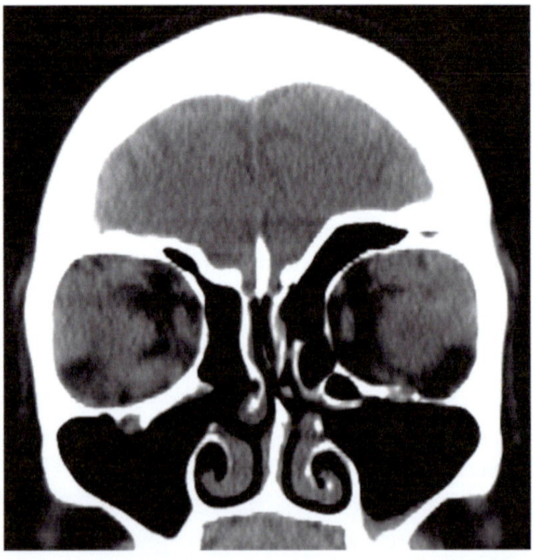

Fig. 4.76 IgG4-related disease. Coronal CT image shows enlargement of the bilateral lacrimal glands and adjacent extraocular muscles with infiltrative margins

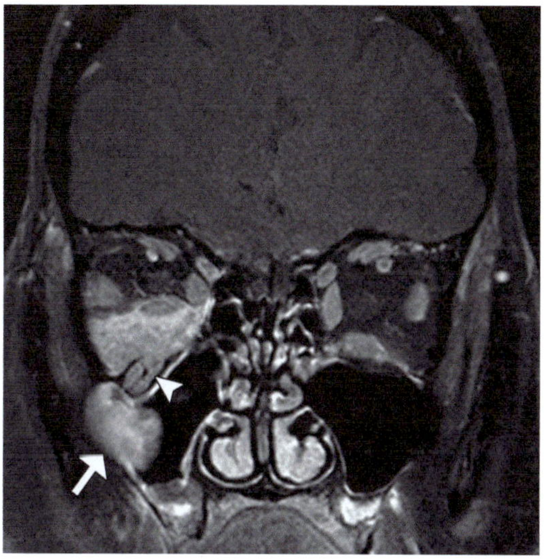

Fig. 4.77 IgG4-related disease. Coronal fat-suppressed post-contrast T1-weighted MRI shows an enhancing mass in the right cheek (arrow) with extension along the inferior orbital nerve (arrowhead) and into the orbit

lesions are also frequently hypermetabolic on ^{18}FDG-PET (Fig. 4.78), which is, therefore, a useful tool for the differential diagnosis of IgG4-RD, and for mapping involved organs, guiding biopsy, and monitoring treatment response. Very hypercellular and more chronic lesions tend to display low signal on T2-weighted MR sequences due to the presence of fibrosis.

Kimura Disease

Overview

Kimura disease is a rare benign chronic inflammatory condition that occurs primarily in Asian individuals, characterized by masses and surrounding tissues that are

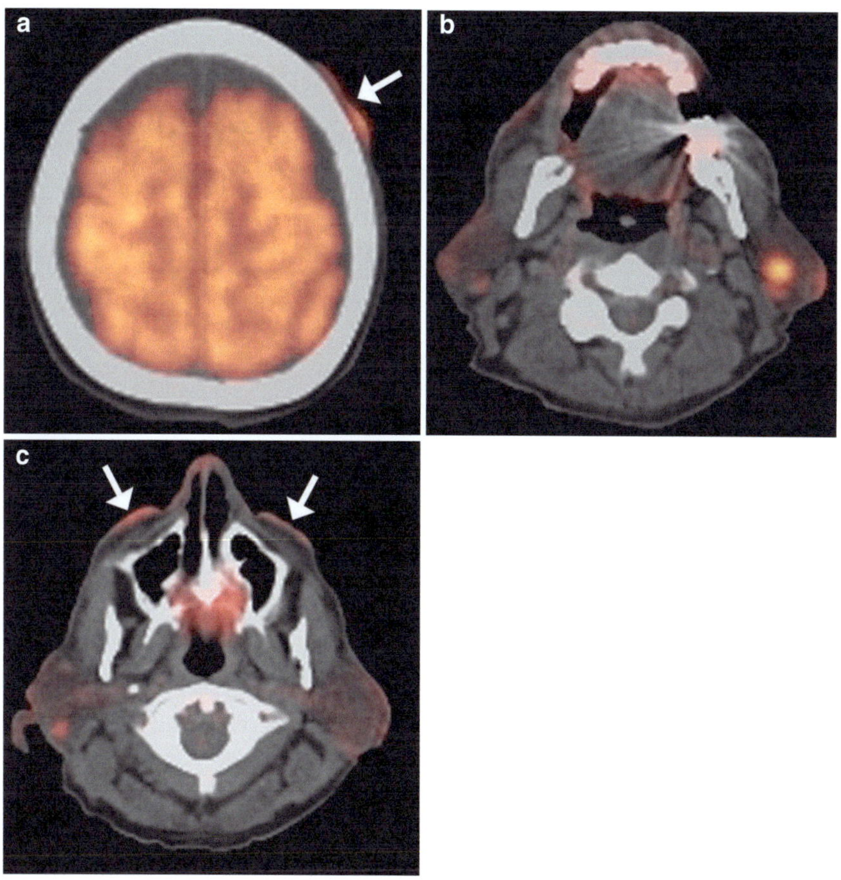

Fig. 4.78 IgG4-related disease. Axial ^{18}FDG-PET/CT images (**a–c**) show multiple hypermetabolic scalp and face lesions (*arrows*) and bilateral parotid lymphadenopathy in the same patient shown in Fig. 4.74

infiltrated by eosinophils, often accompanied by peripheral blood eosinophilia and elevated serum IgE. Most lesions occur in the head and neck, especially in the parotid and submandibular regions.

Clinicopathologic Findings

The typical presentation of Kimura disease is that of a large subcutaneous mass in young Asian males. Moreover, Kimura disease is a systemic immune-mediated process that commonly presents with lymphadenopathy, eosinophilia, increased serum levels of IgE, and may be associated with renal disease. Histologically, lymphoid follicles with germinal center formation, eosinophilic infiltrates, eosinophilic microabscesses, and eosinophilic folliculolysis are salient features of Kimura disease (Fig. 4.79). Treatment for Kimura disease includes surgical resection and regional or systemic steroid therapy with generally excellent prognosis.

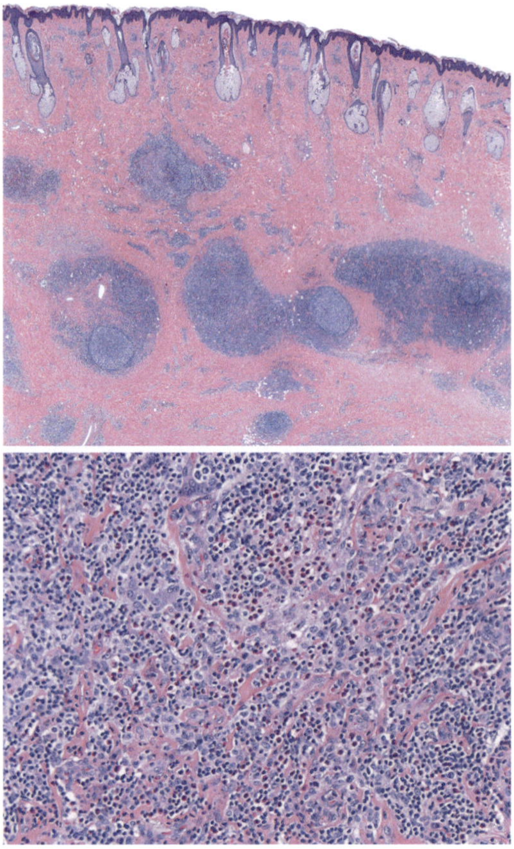

Fig. 4.79 Kimura disease. Low and high power hematoxylin and eosin stained photomicrographs show dermal inflammation composed of lymphoid follicles with germinal centers and proliferation of vessels with associated eosinophils, mononuclear inflammatory cells, and dense eosinophilic collagen

Imaging Findings

On diagnostic imaging, Kimura disease typically manifests as enhancing periparotid subcutaneous masses with associated regional lymphadenopathy (Fig. 4.80), often bilaterally. The lesions can be ill-defined and contain prominent flow voids.

Benign Miliary Osteoma Cutis

Overview

Benign military osteoma cutis is a common benign condition that represents the formation of ossific foci in the skin of the face and is likely secondary to age-related chronic inflammation.

Clinicopathologic Findings

Benign miliary osteoma cutis refers to the variant of morphologically normal bone formation disorder in the skin, presenting as multiple, tiny skin-colored, non-tender, firm papules. Histologically, the lesions contain intramembranous superficial ossification, which may be due to osteoblastic metaplasia of mesenchymal elements. The osteomas tend to accumulate gradually after appearing during middle age.

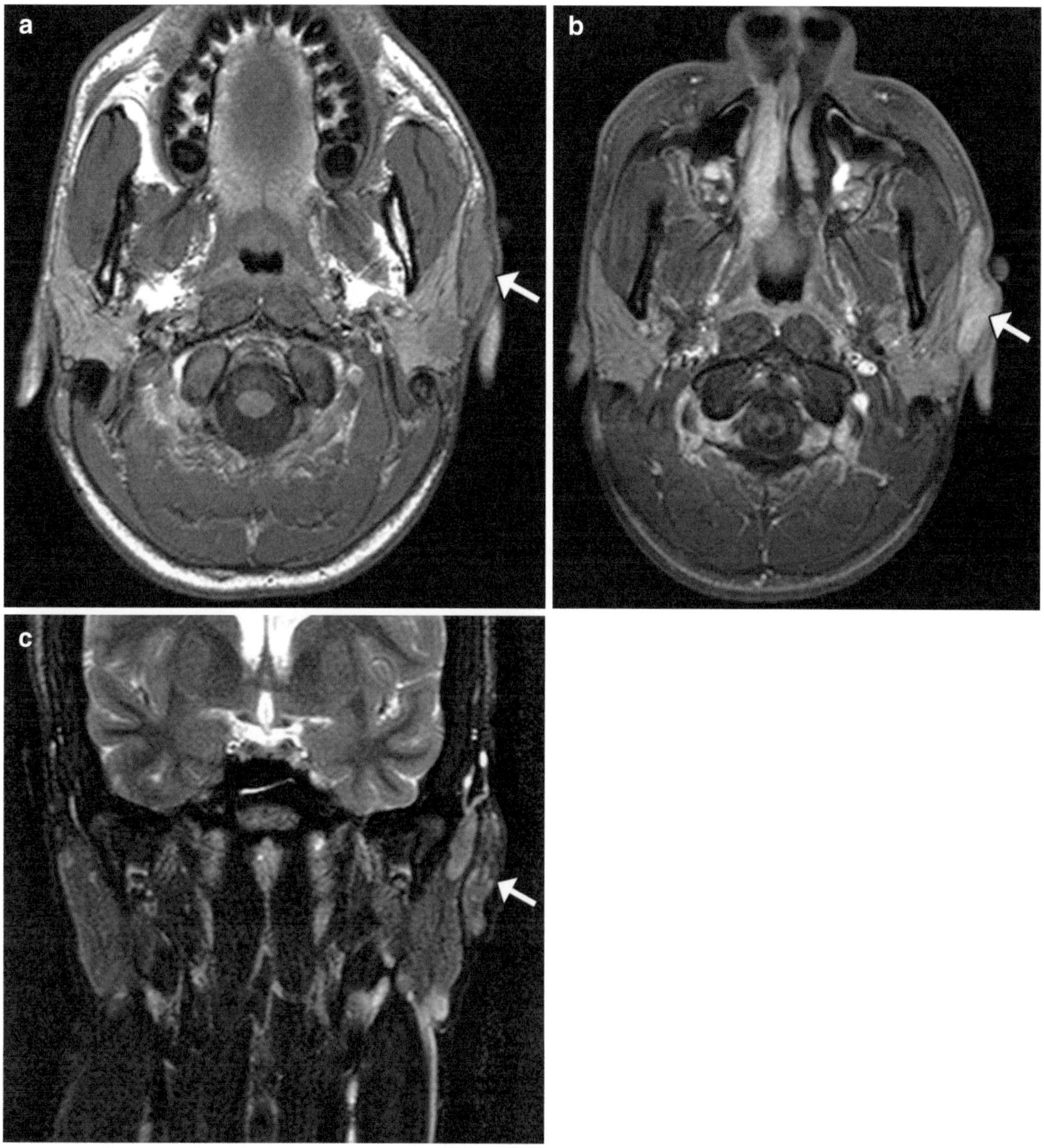

Fig. 4.80 Kimura disease. Axial T1-weighted (**a**), axial fat-suppressed post-contrast T1-weighted (**b**), and coronal STIR (**c**) MR images show a left periparotid subcutaneous mass (arrows) and left parotid lymphadenopathy

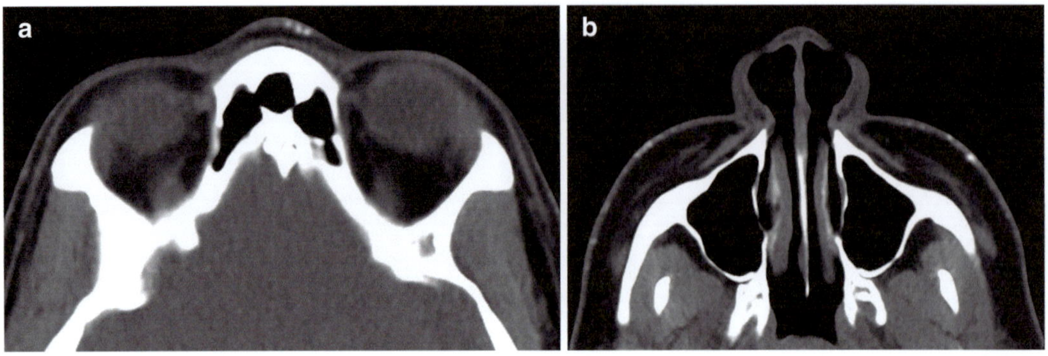

Fig. 4.81 Miliary osteoma cutis. Axial CT images show multiple punctate calcifications in the skin of the face

Imaging Findings

Benign military osteoma cutis is commonly encountered incidentally on CT and appears as punctate calcified/ossified nodules in the skin of the face (Fig. 4.81).

Parry Romberg Syndrome

Overview

Parry Romberg syndrome is characterized by progressive hemifacial atrophy and neurological deficits. This rare disease most commonly begins during childhood and gradually progresses before it suddenly halts. The etiology of Parry Romberg may be attributable to an autoimmune or inflammatory process although the etiology is still not well-elucidated.

Clinicopathologic Findings

Parry Romberg syndrome is characterized by sunken appearance of the affected hemiface (Fig. 4.82). The skin can be dry and there may be dark pigmentation or even vitiligo. Sometimes a sharp demarcation line is present between the normal and abnormal skin, which has been described as "en coup de sabre." Additionally, atrophy of the underlying muscles, cartilage, and bones may also be observed. The most common neurologic complications of Parry Romberg syndrome include trigeminal neuritis, facial paresthesia, severe headache, and seizures.

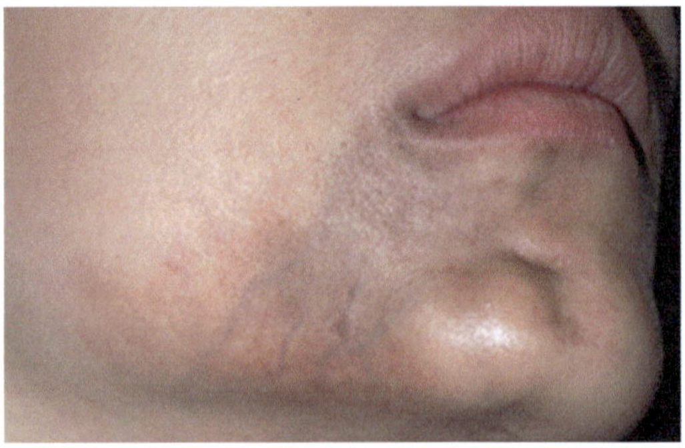

Fig. 4.82 Parry Romberg syndrome. Photograph shows morphea with unilateral atrophy and skin discoloration in the lower face. Courtesy of Vesna Petronic-Rosic, MD, MSc

Imaging Findings

Maxillofacial CT or MRI in patients with Parry Romberg syndrome may demonstrate initial transient swelling and enhancement, following by generalized atrophy of the soft tissues of the affected hemiface, including the mastication muscles, hemitongue, submandibular and parotid glands, and parapharyngeal and subcutaneous tissues (Fig. 4.83). Intracranial abnormalities associated with that may be encountered on neuroimaging include ipsilateral linear or discrete subcortical calcifications white matter lesions (Fig. 4.84), as well as ipsilateral focal or hemispheric brain atrophy, leptomeningeal thickening and contrast enhancement, abnormalities of the thalamus or gray matter, microhemorrhages, and vascular abnormalities.

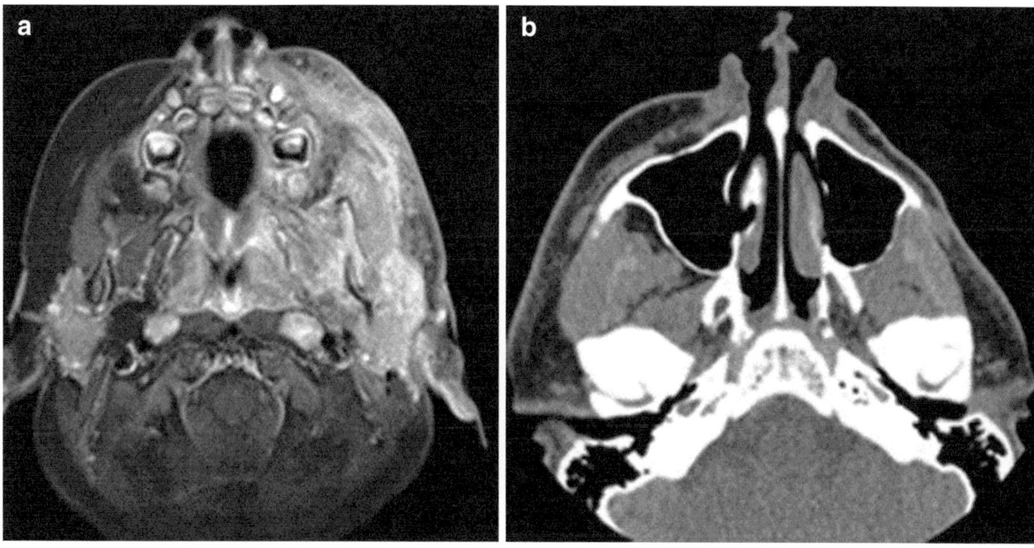

Fig. 4.83 Parry Romberg syndrome. Axial fat-suppressed post-contrast T1-weighted MRI (**a**) shows diffuse enhancement of the skin and subcutaneous tissues of the left face as well as the masticator. Follow-up CT image obtained several years later (**b**) shows atrophy of the left face subcutaneous tissues in the "burned-out phase"

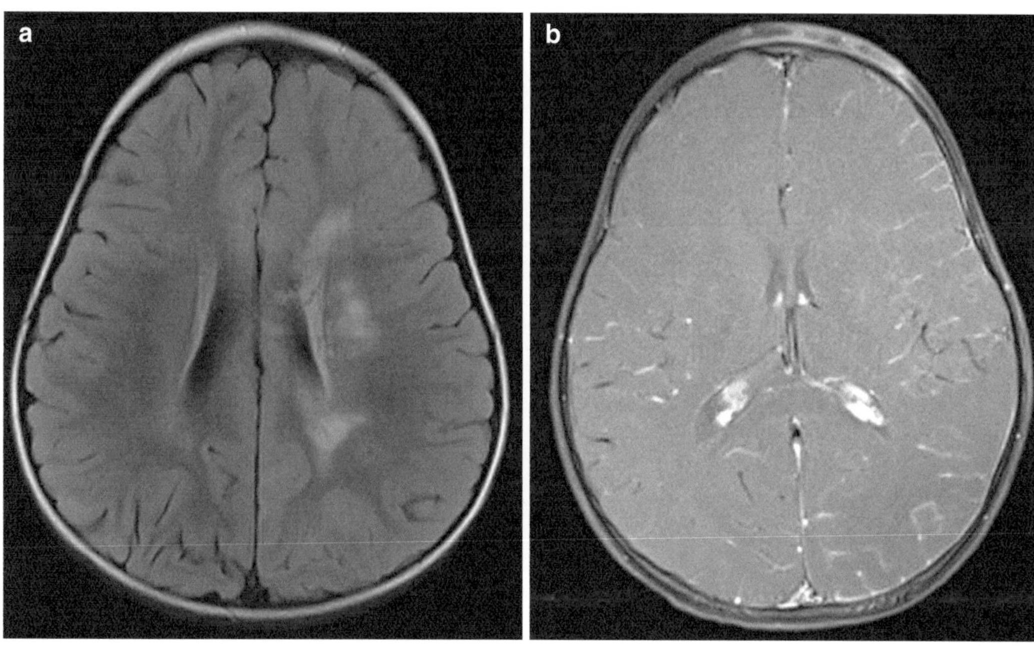

Fig. 4.84 Parry Romberg syndrome. Axial T2-weighted FLAIR (**a**) and post-contrast fat-suppressed T1-weighted (**b**) MR images show white matter lesions and leptomeningeal enhancement in the left cerebral hemisphere. There is also enhancement in the frontal scalp

Acknowledgement Thanks to Joshua Eassa MD for preparing an early draft of this chapter.

Suggested Reading

Abdel Razek AA. Imaging of connective tissue diseases of the head and neck. Neuroradiol J. 2016;29(3):222–30.

Abuel-Haija M, Hurford MT. Kimura disease. Arch Pathol Lab Med. 2007;131(4):650–1.

Agarwal R, Sze G. Neuro-lyme disease: MR imaging findings. Radiology. 2009;253(1):167–73.

Albright JT, Pransky SM. Nontuberculous mycobacterial infections of the head and neck. Pediatr Clin North Am. 2003;50(2):503–14.

Bodey GP, Boktour M, Mays S, Duvic M, Kontoyiannis D, Hachem R, Raad I. Skin lesions associated with Fusarium infection. J Am Acad Dermatol. 2002;47(5):659–66.

Chasset F, Barete S, Charlotte F, Cohen-Aubart F, Arnaud L, Le Pelletier F, Emile JF, Francès C, Amoura Z, Haroche J. Cutaneous manifestations of Erdheim-Chester disease (ECD): clinical, pathological, and molecular features in a monocentric series of 40 patients. J Am Acad Dermatol. 2016;74(3): 513–20.

Christoforidis GA, Spickler EM, Recio MV, Mehta BM. MR of CNS sarcoidosis: correlation of imaging features to clinical symptoms and response to treatment. AJNR Am J Neuroradiol. 1999;20(4):655–69.

Cives M, et al. Erdheim-Chester disease: a systematic review. Crit Rev Oncol Hematol. 2015;95(1):1–11.

Deigendesch N, Stenzel W. Acute and chronic viral infections. Handb Clin Neurol. 2017;145:227–43.

Denton CP, Khanna D. Systemic sclerosis. Lancet. 2017;390(10103):1685–99.

DeQuattro K, Imboden JB. Neurologic manifestations of rheumatoid arthritis. Rheum Dis Clin North Am. 2017;43(4):561–71.

Deshpande V. IgG4 related disease of the head and neck. Head Neck Pathol. 2015;9(1):24–31.

DiCaprio MR, Roberts TT. Diagnosis and management of Langerhans cell histiocytosis. J Am Acad Orthop Surg. 2014;22(10):643–52.

Drier A, Haroche J, Savatovsky J, Godenèche G, Dormont D, Chiras J, Amoura Z, Bonneville F. Cerebral, facial, and orbital involvement in Erdheim-Chester disease: CT and MR imaging findings. Radiology. 2010;255(2):586–94.

Fox RI. Sjögren's syndrome. Lancet. 2005;366(9482): 321–31.

Fujita A, Sakai O, Chapman MN, Sugimoto H. IgG4-related disease of the head and neck: CT and MR imaging manifestations. Radiographics. 2012;32(7): 1945–58.

Garcia Garcia SC, Salas Alanis JC, Flores MG, Gonzalez Gonzalez SE, Vera Cabrera L, Ocampo Candiani J. Coccidioidomycosis and the skin: a comprehensive review. An Bras Dermatol. 2015;90(5):610–9.

García-Carrasco M, Sisó A, Ramos-Casals M, Rosas J, de la Red G, Gil V, Lasterra S, Cervera R, Font J, Ingelmo M. Raynaud's phenomenon in primary Sjögren's syndrome. Prevalence and clinical characteristics in a series of 320 patients. J Rheumatol. 2002;29(4):726–30.

García-Patos V. Rheumatoid nodule. Semin Cutan Med Surg. 2007;26(2):100–7.

Ginat DT, Dhillon G, Almast J. Magnetic resonance imaging of neurosarcoidosis. J Clin Imaging Sci. 2011;1:15.

Ginat DT, Freitag SK, Kieff D, Grove A, Fay A, Cunnane M, Moonis G. Radiographic patterns of orbital involvement in IgG4-related disease. Ophthal Plast Reconstr Surg. 2013;29(4):261–6.

Ginat DT, Vargas SO, Silvera VM, Volk MS, Degar BA, Robson CD. Imaging features of juvenile xanthogranuloma of the pediatric head and neck. AJNR Am J Neuroradiol. 2016;37(5):910–6.

Grana N. Langerhans cell histiocytosis. Cancer Control. 2014;21(4):328–34.

Grois NG, Favara BE, Mostbeck GH, Prayer D. Central nervous system disease in Langerhans cell histiocytosis. Hematol Oncol Clin North Am. 1998;12(2):287–305.

Guarner J, Brandt ME. Histopathologic diagnosis of fungal infections in the 21st century. Clin Microbiol Rev. 2011;24(2):247–80.

Hildenbrand P, Craven DE, Jones R, Nemeskal P. Lyme neuroborreliosis: manifestations of a rapidly emerging zoonosis. AJNR Am J Neuroradiol. 2009;30(6):1079–87.

Howard JE, et al. Langerhans cell sarcoma: a systematic review. Cancer Treat Rev. 2015;41(4):320–31.

Ibrahim F, Khan T, Pujalte GG. Bacterial skin infections. Prim Care. 2015;42(4):485–99.

Jafri K, Patterson SL, Lanata C. Central nervous system manifestations of systemic lupus erythematosus. Rheum Dis Clin North Am. 2017;43(4):531–45.

Joaquim AF, Ghizoni E, Tedeschi H, Appenzeller S, Riew KD. Radiological evaluation of cervical spine involvement in rheumatoid arthritis. Neurosurg Focus. 2015;38(4):E4.

Judson MA. The clinical features of sarcoidosis: a comprehensive review. Clin Rev Allergy Immunol. 2015;49(1):63–78.

Kaafarani HM, King DR. Necrotizing skin and soft tissue infections. Surg Clin North Am. 2014;94(1):155–63.

Kim D, Franco GA, Shigehara H, Asaumi J, Hildenbrand P. Benign miliary osteoma cutis of the face: a common incidental CT finding. AJNR Am J Neuroradiol. 2017;38(4):789–94.

Kittridge A, Routhouska SB, Korman NJ. Dermatologic manifestations of Sjögren syndrome. J Cutan Med Surg. 2011;15(1):8–14.

Koeller KK, Shih RY. Viral and prion infections of the central nervous system: radiologic-pathologic correlation: from the radiologic pathology archives. Radiographics. 2017;37(1):199–233.

Krumholz A, Stern BJ. Neurologic manifestations of sarcoidosis. Handb Clin Neurol. 2014;119:305–33.

Kuhn A, Landmann A. The classification and diagnosis of cutaneous lupus erythematosus. J Autoimmun. 2014;48-49:14–9.

Lessner A, Stern GA. Preseptal and orbital cellulitis. Infect Dis Clin North Am. 1992;6(4):933–52.

Martin-Duverneuil N, et al. MRI features of neurodegenerative Langerhans cell histiocytosis. Eur Radiol. 2006;16(9):2074–82.

Mathur M, Johnson CE, Sze G. Fungal infections of the central nervous system. Neuroimaging Clin N Am. 2012;22(4):609–32.

May AK. Skin and soft tissue infections. Surg Clin North Am. 2009;89(2):403–20, viii.

Müllegger RR, Glatz M. Skin manifestations of lyme borreliosis: diagnosis and management. Am J Clin Dermatol. 2008;9(6):355–68.

Murthy JM, Sundaram C. Fungal infections of the central nervous system. Handb Clin Neurol. 2014;121:1383–401.

Myllylä RM, Haapasaari KM, Palatsi R, Germain-Lee EL, Hägg PM, Ignatius J, Tuukkanen J. Multiple miliary osteoma cutis is a distinct disease entity: four case reports and review of the literature. Br J Dermatol. 2011;164(3):544–52.

Niemelä RK, Pääkkö E, Suramo I, Takalo R, Hakala M. Magnetic resonance imaging and magnetic resonance sialography of parotid glands in primary Sjogren's syndrome. Arthritis Rheum. 2001;45(6):512–8.

Park SW, Kim HJ, Sung KJ, Lee JH, Park IS. Kimura disease: CT and MR imaging findings. AJNR Am J Neuroradiol. 2012;33(4):784–8.

Postal M, Lapa AT, Reis F, Rittner L, Appenzeller S. Magnetic resonance imaging in neuropsychiatric systemic lupus erythematosus: current state of the art and novel approaches. Lupus. 2017;26(5):517–21.

Raman Sharma R. Fungal infections of the nervous system: current perspective and controversies in management. Int J Surg. 2010;8(8):591–601.

Ramdass P, Mullick S, Farber HF. Viral skin diseases. Prim Care. 2015;42(4):517–67.

Ribero S, Sciascia S, Borradori L, Lipsker D. The cutaneous spectrum of lupus erythematosus. Clin Rev Allergy Immunol. 2017;53(3):291–305.

Robson CD, Hazra R, Barnes PD, Robertson RL, Jones D, Husson RN. Nontuberculous mycobacterial infection of the head and neck in immunocompetent children: CT and MR findings. AJNR Am J Neuroradiol. 1999;20(10):1829–35.

Saidha S, Sotirchos ES, Eckstein C. Etiology of sarcoidosis: does infection play a role? Yale J Biol Med. 2012;85(1):133–41.

Sangüeza OP, Salmon JK, White CR Jr, Beckstead JH. Juvenile xanthogranuloma: a clinical, histopathologic and immunohistochemical study. J Cutan Pathol. 1995;22(4):327–35.

Sayah A, English JC III. Rheumatoid arthritis: a review of the cutaneous manifestations. J Am Acad Dermatol. 2005;53(2):191–209, quiz 210–2.

Shah R, Roberson GH, Curé JK. Correlation of MR imaging findings and clinical manifestations in neurosarcoidosis. AJNR Am J Neuroradiol. 2009;30(5):953–61.

Shih RY, Koeller KK. Bacterial, fungal, and parasitic infections of the central nervous system: radiologic-pathologic correlation and historical perspectives. Radiographics. 2015;35(4):1141–69.

Soares BP, Provenzale JM. Imaging of herpesvirus infections of the CNS. AJR Am J Roentgenol. 2016;206(1):39–48.

Stone J. Parry-Romberg syndrome: a global survey of 205 patients using the Internet. Neurology. 2003;61(5):674–6.

Strle F, Stanek G. Clinical manifestations and diagnosis of lyme borreliosis. Curr Probl Dermatol. 2009;37:51–110.

Sukumaran V, Senanayake S. Bacterial skin and soft tissue infections. Aust Prescr. 2016;39(5):159–63.

Sun Z, Zhang Z, Fu K, Zhao Y, Liu D, Ma X. Diagnostic accuracy of parotid CT for identifying Sjögren's syndrome. Eur J Radiol. 2012;81(10):2702–9.

Swanson PA 2nd, McGavern DB. Viral diseases of the central nervous system. Curr Opin Virol. 2015;11:44–54.

Tahan SR, Pastel-Levy C, Bhan AK, Mihm MC Jr. Juvenile xanthogranuloma. Clinical and pathologic characterization. Arch Pathol Lab Med. 1989;113(9):1057–61.

Thrasher RD, Kingdom TT. Fungal infections of the head and neck: an update. Otolaryngol Clin North Am. 2003;36(4):577–94.

Tilstra JS, Lienesch DW. Rheumatoid nodules. Dermatol Clin. 2015;33(3):361–71.

Tokura Y, Yagi H, Yanaguchi H, Majima Y, Kasuya A, Ito T, Maekawa M, Hashizume H. IgG4-related skin disease. Br J Dermatol. 2014;171(5):959–67.

Toledano P, Sarbu N, Espinosa G, Bargalló N, Cervera R. Neuropsychiatric systemic lupus erythematosus: magnetic resonance imaging findings and correlation with clinical and immunological features. Autoimmun Rev. 2013;12(12):1166–70.

Umehara H, Okazaki K, Masaki Y, Kawano M, Yamamoto M, Saeki T, Matsui S, Yoshino T, Nakamura S, Kawa S, Hamano H, Kamisawa T, Shimosegawa T, Shimatsu A, Nakamura S, Ito T, Notohara K, Sumida T, Tanaka Y, Mimori T, Chiba T, Mishima M, Hibi T, Tsubouchi H, Inui K, Ohara H. Comprehensive diagnostic criteria for IgG4-related disease (IgG4-RD), 2011. Mod Rheumatol. 2012;22(1):21–30.

van Burik JA, Colven R, Spach DH. Cutaneous aspergillosis. J Clin Microbiol. 1998;36(11):3115–21.

Wang SH, Pancholi P. Mycobacterial skin and soft tissue infection. Curr Infect Dis Rep. 2014;16(11):438.

Wigley FM, Flavahan NA. Raynaud's phenomenon. N Engl J Med. 2016;375(6):556–65.

Wijdicks EF, Klein CJ. Guillain-Barré syndrome. Mayo Clin Proc. 2017;92(3):467–79.

Wong M, Phillips CD, Hagiwara M, Shatzkes DR. Parry Romberg syndrome: 7 cases and literature review. AJNR Am J Neuroradiol. 2015;36(7):1355–61.

Wortsman X. Imaging of hidradenitis suppurativa. Dermatol Clin. 2016;34(1):59–68.

Zhao Z, Wang Y, Guan Z, Jin J, Huang F, Zhu J. Utility of FDG-PET/CT in the diagnosis of IgG4-related diseases. Clin Exp Rheumatol. 2016;34(1):119–25. Epub 2016 Feb 2.

Benign Cysts, Tumors, and Tumor-Like Non-vascular Lesions of the Skin and Subcutaneous Tissues

5

Daniel Thomas Ginat, Nicole A. Cipriani, Joshua Eassa, and Vesna Petronic-Rosic

Contents

D. T. Ginat (✉)
Department of Radiology, University of Chicago, Pritzker School of Medicine, Chicago, IL, USA
e-mail: dtg1@uchicago.edu

N. A. Cipriani
Department of Pathology, University of Chicago, Chicago, IL, USA

J. Eassa
Prtizker School of Medicine, University of Chicago, Chicago, IL, USA

V. Petronic-Rosic
Section of Dermatology, Department of Medicine, University of Chicago, Chicago, IL, USA

Abstract

There is a wide variety of benign tumors and tumor-like lesions that can involve the skin and subcutaneous tissues in the head and neck regions. This chapter reviews the characteristic clinicopathological and imaging findings of benign keratinocytic and adnexal lesions, benign lipomatous tumors, and benign and "borderline" fibrous tumors and proliferations.

D. T. Ginat (ed.), *Neuroradiological Imaging of Skin Diseases and Related Conditions*,
https://doi.org/10.1007/978-3-319-90931-8_5

Benign Keratinocytic and Adnexal Lesions

Pilomatrixoma

Overview

Pilomatrixoma (formerly known as calcifying epithelioma of Malherbe) is a benign dermal tumor of ectodermal hair follicle matrix cells (cortical cells) found mainly in children and young adults, with a smaller proportion also being found in the elderly. Most cases are sporadic and solitary, but tumors may be associated with other conditions, such as Gardner syndrome, myotonic muscular dystrophy, sarcoidosis, skull dysostosis, Rubinstein-Taybi syndrome, and Turner syndrome. The lesions can be effectively treated by complete surgical resection.

Clinicopathologic Findings

Pilomatrixomas typically present as painless, superficial dermal tumors that are freely mobile under the skin. The lesions are hard nodules (Fig. 5.1). Additionally, the overlying skin color may change to a bluish hue and skin ulceration may be present. Yellow or white flecks representing calcifications may also be visible through the skin. Histologically, the tumor consists of basophilic epithelial cells in the periphery and shadow or ghost cells without nuclei in the tumor center (Fig. 5.2). The ghost cell keratin frequently undergoes calcification.

Imaging Findings

Pilomatrixomas are well-circumscribed subcutaneous nodules with partial attachment to the overlying skin. On ultrasound, the lesions are mostly hyperechoic with posterior acoustic shadowing and a hypoechoic rim. On CT, the lesions appear as enhancing soft-tissue masses with varying amounts of calcification (Fig. 5.3). MRI can demonstrate internal reticulations and patchy areas of high T2 signal within the pilomatrixomas (Fig. 5.4), corresponding to edematous

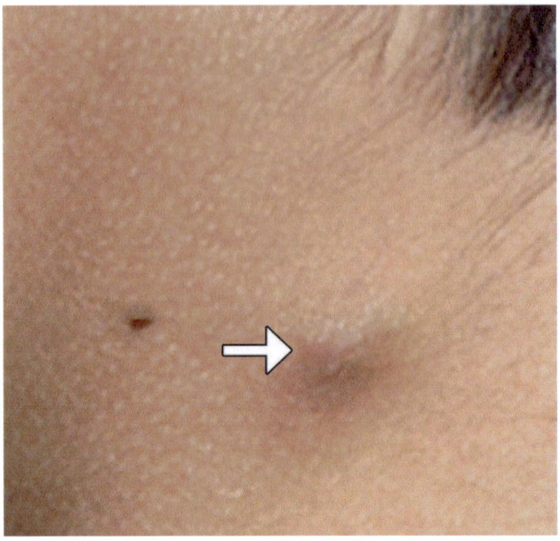

Fig. 5.1 Pilomatrixoma. The photograph shows a nodular lesion on the neck with slight bluish discoloration of the skin (arrow)

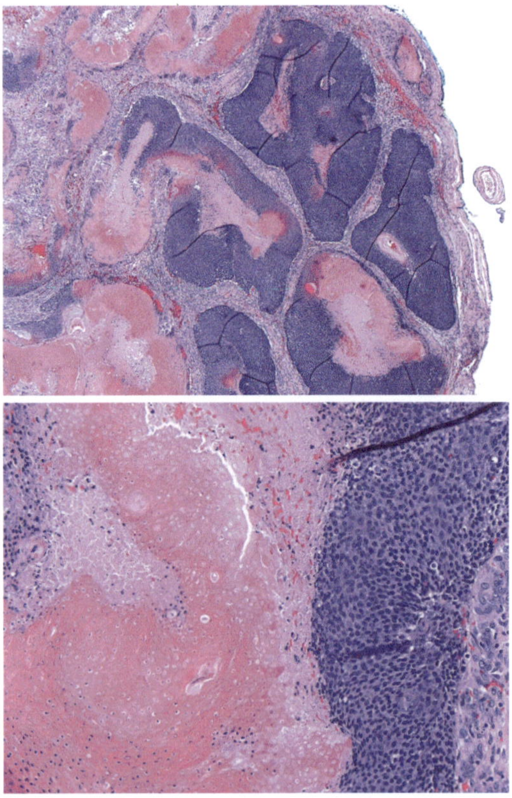

Fig. 5.2 Pilomatrixoma. Low and high power hematoxylin and eosin stained histologic section show dark blue basaloid cells towards the periphery of tumor islands and pale eosinophilic anucleate ghost cells towards the center of tumor islands

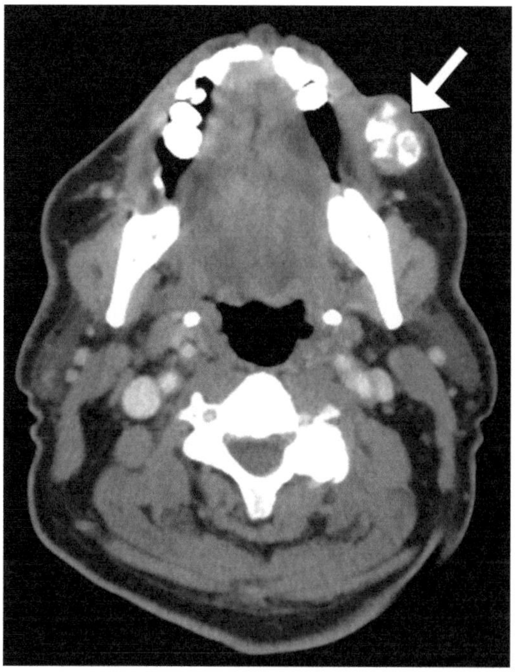

Fig. 5.3 Pilomatrixoma. Axial CT image shows a partially calcified mass in the subcutaneous tissues of the anterior left face (arrow)

stroma on pathology. Peritumoral inflammatory changes and the presence of a connective capsule may have corresponding imaging manifestations, including peripheral enhancement. The lesions tend not display restricted diffusion.

Epidermoid Cyst

Overview

Epidermoid cyst is a generic term that refers to either epidermal cyst (epidermal inclusion cyst, infundibular cyst, and keratin cyst) or pilar (trichilemmal or isthmus-catagen) cyst. Epidermoid cysts can be congenital or acquired and are most common cutaneous cystic lesions of the head and neck and tend to be located in the neck, cheeks, periauricular area, and the nasal area. The cysts are typically asymptomatic unless they become infected or inflamed. Surgical excision with complete removal of the cyst wall or capsule is a treatment option in symptomatic cases.

Clinicopathologic Findings

Epidermoid cysts usually appear as sessile protuberances of the skin with diameters ranging from a few millimeters to several centimeters. The cysts are fluctuant and can be erythematous and painful if infected or inflamed. Epidermoid cysts often have a central punctum and are freely moveable on palpation. The cyst wall is composed of stratified squamous epithelium with a granular layer and intraluminal loose keratin debris (Fig. 5.5).

Imaging Findings

Ultrasound of epidermoid cysts typically demonstrates hypoechoic or heterogeneoues nodules with thin and irregular walls (Fig. 5.6). CT often demonstrates fluid attenuation within the cyst (Fig. 5.7), but cysts are occasionally of higher attenuation. On MRI, the cysts may vary from low to high signal intensity on T1-weighted sequences, often display high signal on T2-weighted sequences, and do not enhance (Fig. 5.8). Epidermoid cysts tend to be brighter than other cysts on DWI. Infected or inflamed epidermoid cysts can mimic dermal neoplasms on PET due to the presence of hypermetabolism (Figs. 5.8 and 5.9). Dermatobia hominis (botfly), which causes furuncular myiasis endemic to South America, is another exotic differential consideration.

Pilar Cysts

Overview

Pilar cysts (trichilemmal or isthmus-catagen cysts) arise from the outer hair root sheath or trichilemma. The lesions are more common in women than men, mostly occur in individuals over 60 years of age and are usually located on the scalp.

Clinicopathologic Findings

Pilar cysts are typically found on the scalp as a smooth, skin-colored, dome-shaped protrusion,

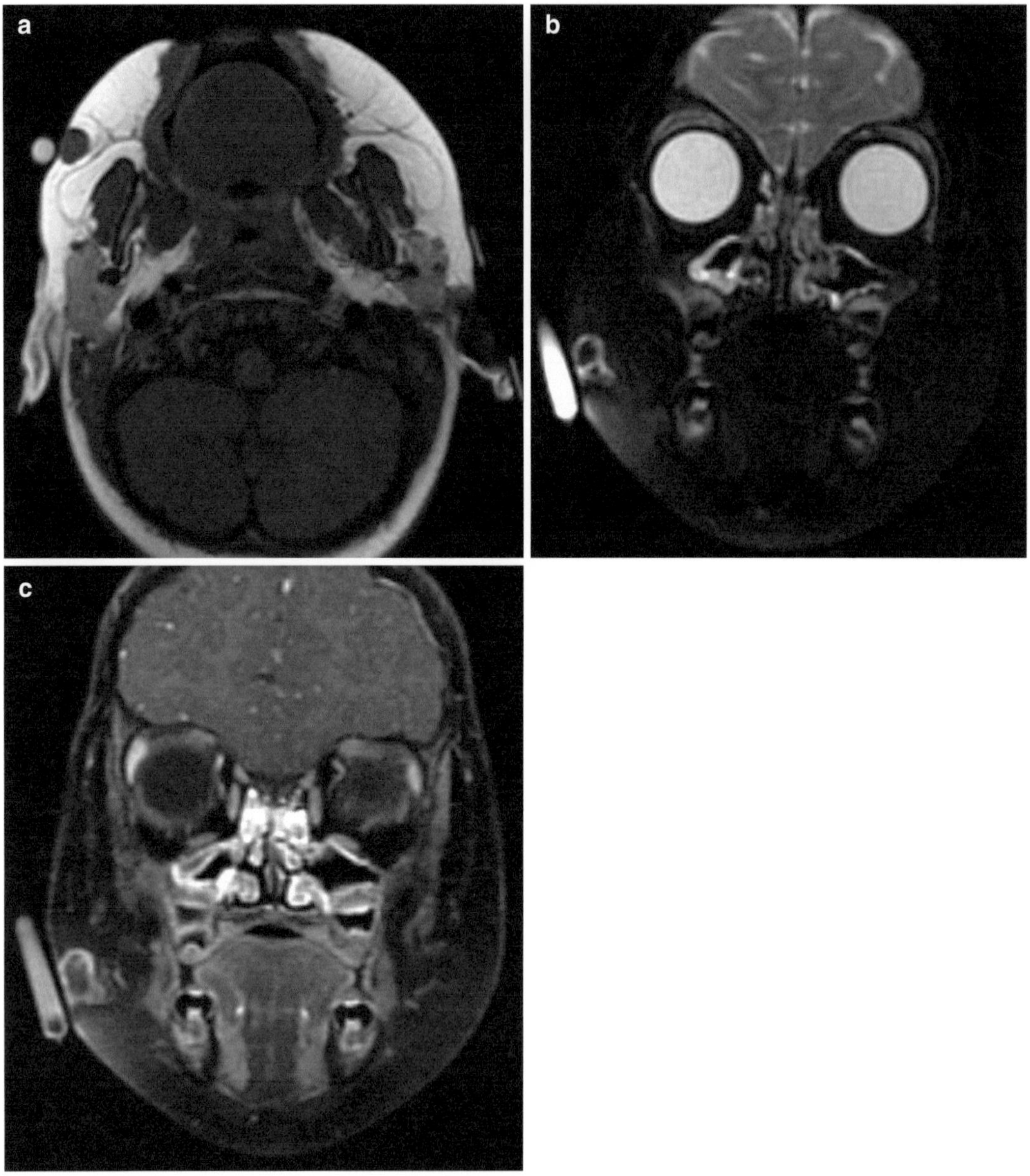

Fig. 5.4 Pilomatrixoma. Axial T1-weighted (**a**), coronal fat-suppressed T2-weighted (**b**), and coronal post-contrast T1-weighted (**c**) MR images show a nodule in the right cheek of an infant with mild peritumoral edema and enhancement. An overlying vitamin E marker is present

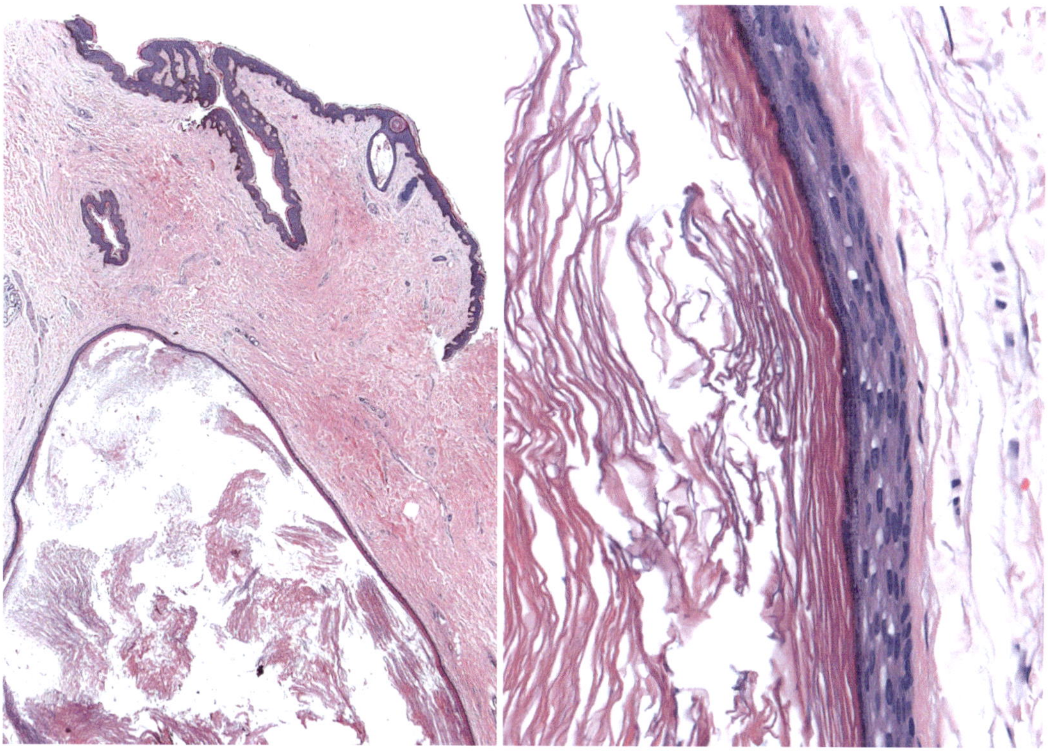

Fig. 5.5 Epidermoid cyst. Low power (left) hematoxylin and eosin stained histological section shows skin with a dermal-based cystic lesion. High power (right) hematoxylin and eosin stained histological section demonstrates a stratified squamous epithelial lining with a granular layer and loose intraluminal keratin debris

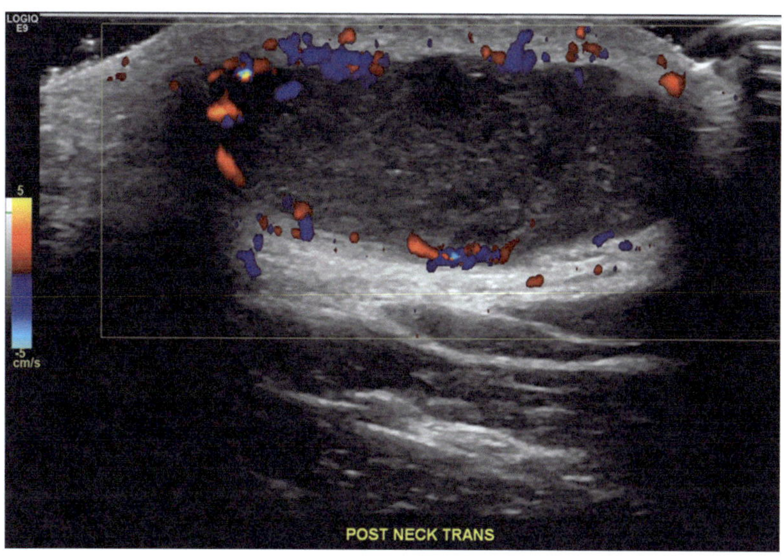

Fig. 5.6 Epidermoid cyst. Doppler ultrasound shows a heterogeneous hypoechoic subcutaneous lesion with enhanced through transmission and no internal vascularity

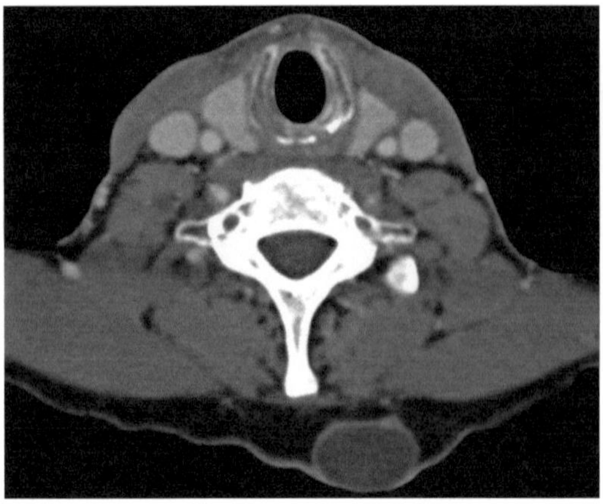

Fig. 5.7 Epidermoid cyst. Axial CT image shows a well-defined fluid attenuation lesion with a thin wall in the subcutaneous tissues that contacts the skin of the posterior left neck

often devoid of hair (partial or complete alopecia). Pilar cysts present as firm subcutaneous nodules, most frequently in the hair-bearing scalp, but can be found elsewhere. The lesions typically measure 1–3 cm in diameter, and range in color from tan to pink or red (Fig. 5.10). Pilar cysts do not have an overlying punctum, as can be found with epidermoid cysts. On histology, pilar cysts are filled with dense eosinophilic keratin debris and the cyst wall displays trichilemmal differentiation, as occurs in the outer root sheath of the hair follicle (Fig. 5.11). Focal rupture of the cyst can occur and lead to giant cell reaction.

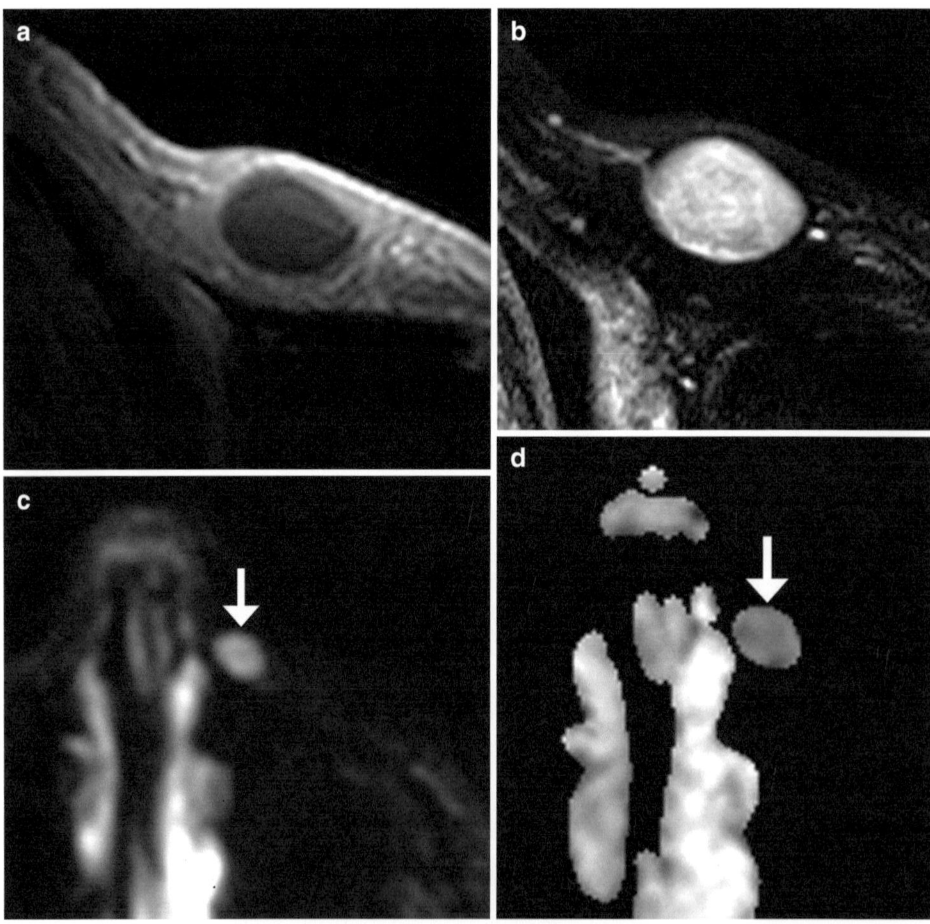

Fig. 5.8 Epidermoid cyst. Axial post-contrast fat-suppressed T1-weighted (**a**), axial fat-suppressed T2 (**b**) MRI images obtained with microscopy coil and axial DWI (**c**) and ADC map (**d**) show a well-defined non-enhancing lesion in the left cheek subcutaneous tissues with some restricted diffusivity (arrows)

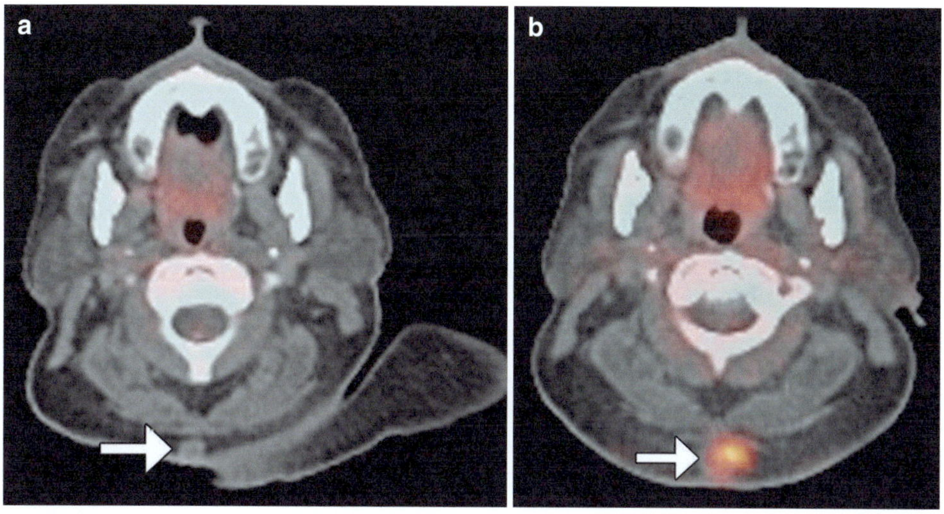

Fig. 5.9 Ruptured epidermoid cyst with inflammation. The patient has a history of melanoma. The initial [18]FDG-PET-CT (**a**) shows a nodule in the subcutaneous tissues of the posterior neck (arrow). Follow-up PET-CT (**b**) shows interval hypermetabolism associated with the lesion (arrow), which developed purulent drainage

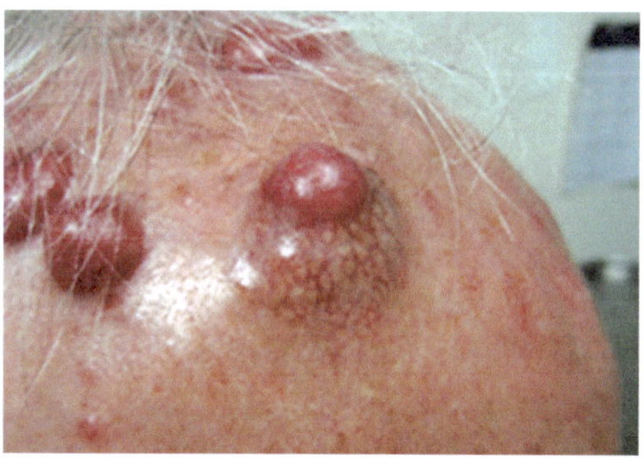

Fig. 5.10 Pilar cyst. Photograph shows multiple red nodules in the hair-bearing scalp

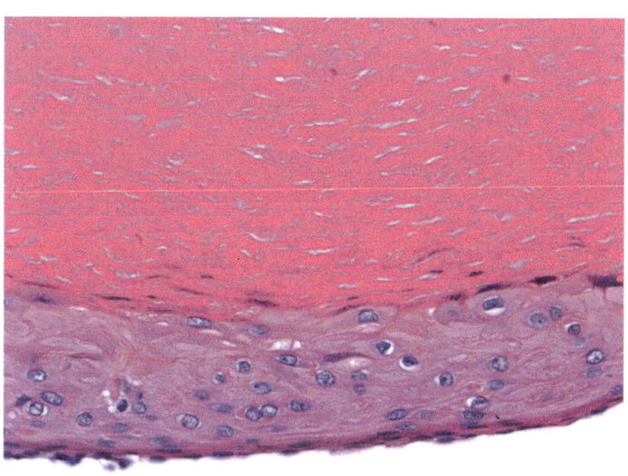

Fig. 5.11 Pilar cyst. High power hematoxylin and eosin stained histological section of a pilar cyst wall shows stratified squamous epithelium with pale eosinophilic cytoplasm, without a granular layer. Densely packed brightly eosinophilic keratin fills the cyst

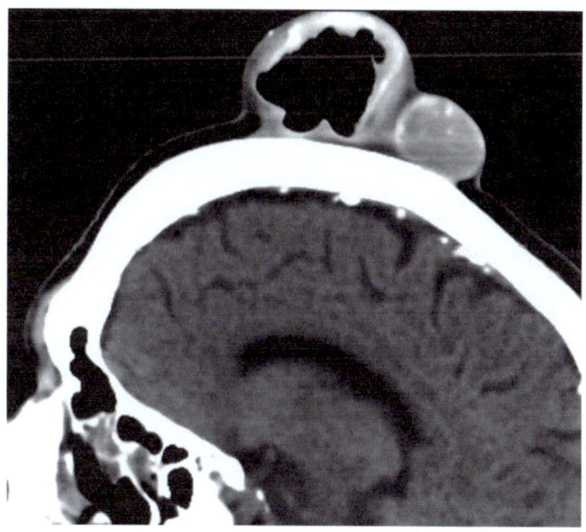

Fig. 5.12 Pilar cysts. Sagittal CT image shows two cystic scalp lesions with peripheral calcifications in the irregular, thick walls, one of which has ruptured and contains gas

Imaging Findings

Pilar cyst contents are frequently hyperattenuating on CT and calcifications are often present within the irregular walls of the cysts (Fig. 5.12). On MRI, the cysts can display variable and heterogeneous T1 and T2 signal characteristics. Additionally, pilar cysts can display contrast enhancement and internal hemorrhage (Fig. 5.13).

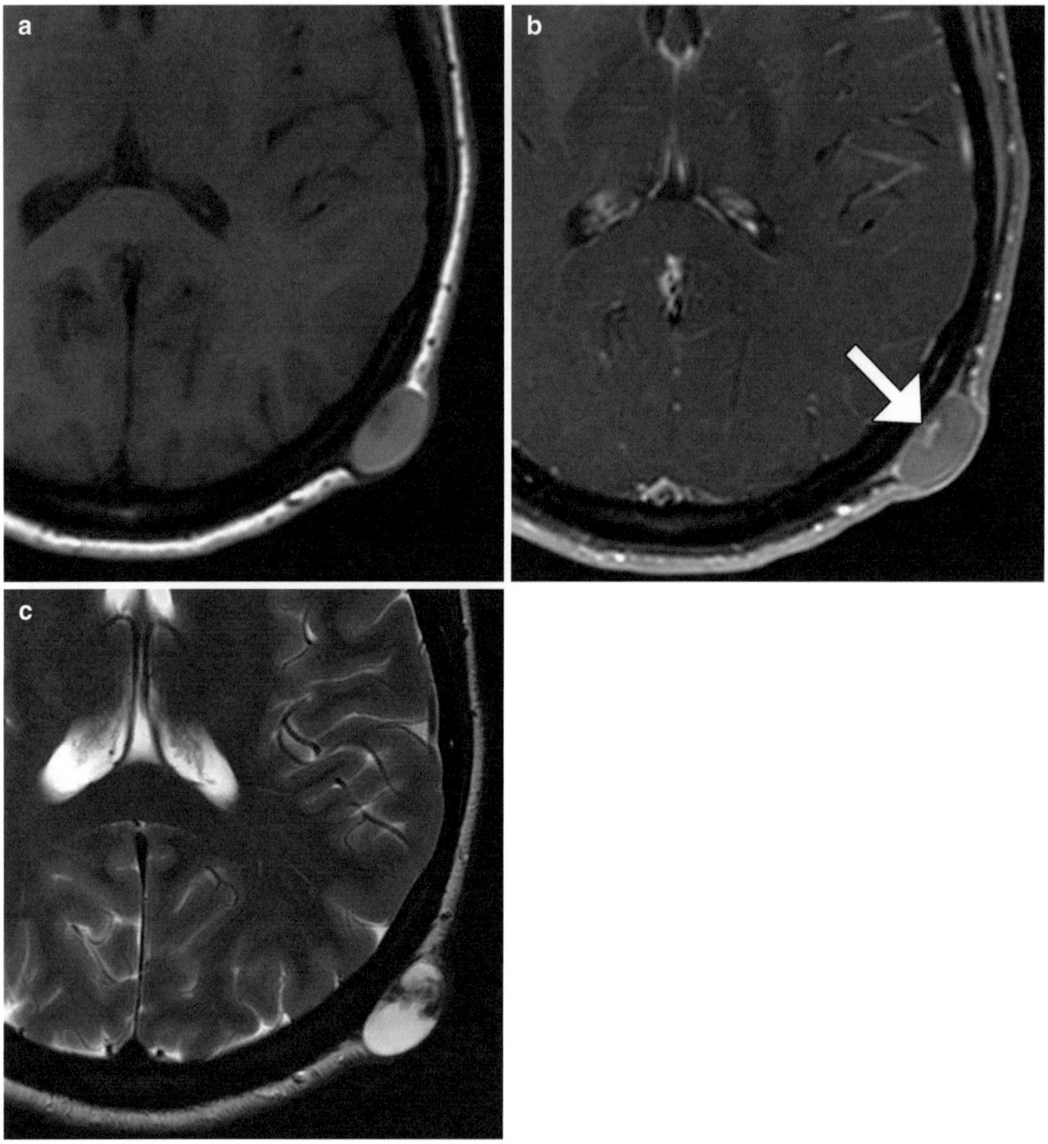

Fig. 5.13 Pilar cyst. The patient presented with an enlarging left scalp mass. Axial T1-weighted (**a**), post-contrast fat-suppressed T1-weighted (**b**), and axial T2-weighted (**c**) MR images show a mildly T1 hyperintense well-defined lesion in the left parietal scalp subcutaneous tissues with a focus of enhancement (arrow) and streaky areas of T2 hypointensity due to hemorrhage

Hidrocystoma

Overview

Hidrocystomas are cystic tumors that can be of two main types: apocrine and eccrine. Apocrine hidrocystomas are benign cystic tumors of apocrine glands found most commonly near the eyelid margins and on the cheeks. The lesions are more commonly found in females between 30 and 70 years of age.

Clinicopathologic Findings

Hidrocystomas present as dome-shaped lesions that are smooth, clear, and cystic (Fig. 5.14). The color can vary from tan to blue to black and its size ranges from 3 to 15 mm. Although usually solitary, apocrine hidrocystomas may appear as multiple lesions. Hidrocystomas are usually are usually found in the head and neck, particularly the eyelid. Apocrine hidrocystomas are composed of secretory columnar epithelium, while eccrine hidrocystomas result from dilation of the eccrine duct (Fig. 5.15).

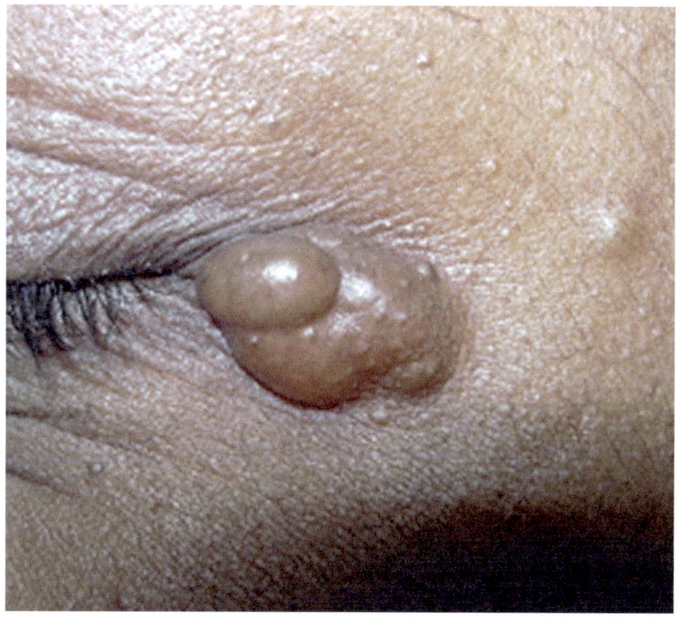

Fig. 5.14 Apocrine hidrocystoma. Photograph shows dome-shaped lesions that classically arise in the lateral canthus

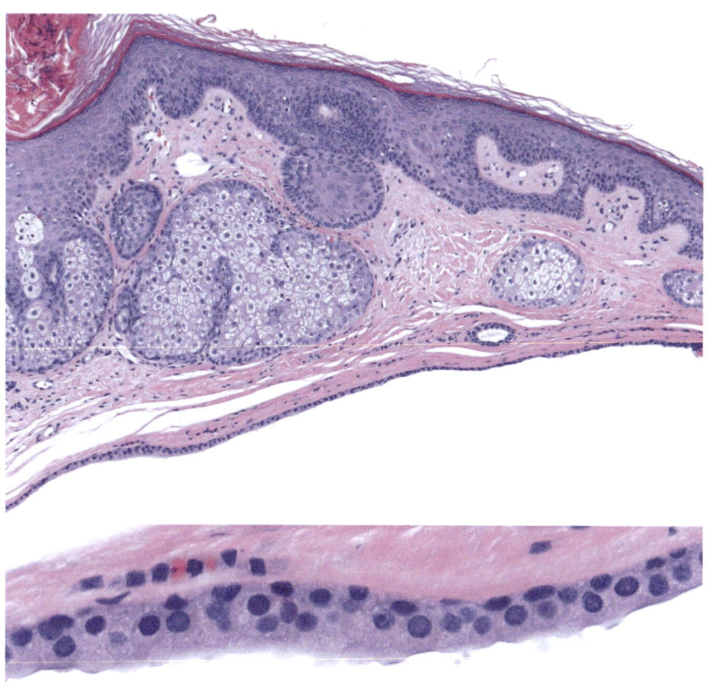

Fig. 5.15 Hidrocystoma. Low and high power hematoxylin and eosin stained histological sections of a dermal cyst lined by a bilayered epithelium comprised of flattened basally located cells and plump cuboidal luminally located cells with apical blebs, typical of apocrine hidrocystoma

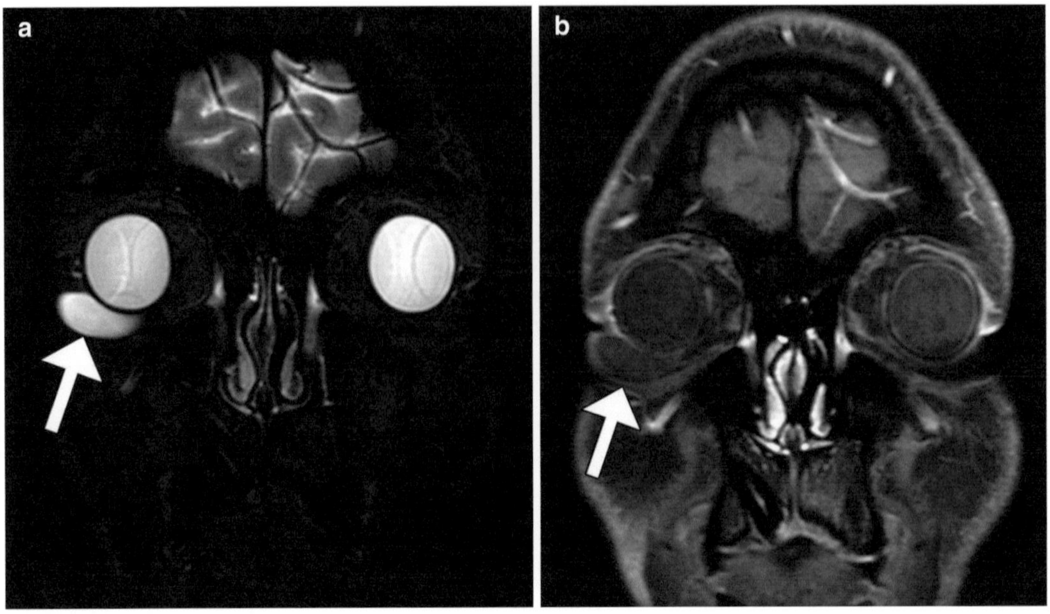

Fig. 5.16 Eccrine hidrocystoma. Coronal STIR (**a**) and fat-suppressed post-contrast T1-weighted (**b**) MR images show a cystic lesion in the right inferolateral eyelid (arrows)

Imaging

Hidrocystomas may be encountered incidentally on diagnostic imaging. MRI and CT demonstrate small cystic lesions in the lateral periorbital regions, without deep connections to the orbital contents (Fig. 5.16). The characteristic location and lack of enhancement is suggestive of this benign entity. The imaging differential diagnosis may nevertheless include inclusion cysts, although hidrocystomas do not tend to display restricted diffusion, and abscess, although uncomplicated cysts do not have associated inflammatory changes.

Syringocystadenoma Papilliferum

Overview

Syringocystadenoma papilliferum is a ceruminous gland tumor that most commonly occurs in the head and neck. Ceruminous glands are related to apocrine glands. Other benign ceruminous gland tumors include ceruminous adenoma and ceruminous pleomorphic adenoma.

Clinicopathology Findings

Syringocystadenoma papilliferum can present as a plaque or as a papule. The popular form often has an umbilication that may discharge fluid or keratinous debris (Fig. 5.17). The lesions tend to be skin-colored or pink, are often moist, and there may lack overlying hair. When multiple papules are present, they tend to be arranged in a linear configuration.

Microscopically, the surface of syringocystadenoma papilliferum is variable, ranging from smooth to papillomatous to a cup-like depression of small papillations, but the presence of ducts connecting the surface to the main body of the lesion is a common feature of these tumors. Histologically, the lesions characteristically contain papillary fronds, and cyst-like spaces lined by myoepithelial cells and columnar epithelial cells (Fig. 5.18). The connective tissue stroma that surrounds the duct-like structures projects into the papillations and often contains inflammatory cells. Although syringocystadenoma papilliferum is typically benign, like all ceruminous gland tumors, it can potentially be malignant.

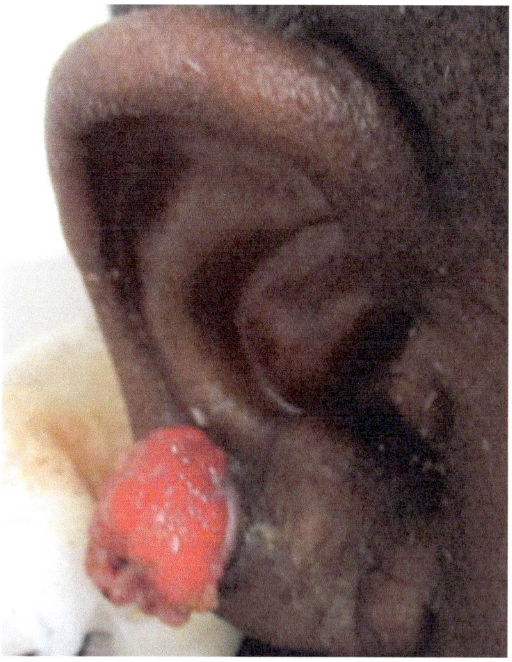

Fig. 5.17 Syringocystadenoma papilliferum. Photograph shows a moist pinkish papule with central umbilication arising from the lower ear

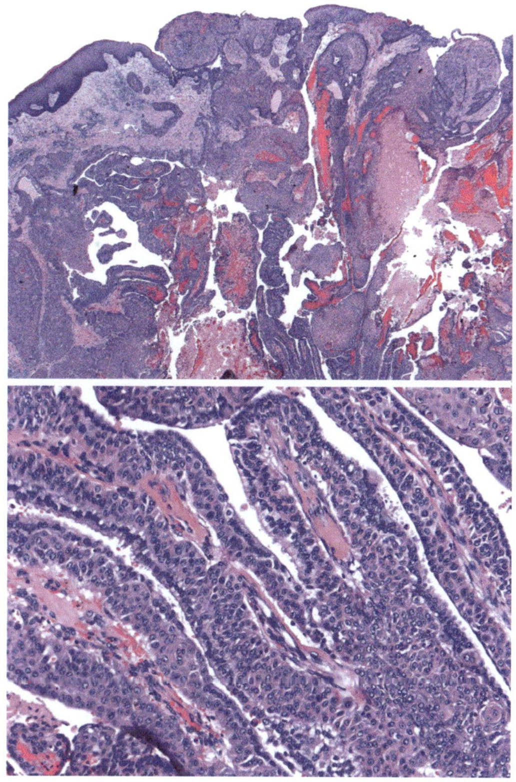

Fig. 5.18 Syringocystadenoma papilliferum. Low power image (top) shows a cellular, tumor with connection to the surface epithelium and invaginations composed of solid areas, papillary fronds, and cyst-like spaces. Higher power image (bottom) shows papillary fronds lined by a double layer of cells: flattened to cuboidal myoepithelial cells and plump columnar epithelial cells

Imaging Findings

Syringocystadenoma papilliferum tends to appear as lobulated soft-tissue tumors with well-defined margins. The lesions tend to have high signal on T2-weighted sequences, intermediate signal on T1-weighted sequences and enhance (Fig. 5.19).

Benign Lipomatous Tumors

Overview

Benign lipomatous tumors that may be encountered in the subcutaneous tissues of the head and neck include the following entities: lipoma, lipomatosis, lipoblastoma, angiolipoma, angiolipoma, chondroid lipoma, spindle cell lipoma, and hibernoma. Some of these conditions are discussed further below:

- *Lipoma* is a very common neoplasm that comprises nearly 50% of soft-tissue tumors overall and is often located in the posterior neck and upper back. Superficial lipomas are smaller than 5 cm in 80% of cases, with only 1% of lesions greater than 10 cm in size. A lipoma typically manifests as a discrete mobile palpable doughy, solitary soft-tissue mass.
- *Infiltrating lipomatosis* mainly occurs in infants and is a proliferation of mature adipose tissue that infiltrates muscle and soft tissue. Consequently, surgical excision is technically difficult and recur-

rence is common. The facial nerve is usually involved, and paralysis commonly results after surgery.

- *Spindle cell lipoma* has a predilection for the posterior neck and shoulder in middle-aged men.
- *Lipoblastoma* is a rare benign mesenchymal tumor of embryonal white fat that is present during infancy and early childhood. Lipoblastomas tend to evolve into mature lipomas.

Clinicopathologic Findings

Lipomas tend to grow insidiously large without any symptoms and cause few problems other than those of localized mass and cosmetic concerns. A lipoma typically manifests as a discrete solitary, mobile, palpable, doughy, soft-tissue mass. Typically, these tumors are encapsulated by a fibrous shell, smooth or lobulated, are easy to remove, and rarely recur. A lipoma is composed of mature adipocytes with uniform nuclei (Fig. 5.20).

Infiltrating facial lipomatosis presents at birth, typically unilaterally in one cheek. Additionally, the underlying bone may be hypertrophied. Hemifacial hypertrophy and a facial mass are the presenting symptoms in patients with infiltrating facial lipomatosis. Structures ipsilateral to the lesion, such as the eye, nose, and lips, may be distorted due to mass effect from the lipomatous tumor. The mass may cause early eruption of deciduous and permanent teeth and be associated with cutaneous capillary blush.

Spindle cell lipomas are slow-growing tumors comprised of spindled cells with blunt nuclei admixed with fat cells and ropey collagen bundles. Mast cells, lymphocytes, myxoid tissue, and vascular elements may also be present to varying degrees. The presence of scattered bizarre multinucleated giant cells with radially arranged nuclei (floret cells) is indicative of a related lesion, pleomorphic lipoma (Fig. 5.21). Cytogenetic analysis often reveals monosomy or partial loss of chromosome 13 or 16.

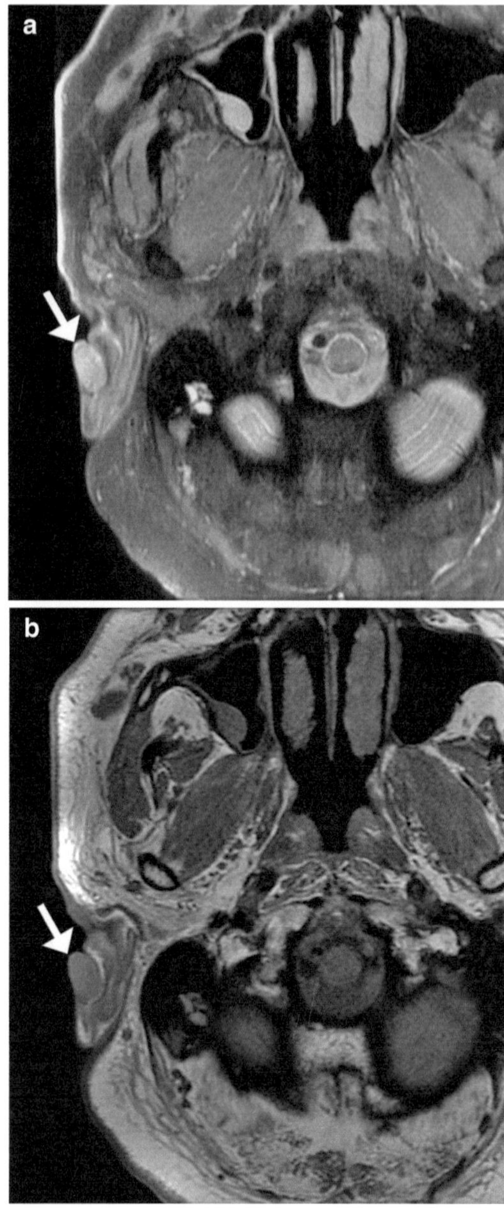

Fig. 5.19 Syringocystadenoma papilliferum. Axial T2-weighted (**a**) and T1-weighted (**b**) show an exophytic nodule arising from right auricle (arrows)

Lipoblastomas are composed of monovacuolated and multivacuolated lipoblasts, spindled to stellate mesenchymal cells, a plexiform capillary network, myxoid stroma, and mature adipocytes organized into lobules separated by fibrous septa (Fig. 5.22). A "signet ring" appearance may be encountered when lipoblasts are relatively small

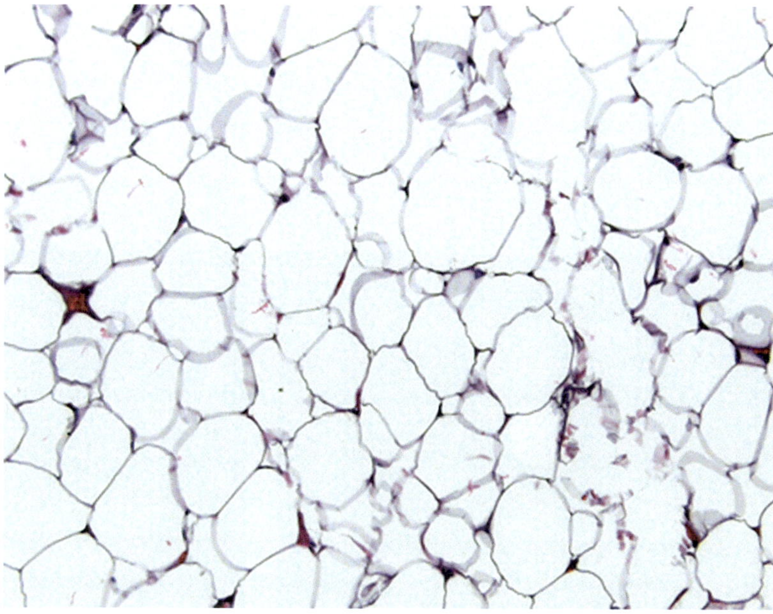

Fig. 5.20 High power hematoxylin and eosin stained histological section image showing mature adipocytes with compressed nuclei at the periphery of fat cells, characteristic of lipoma

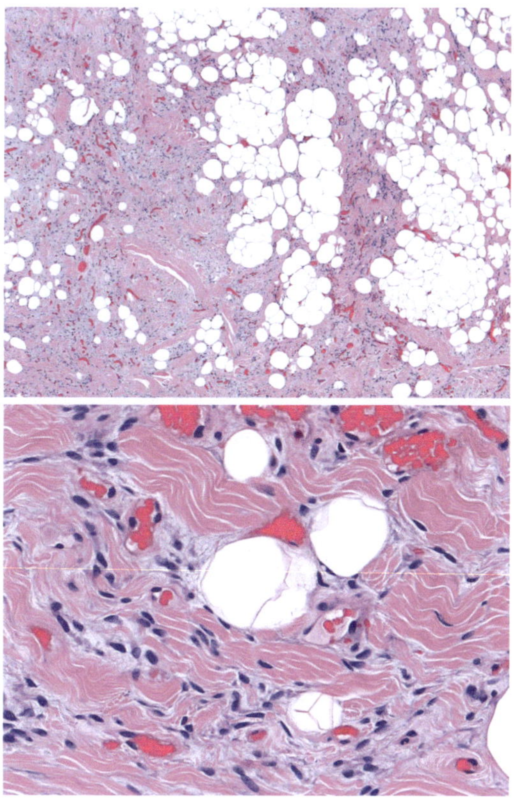

Fig. 5.21 Spindle cell lipomas. Low power (top) hematoxylin and eosin stained histological section image showing admixed mature adipocytes and cellular fibrous tissue. High power (bottom) image demonstrates ropey collagen bundles and spindle cells with bland oval nuclei, characteristic of spindle cell lipoma

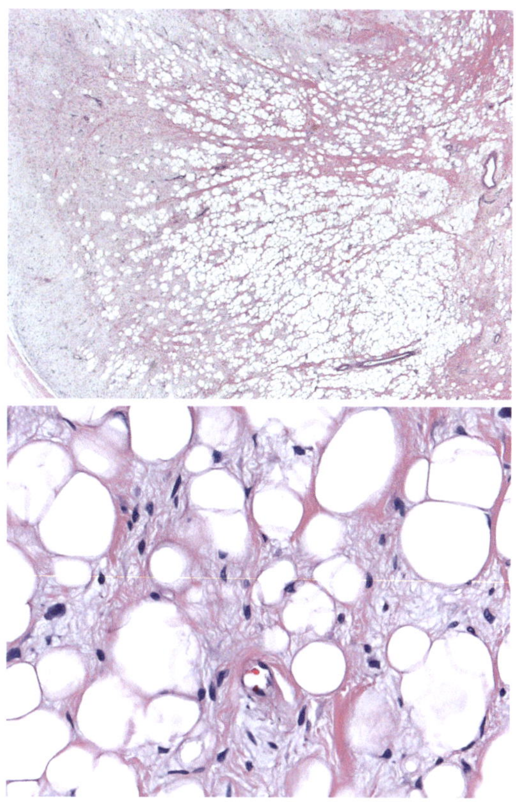

Fig. 5.22 Lipoblastomas. Low (top) and high (bottom) power hematoxylin and eosin stained histological section images show an adipocytic neoplasm with focally myxoid stroma, interspersed fibrous septae, and variably sized adipocytes. Lipoblastomas may have variable numbers of actual lipoblasts, depending on the maturity of the lesion

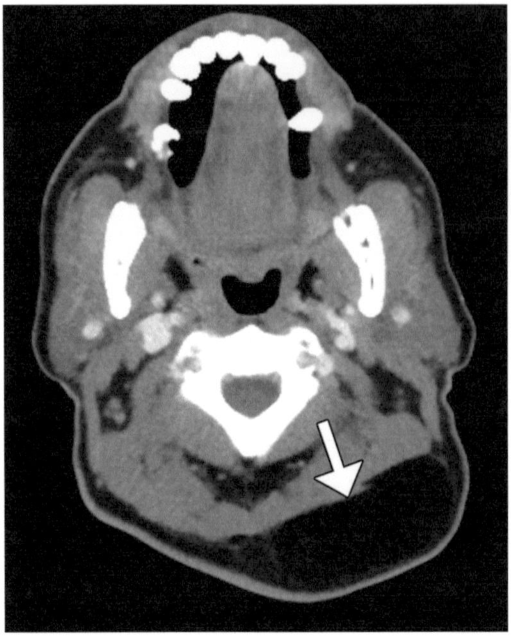

Fig. 5.23 Lipoma. Axial CT image shows an encapsulated fat-attenuation mass in the posterior left neck subcutaneous tissues (arrow)

and round with a single vacuole-like fat droplet. The tumors feature characteristic cytogenetic abnormalities, including deletions and rearrangement of 8q11–13. These lesions do not have a tendency to metastasize.

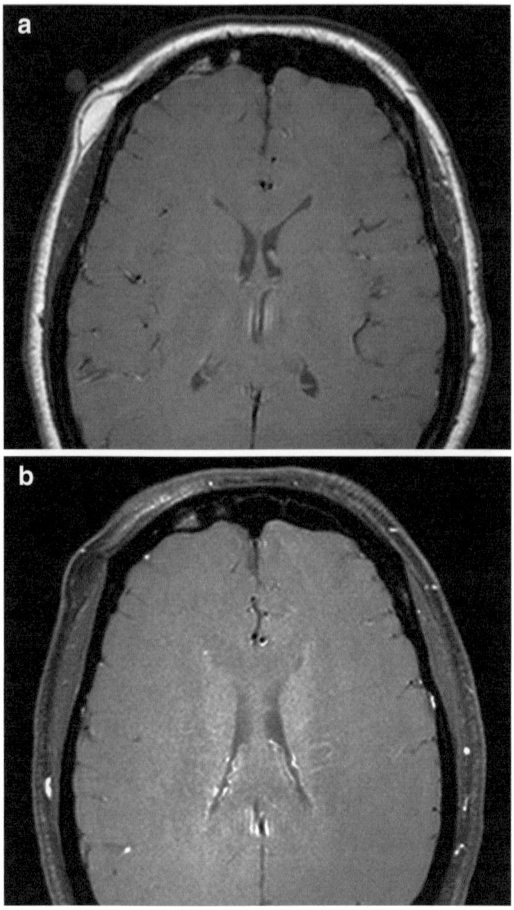

Fig. 5.24 Lipoma. Axial T1 (**a**) and fat-suppressed post-contrast T1 (**b**) MR images show a right frontal scalp lipoma

Imaging Findings

Imaging features of benign lipomatous lesions are often pathognomonic. In general, both CT and MRI exams are useful for detecting lipomatous lesions and planning surgical resection. In particular, intravenous administration of contrast helps to depict the tumor margins and vascularization. Ultrasound can also be useful for the assessment of suspected superficial lipomas, particularly in young children because there is no ionizing radiation exposure and no need for sedation.

Lipomas commonly appear as well-defined homogeneous masses although septations of variable thickness may be present. The tumors have CT attenuation values ranging from −60 to −120 HU (Fig. 5.23), display fat-suppression on MRI (Fig. 5.24), and do not typically containing enhancing components. The tumors are typically hyperechoic on ultrasound.

Infiltrating facial lipomatosis appears as an expansive, ill-defined process with predominantly fat characteristics, although they may appear somewhat heterogeneous, particular due to the engulfed and deformed normal tissues (Fig. 5.25). There can be involvement of the salivary glands, muscles, and nerves. In addition, bone hypertrophy may also be observed.

Spindle cell lipomas may display variable imaging features, but often appear as well defined, complex tumors that display significant enhancement with relatively minimal adipose tissue components mostly located in the periphery

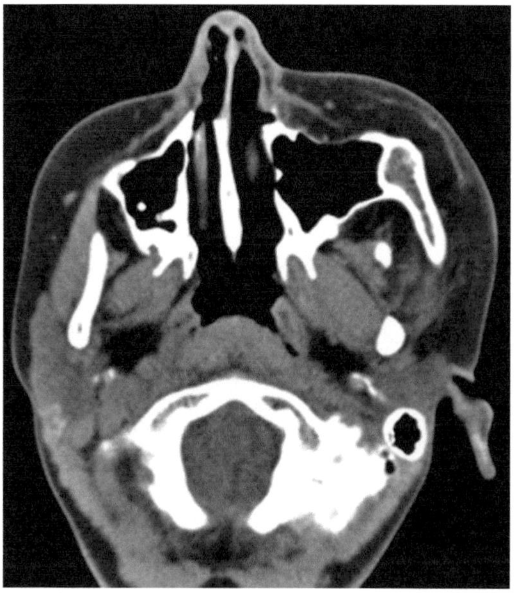

Fig. 5.25 Infiltrating facial lipomatosis. Axial CT image shows diffuse enlargement of the subcutaneous fat in the left cheek and hypertrophy of the zygoma

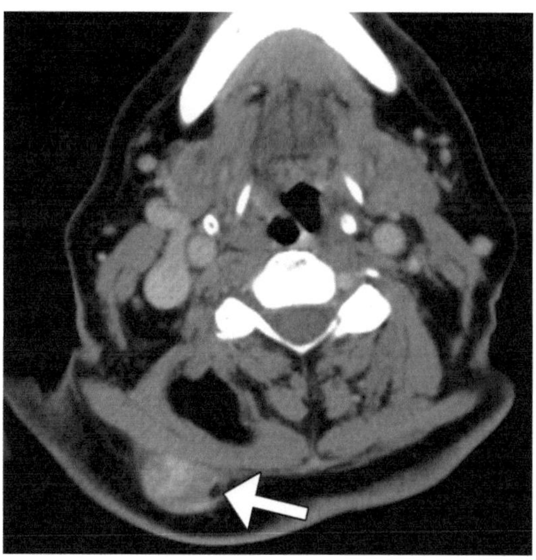

Fig. 5.26 Spindle cell lipoma. Axial post-contrast CT image shows a heterogeneously enhancing ovoid mass in the posterior right neck subcutaneous tissues with a small peripheral focus of fat attenuation (arrow). There is also a right paraspinal intramuscular lipoma

of the lesion (Fig. 5.26). The degree of contrast enhancement of the non-adipose components in spindle cell lipomas tends to be more intense than in liposarcomas.

Lipoblastomas are often well defined and contain internal septations that are visible on ultrasound, CT, and MRI (Fig. 5.27). Early on, there may be prominent myxoid areas within the tumor, which are hypoechoic on ultrasound (Fig. 5.28), low attenuation on CT, and on MR imaging are low signal intensity with T1-weighted sequences and high signal intensity with T2-weighted sequences, reflecting their high water content.

Benign and "Borderline" Fibrous Tumors and Proliferations

Overview

Benign fibrous soft-tissue tumors constitute a large, heterogeneous group of lesions. Some of the lesions, such as nodular fasciitis and acrochordons, have a self-limited course, small size, and superficial location and rarely recur after excision. Other lesions, such as extra-abdominal desmoid tumor, demonstrate a tendency towards aggressive behavior, large size, and intramuscular extension, and have high local recurrence rates, which may prompt the use of adjuvant therapies in addition to surgery. Therefore, when interpreting diagnostic imaging of soft-tissue masses in adults, the radiologists should be aware of lesion behavior, common sites of occurrence, and the pathologic characteristics that correlate with the imaging features of benign fibrous tumors and proliferations, of which selected examples are discussed further in the subsequent sections.

Clinicopathologic Findings

Solitary fibrous tumors rarely occur in the skin, but when they do, the favored sites of involvement include the cheek, scalp, lip, and temple. The histologic features of this lesion may be confounded with a variety of other spindle cell tumors. Histologically, the tumor is composed of

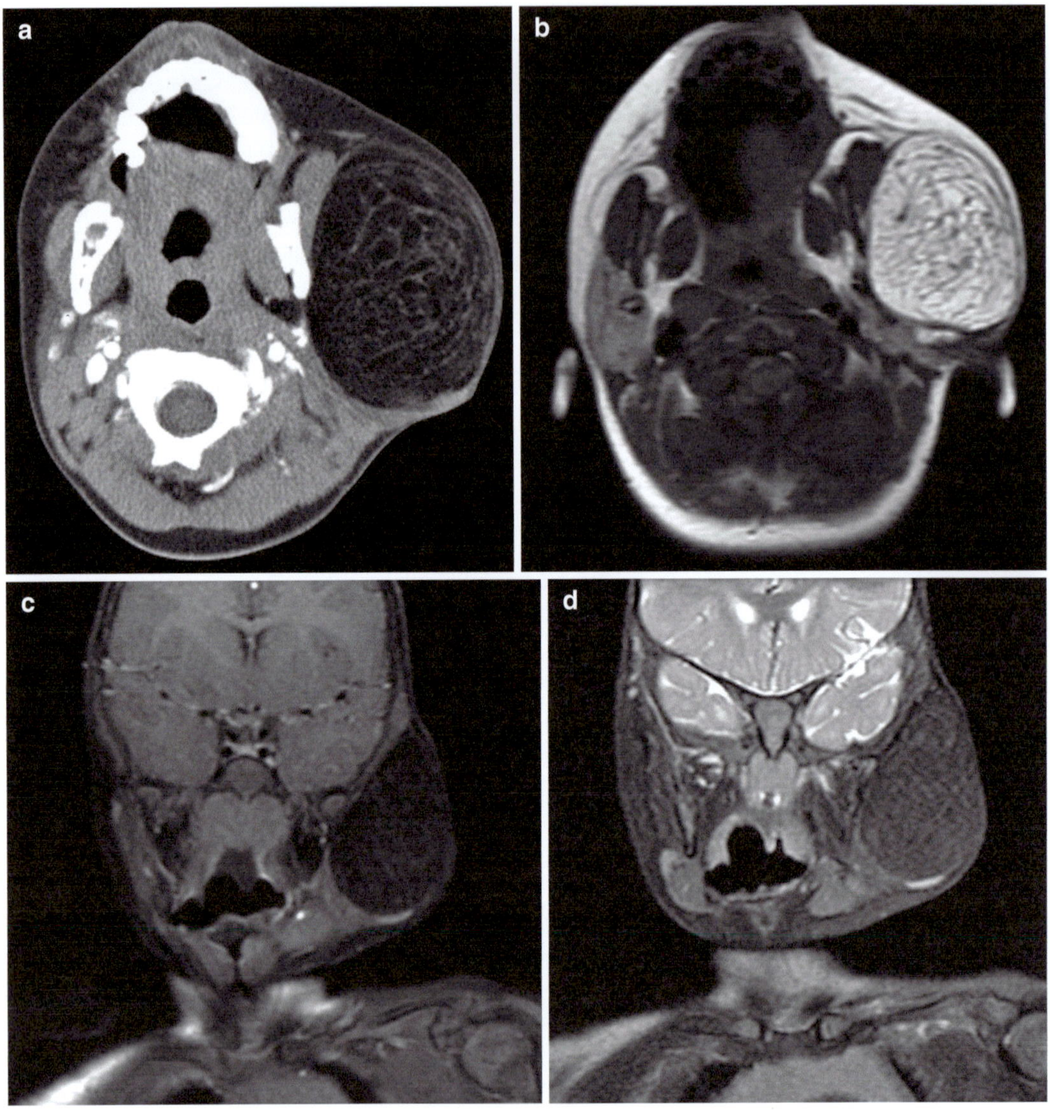

Fig. 5.27 Lipoblastoma. Axial CT image (**a**) and corresponding axial T1 (**b**), coronal post-contrast fat-suppressed T1 (**c**), and coronal fat-suppressed T2 (**d**) MR images show a bulky well-defined predominantly fat-attenuation mass in the left face with multiple linear septations in an infant

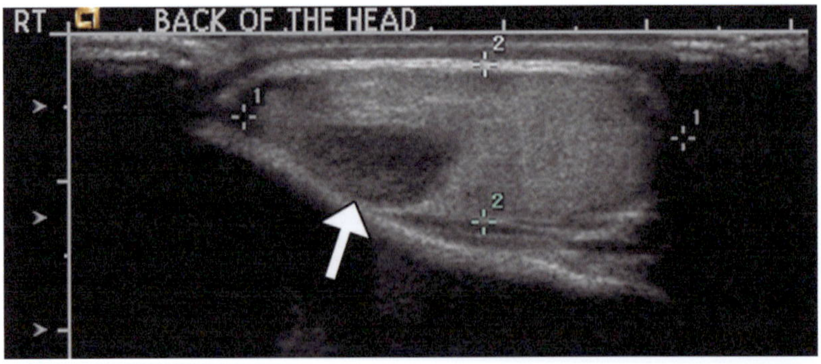

Fig. 5.28 Lipoblastoma. Ultrasound image shows a predominantly hyperechoic mass in the scalp of an infant with a hypoechoic component (arrow)

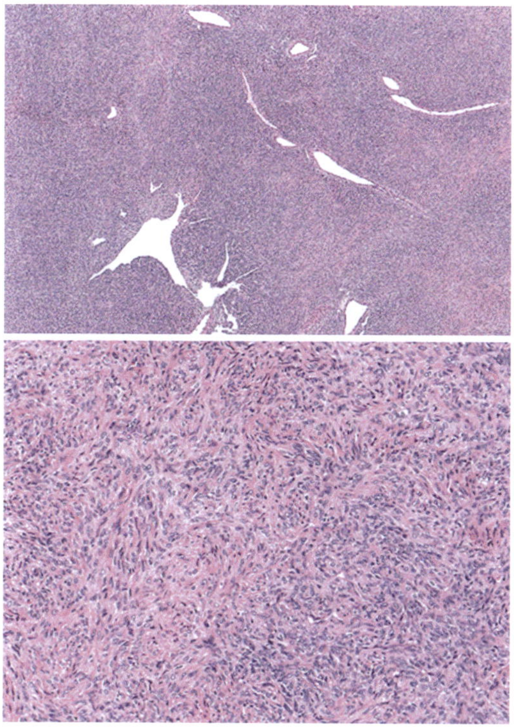

Fig. 5.29 Solitary fibrous tumor. Low power (top) hematoxylin and eosin stained histological section image shows sheets of monotonous spindle cells with numerous admixed thin-walled, dilated, branching blood vessels (also called staghorn or hemangiopericytoma). High power (bottom) image showing bland spindle cells arranged in short fascicles and whorls with stromal collagen

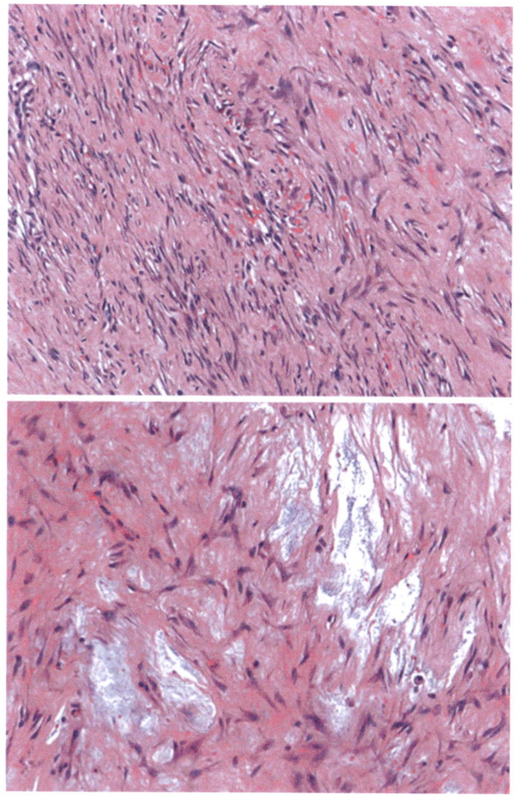

Fig. 5.30 Nodular fasciitis. High power hematoxylin and eosin stained histological section images show "tissue-culture" like myofibroblasts with vesicular nuclei and stellate-shaped cytoplasm, arranged in varying degrees of cellularity. Frequently, extravasated red blood cells (top) and myxoid cystic degeneration of stroma (bottom) are appreciated

spindle-shaped cells arranged in the so-called pattern of short and narrow fascicles with interspersed bundles of thick collagen and numerous thin-walled dilated branching blood vessels (frequently referred to as hemangiopericytoma-like) (Fig. 5.29). Immunostains show reactivity for CD34 and CD99, and occasionally for bcl-2, smooth-muscle actin, and EMA. The lesions do not stain for factor XIIIa, keratin, desmin, or S100. Positive nuclear stain for STAT6 is reflective of the underlying NAB2-STAT6 rearrangement recently described in these tumors. Ultimately, solitary fibrous tumors appear to be "borderline" neoplasms that uncommonly recur and metastasize although malignant features such as hypercellularity and increased mitoses may portend worse prognosis.

Nodular fasciitis is comprised of benign proliferations of fibroblasts and myofibroblasts that may be categorized as myxoid, cellular, or fibrous, based on the predominant histologic feature of the lesion (Fig. 5.30). These lesions can potentially mimic sarcomas. Most cases of nodular fasciitis involve the subcutaneous tissues and are circumscribed.

Keloids often occur after an injury or in association with connective tissues disease particularly in areas of skin tension. Keloids are hypocellular and composed of abundant type I collagen (Fig. 5.31). Unlike hypertrophic scars, keloids grow beyond the margins of an injury site, contain keloidal collagen, contain less

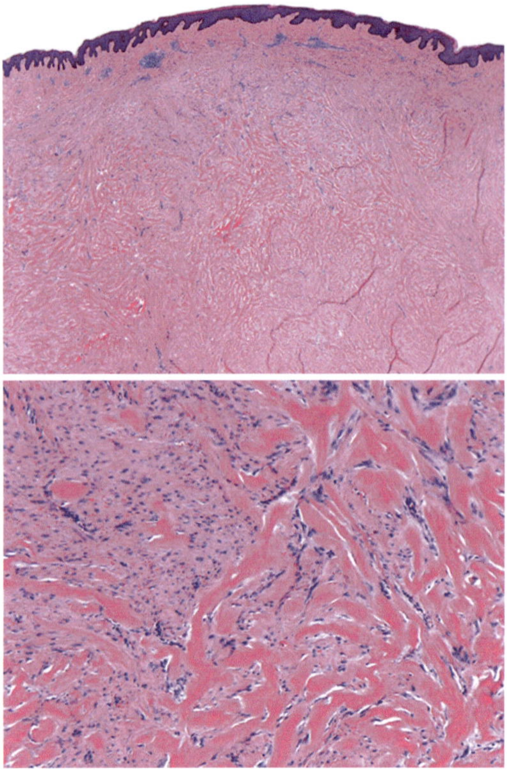

Fig. 5.31 Keloid. Low power (top) hematoxylin and eosin stained histological section shows a hypocellular dermal proliferation of spindle cells and ropey (keloidal) collagen (high power, bottom)

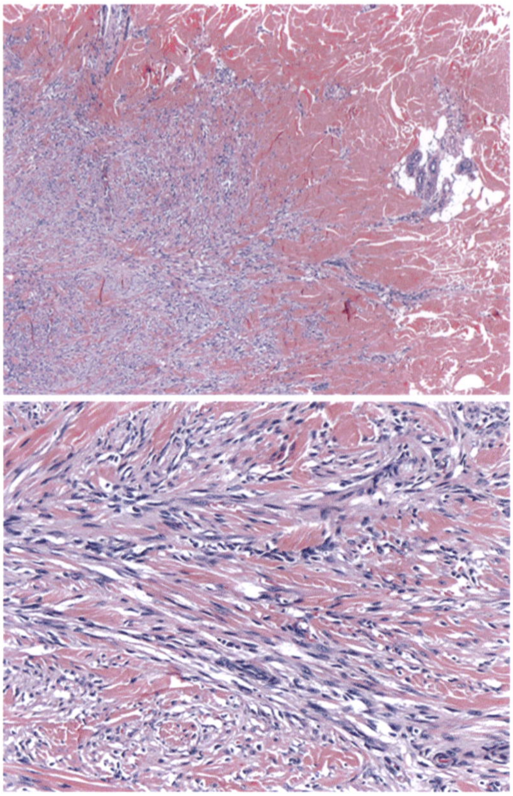

Fig. 5.32 Benign fibrous histiocytoma. Low power (top) hematoxylin and eosin stained histological section demonstrates a dense spindle cell tumor with peripheral infiltration and trapping of dermal collagen bundles. Skin adnexal structures (eccrine glands) are seen on the right. High power (bottom) hematoxylin and eosin stained histological section shows fascicles of spindle cells amongst eosinophilic dermal collagen fibers

smooth-muscle actin, and have higher recurrence rates after surgery.

Benign fibrous histiocytoma is also known as dermatofibroma, fibrous dermatofibroma, fibrous histiocytoma, fibroma simplex, nodular subepidermal fibrosis, and sclerosing hemangioma. These lesions consist of spindled fibroblasts and admixed histiocytes arranged in short fascicles (Fig. 5.32). Benign fibrous histiocytomas contain a significant population of factor XIIIa-positive dendritic cells, which is a distinguishing feature from dermatofibrosarcoma protuberans.

Acrochordons (also known as skin tags or fibroepithelial polyps) are small skin outgrowths that are often located in areas of skin friction. Acrochordons are a defining feature of Birt-Hogg-Dubé syndrome, along with fibrofolliculomas and trichodiscomas. Acrochordons appear as pedunculated polypoid lesions that may be hyperpigmented (Fig. 5.33). The lesions are covered by epidermis and contain a fibrous core (Fig. 5.34).

Imaging Findings

Variations in the histopathologic features of fibrous tumors with regard to the amount and distribution of cells and extracellular matrix often correlate with the MR imaging appearance of the lesions, particularly on T2-weighted images. In general, hypocellular fibrous tumors with abun-

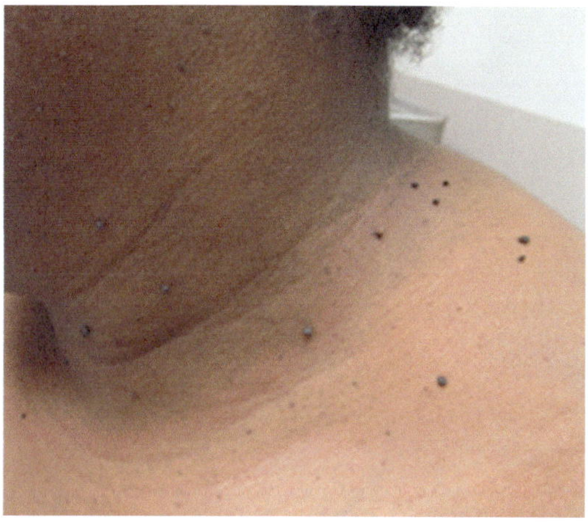

Fig. 5.33 Acrochordon, Photograph shows multiple hyperpigmented skin tags of the neck and upper chest

dant collagenous components tend to display lower signal intensity on T2-weighted images than more cellular lesions and lesions that contain greater amounts of extracellular myxoid matrix. MRI provides an accurate assessment of the size and extent of fibrous lesions before biopsy or excision. In addition, MRI can be useful for post-treatment assessment, especially for infiltrative tumors that involve major neurovascular structures and that are treated with adjuvant radiation or chemotherapy.

Solitary fibrous tumors appear as well-defined soft-tissue masses that tend to display avid enhancement on imaging (Fig. 5.35). Often, MRI also demonstrates low T2 signal intensity components that correspond to the rich fibrous content of the tumors.

Benign fibrous histiocytomas predominantly appear as enhancing solid lesions that characteristically demonstrate skin retraction (Fig. 5.36). Otherwise, the imaging features of these rare lesions are not thoroughly described in the literature.

Nodular fasciitis has a variable imaging appearance, in which highly collagenous lesions have hypointense signal on all MRI sequences, while tumors with low collagen content tend to display high T2 signal (Fig. 5.37). Contrast enhancement is typically diffuse, but may be peripheral in lesions with a greater extracellula myxoid matrix and central fluid-filled spaces. The differential diagnosis on imaging includes extra-abdominal desmoid tumor, neurofibroma, fibrous histiocytoma, and soft-tissue sarcoma.

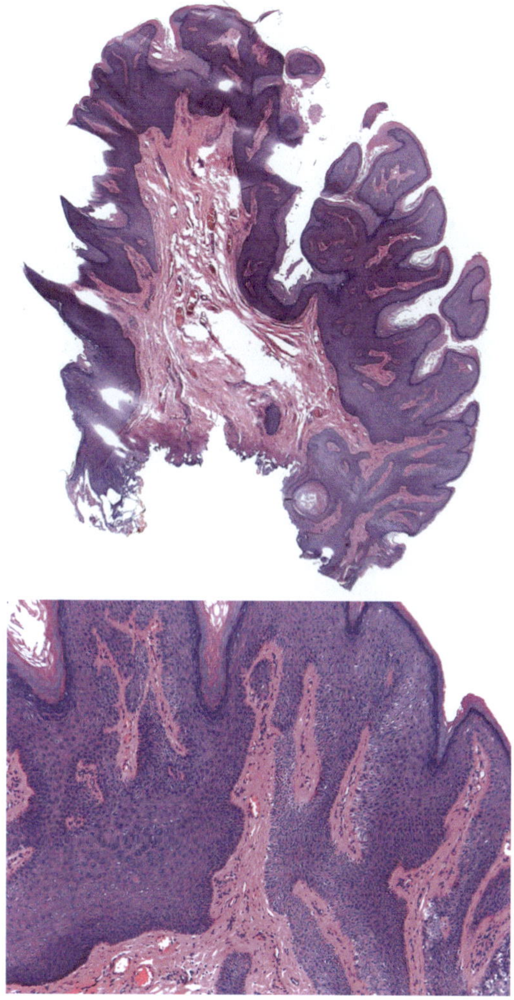

Fig. 5.34 Acrochordon. Low (top) and high power (bottom) hematoxylin and eosin stained histological sectiona show a polypoid, exophytic lesion covered by stratified squamous epithelium with a fibrous and vascular core

Keloids typically appear as well-defined, homogeneous soft-tissues mass that protrude from the skin surface, are markedly T2 hypointense, and display mild enhancement (Fig. 5.38).

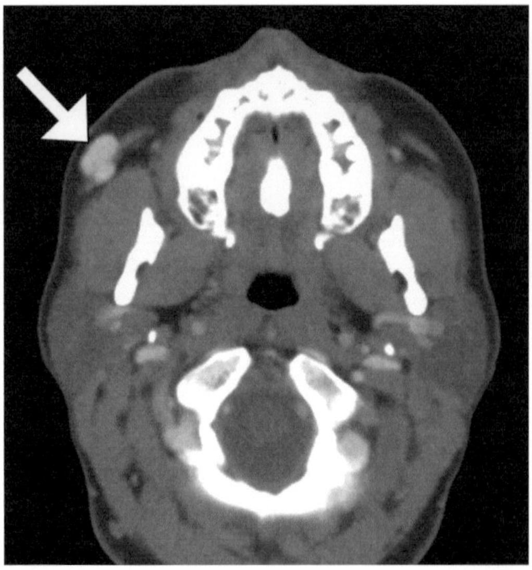

Fig. 5.35 Solitary fibrous tumor. Axial post-contrast CT image shows an avidly enhancing mass in the right cheek subcutaneous tissues (arrow), alongside the zygomatic major muscle

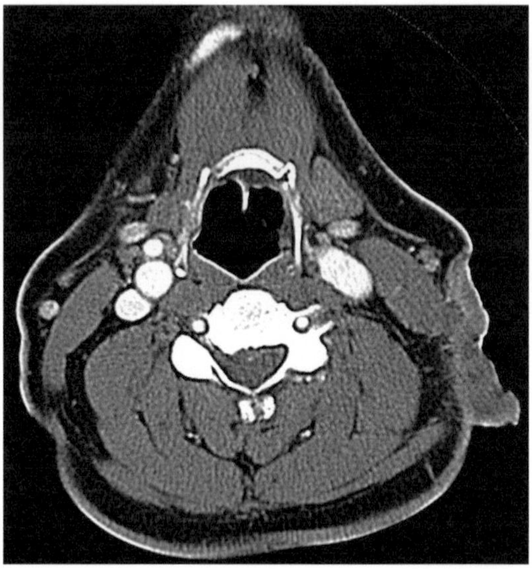

Fig. 5.36 Benign fibrous histiocytoma. Axial CT image shows a flat superficial left neck soft-tissue mass with central retraction. Courtesy of Charles Schatz MD, FACR

Acrochordons appear as small soft-tissue attenuation pedunculated lesions arising from the skin on CT (Fig. 5.39). On ultrasound, acrochordons are hypoechogenic. These lesions are often incidental and should not confounded with more ominous-appearing skin malignancies on imaging. Otherwise, head and neck imaging may be performed in patients with Birt-Hogg-Dubé syndrome to assess for tumors, such as basal cell and squamous cell carcinoma of the skin, dermatofibrosarcoma protuberans, meningiomas, and thyroid nodules (Fig. 5.40).

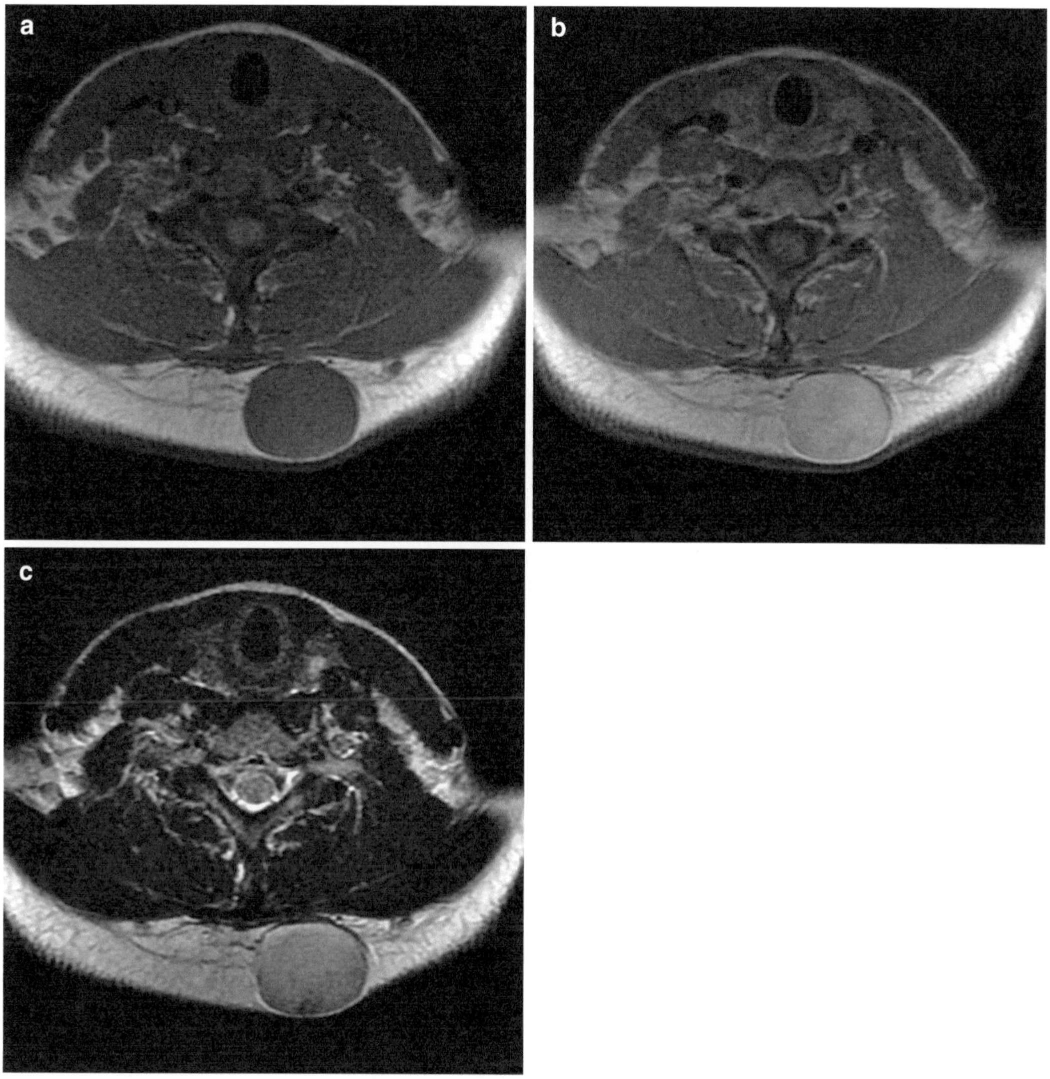

Fig. 5.37 Nodular fasciitis. Axial T1-weighted, axial post-contrast T1-weighted (**b**), and axial T2-weighted (**c**) MR images show a well-defined ovoid mass with predominantly high T2 signal with minimal low T2 signal posteriorly and homogeneous enhancement in the left posterior neck subcutaneous tissues

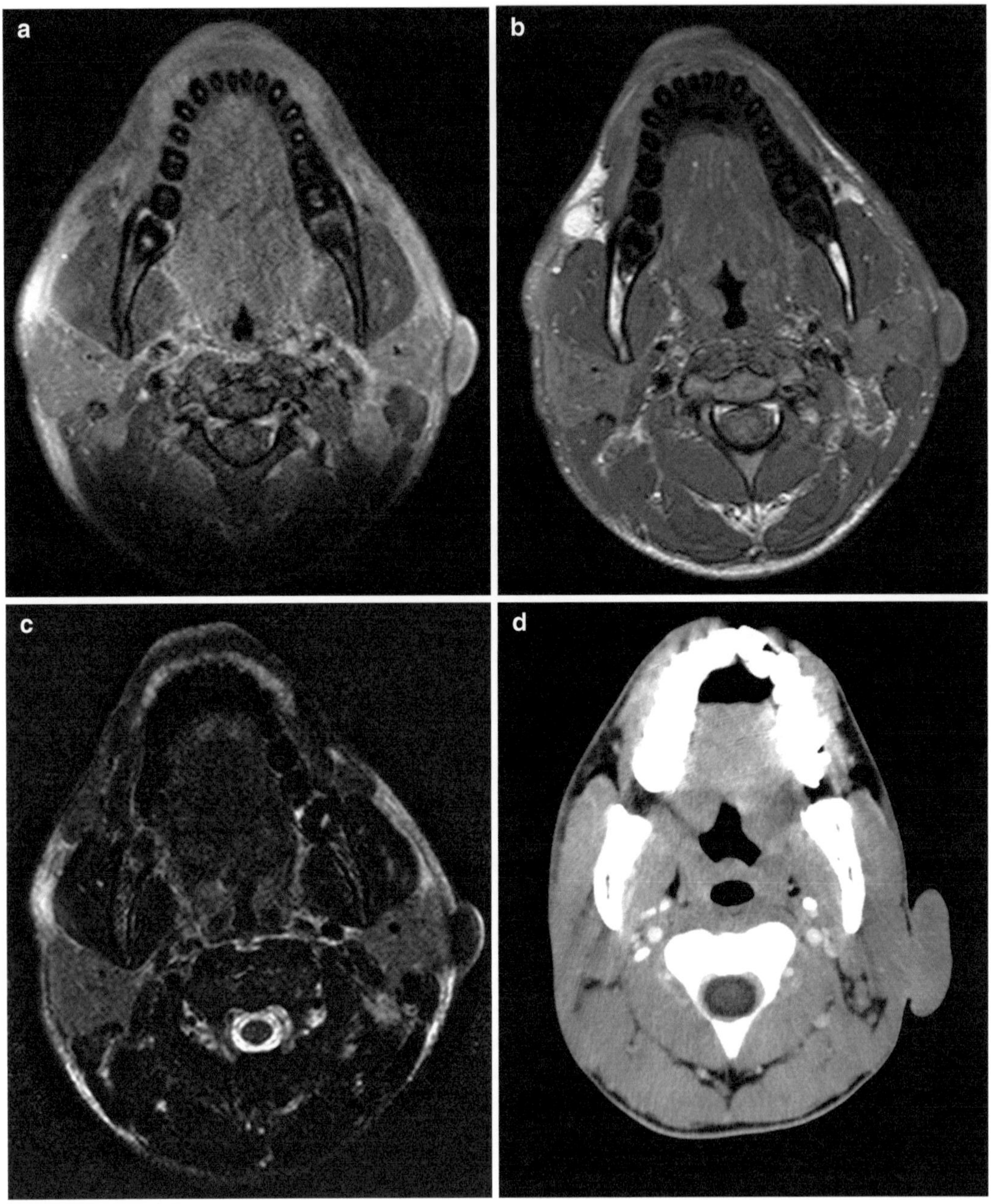

Fig. 5.38 Keloid. Axial T1-weighted (**a**), fat-suppressed post-contrast T1-weighted (**b**), axial T2-weighted (**c**) MR images show a homogeneous, mildly enhancing, markedly T2 hypointense exophytic left neck skin lesion. The axial CT image (**d**) obtained 2 years later for surgical planning shows that the soft-tissue lesion has increased in size

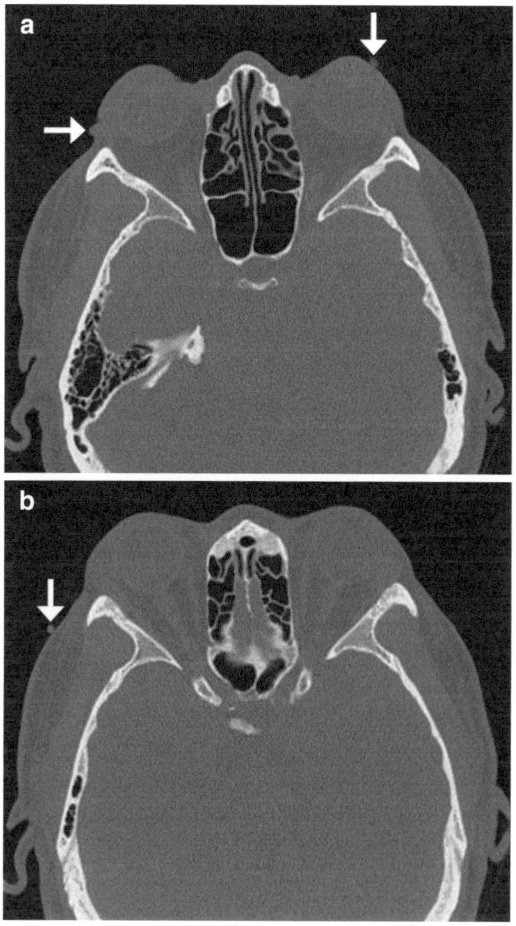

Fig. 5.39 Acrochordon. Axial CT images (**a**, **b**) show a polypoid skin excrescences in the face (arrows)

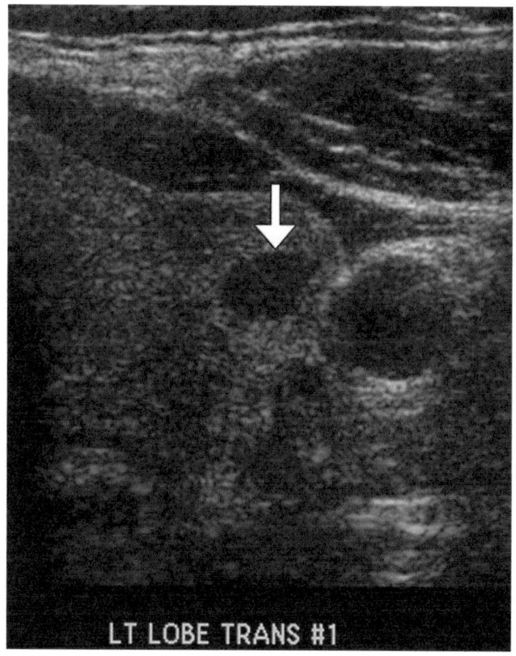

Fig. 5.40 Birt-Hogg-Dubé syndrome with thyroid nodules. Ultrasound shows a hypoechoic nodule in the left lobe of the thyroid. There were several such lesions in the patient's thyroid, which proved to be follicular adenomas

Suggested Reading

Abdelkader M, Riad M, Williams A. Aggressive fibromatosis of the head and neck (desmoid tumours). J Laryngol Otol. 2001;115(10):772–6.

Al-Khateeb TH, Al-Masri NM, Al-Zoubi F. Cutaneous cysts of the head and neck. J Oral Maxillofac Surg. 2009;67(1):52–7.

Bondi R, Urso C. Syringocystadenoma papilliferum. Histopathology. 1996;28:475–7.

Bord A, Valsky DV, Yagel S. Prenatal sonographic diagnosis of congenital perineal skin tag: case report and review of the literature. Prenat Diagn. 2006;26(11):1065–7.

Bowe SN, Wakely PE Jr, Ozer E. Head and neck solitary fibrous tumors: diagnostic and therapeutic challenges. Laryngoscope. 2012;122(8):1748–55.

Bulman JC, Ulualp SO, Rajaram V, Koral K. Pilomatricoma of childhood: a common pathologic diagnosis yet a rare radiologic one. AJR Am J Roentgenol. 2016;206(1):182–8.

Cappabianca S, Colella G, Pezzullo MG, Russo A, Iaselli F, Brunese L, Rotondo A. Lipomatous lesions of the head and neck region: imaging findings in comparison with histological type. Radiol Med. 2008;113(5):758–70.

Choi JW, Kim HJ, Kim J, Kim HJ, Cha JH, Kim ST. Spindle cell lipoma of the head and neck: CT and MR imaging findings. Neuroradiology. 2013;55(1):101–6.

Collins BJ, Fischer AC, Tufaro AP. Desmoid tumors of the head and neck: a review. Ann Plast Surg. 2005;54(1):103–8.

De Beuckeleer LH, De Schepper AM, Neetens I. Magnetic resonance imaging of pilomatricoma. Eur Radiol. 1996;6(1):72–5.

Dinauer PA, Brixey CJ, Moncur JT, Fanburg-Smith JC, Murphey MD. Pathologic and MR imaging features of benign fibrous soft-tissue tumors in adults. Radiographics. 2007;27(1):173–87.

Drevelegas A, Pilavaki M, Chourmouzi D. Lipomatous tumors of soft tissue: MR appearance with histological correlation. Eur J Radiol. 2004;50(3):257–67.

Erdag G, Qureshi HS, Patterson JW, Wick MR. Solitary fibrous tumors of the skin: a clinicopathologic study of 10 cases and review of the literature. J Cutan Pathol. 2007;34(11):844–50.

Ganly I, Patel SG, Stambuk HE, Coleman M, Ghossein R, Carlson D, Edgar M, Shah JP. Solitary fibrous tumors of the head and neck: a clinicopathologic and radiologic review. Arch Otolaryngol Head Neck Surg. 2006;132(5):517–25.

Golden BA, Zide MF. Cutaneous cysts of the head and neck. J Oral Maxillofac Surg. 2005;63(11):1613–9.

Hardisson D, Cuevas-Santos J, Contreras F. Solitary fibrous tumor of the skin. J Am Acad Dermatol. 2002;46(2 Suppl Case Reports):S37–40.

Ibrahim AE, Barikian A, Janom H, Kaddoura I. Numerous recurrent -trichilemmal cysts of the scalp: differential diagnosis and surgical management. J Craniofac Surg. 2012;23(2):e164–8.

Kamakura T, Horii A, Mishiro Y, Takashima S, Kubo T. Magnetic resonance imaging of syringocystadenoma papilliferum of the external auditory canal. Auris Nasus Larynx. 2006;33(1):53–6.

Kuwano Y, Ishizaki K, Watanabe R, Nanko H. Efficacy of diagnostic ultrasonography of lipomas, epidermal cysts, and ganglions. Arch Dermatol. 2009;145(7):761–4.

Lim HW, Im SA, Lim GY, Park HJ, Lee H, Sung MS, Kang BJ, Kim JY. Pilomatricomas in children: imaging characteristics with pathologic correlation. Pediatr Radiol. 2007;37(6):549–55.

Mammino JJ, Vidmar DA. Syringocystadenoma papilliferum. Int J Dermatol. 1991;30:763–6.

Nguyen T, Zuniga R. Skin conditions: benign nodular skin lesions. FP Essent. 2013;407:24–30.

Rosmaninho A, Caetano M, Oliveira A, Pinto de Almeida T, Selores M, Alves R. Proliferating trichilemmal tumor of the nose. An Bras Dermatol. 2012;87(6):914–6.

Sarabi K, Khachemoune A. Hidrocystomas—a brief review. MedGenMed. 2006;8(3):57.

Satyaprakash AK, Sheehan DJ, Sangueza OP. Proliferating trichilemmal tumors: a review of the literature. Dermatol Surg. 2007;33(9):1102–8.

Shah R, Jindal A, Patel N. Acrochordons as a cutaneous sign of metabolic syndrome: a case-control study. Ann Med Health Sci Res. 2014;4(2):202–5.

Skoulakis CE, Papadakis CE, Datseris GE, Drivas EI, Kyrmizakis DE, Bizakis JG. Subcutaneous benign fibrous histiocytoma of the cheek. Case report and review of the literature. Acta Otorhinolaryngol Ital. 2007;27(2):90–3.

Vignes JR, Franco-Vidal V, Eimer S, Liguoro D. Intraorbital apocrine hidrocystoma. Clin Neurol Neurosurg. 2007;109(7):631–3.

Vincent A, Farley M, Chan E, James WD. Birt-Hogg-Dube syndrome: a review of the literature and the differential diagnosis of firm facial papules. J Am Acad Dermatol. 2003;49(4):698–705.

Malignant Skin Neoplasms and Associated Conditions

6

Daniel Thomas Ginat, Nicole A. Cipriani, Carson Barnes, Judy Wu, and Elizabeth Blair

Contents

D. T. Ginat (✉)
Department of Radiology, University of Chicago, Pritzker School of Medicine, Chicago, IL, USA
e-mail: dtg1@uchicago.edu

N. A. Cipriani
Department of Pathology, University of Chicago, Chicago, IL, USA

C. Barnes
Medical University of South Carolina, Charleston, SC, USA

J. Wu
Department of Radiology, University of Chicago, Chicago, IL, USA

E. Blair
Department of Surgery, Section of Otolaryngology, University of Chicago, Chicago, IL, USA

D. T. Ginat (ed.), *Neuroradiological Imaging of Skin Diseases and Related Conditions*,
https://doi.org/10.1007/978-3-319-90931-8_6

Abstract

There are many types of cutaneous malignant neoplasms and associated conditions that can involve the head and neck regions. This chapter reviews the characteristic clinicopathological and imaging findings of basal cell carcinoma, squamous cell carcinoma, melanoma, cutaneous lymphomas, dermatofibrosarcoma protuberans, Kaposi sarcoma, Merkel cell carcinoma, microcystic adnexal carcinoma, sebaceous carcinoma, adenoid cystic carcinoma, angiosarcoma, and metastases.

Basal Cell Carcinoma

Overview

Basal cell carcinoma is the most common type of skin cancer and arises from the non-keratinizing basal layer of the epidermis. The primary risk factor for the development of basal cell carcinoma is exposure to ultraviolet light, including tanning beds. Additional risk factors include light skin and hair color, exposure to toxins (arsenic, ionizing radiation, coal tar), and immunosuppression. The majority of cases occur in the head and neck, particularly the nose, cheeks, and nasolabial folds. There is a tendency for gradual local invasion, but basal cell carcinoma rarely metastasizes or undergoes perineural spread. Treatment includes surgical approaches such as curettage and electrodissection, cryosurgery, conventional excision and Mohs surgery, and non-surgical modalities such as radiotherapy, injectable therapy, and photodynamic therapy approaches. Treatment modality depends on the extent of the tumor.

Clinicopathological Findings

There are multiple subtypes of basal cell carcinoma, as well as mixed tumors that show characteristics of multiple subtypes. The nodular subtype comprises over 50% of basal cell carcinoma and can appear as a raised papule or nodule with telangiectasia and can also resemble a large pore (Fig. 6.1). Each nodule contains cells with large oval nuclei, minimal cytoplasm, and a peripheral palisading pattern (Fig. 6.2). The superficial form makes up about 15% of basal

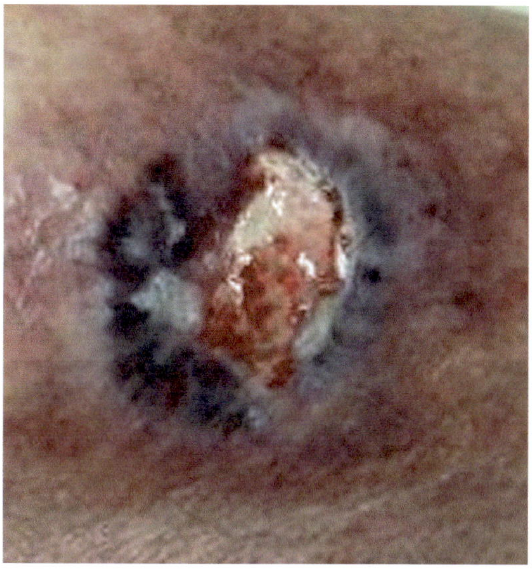

Fig. 6.1 Basal cell carcinoma. Photograph shows a dome-shaped hyperpigmented lesion with a central ulceration

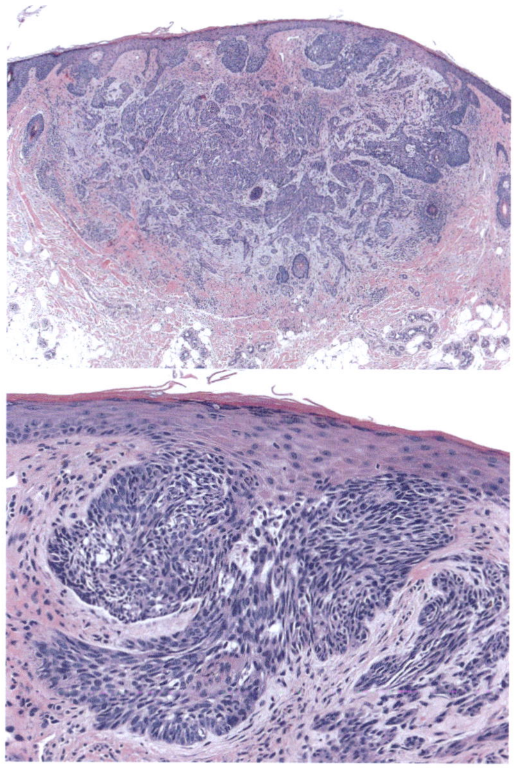

Fig. 6.2 Basal cell carcinoma. Low (top) and high (bottom) power views of basal cell carcinoma show nested tumor that attaches to the surface epithelium, peripheral palisading and invasion into the dermis

cell carcinoma cases and appears like a scaly plaque. This subtype is characterized by many centers of proliferation and is also called multifocal/multicentric. Pigmentation may be present in both the nodular and superficial subtypes. The infiltrative subtype is characterized by thin cords and nests of cells infiltrating the dermis, often with deep invasion. On physical exam, the neoplasm can appear as a scar-like plaque with ill-defined margins. The basosquamous or metatypical basal cell carcinoma has areas of prominent squamous differentiation and may be confused for squamous cell carcinoma. Infiltrative, metatypical, and morpheaform (sclerosing) variants are usually more aggressive. For details regarding staging, please refer to the eighth edition of the American Joint Committee on Cancer (AJCC).

Imaging Findings

Imaging for cases of head and neck basal cell carcinoma is mainly indicated if there is the clinical suspicion of perineural spread, bone involvement, periorbital tumor location, metastasis, or for preoperative planning. CT is particularly useful for identifying involvement of underlying cortical bone (Fig. 6.3). On CT, basal cell carcinomas appear as soft tissue masses. The primary skin tumor is not particularly hypermetabolic on ^{18}FDG-PET-CT in up to 50% of cases although this modality can be more useful for the evaluation of metastases. MRI can be useful for defining the depth of invasion, perineural spread, and involvement of osseous and cartilaginous structures. Lesions are typically iso- to hyperintense on T1-weighted imaging and hyperintense on T2-weighted imaging compared to muscle and display contrast enhancement. High-frequency ultrasound has also proven to be useful in evaluating the depth of tumor invasion in the dermal tissue, but is limited for evaluating underlying bone involvement.

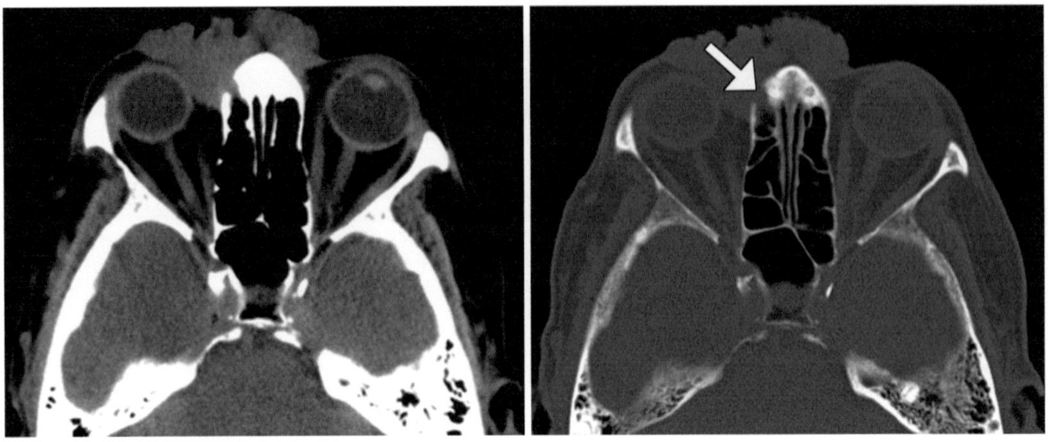

Fig. 6.3 Basal cell carcinoma. Axial CT mages in soft tissue and bone windows show an irregular mass with associated bone erosion (*arrow*)

Squamous Cell Carcinoma

Overview

Squamous cell carcinoma (SCC) is the second most common skin malignancy. It arises from keratinizing epithelium and accounts for 85% of head and neck malignancies. These tumors are often classified as high risk or low risk based upon histologic evaluation. Features that make SCC high risk are invasive tumor phenotype, histologic level of keratinization, diameter larger than 2 cm, thickness deeper than 6 mm, and perineural or lymphovascular invasion. These criteria may also include Clark level and primary tumor location on ear or hair-bearing lip. Low risk SCC has a smaller incidence of metastasis and can often be cured by surgical excision, cryotherapy, radiation therapy, or even topical treatments. High risk SCC may require Mohs surgery, more extensive traditional excision with margin assessment, radiation therapy, and even chemotherapy. The prevalence of metastases is been estimated to be between 2 and 5% overall. Risk factors for developing cutaneous SCC include fair skin, chronic sun exposure, old age, and chronic inflammation. The largest prognostic indicator is lymph node involvement. Disease confined to the primary lesion has an overall 5 year survival of over 90%, while lymph node involvement drops the 5 year survival to less than 40%. There is a tendency for lymph node metastases and perineural spread, for which CT and MRI are useful to interrogate. The most common sites for metastasis include the lymph nodes, brain, liver, lung, and bone although the incidence of metastases is under 5% overall. Primary tumors arising from the ear or lip have a relatively higher risk for metastases.

Clinicopathological Findings

The clinical presentation varies based on how far the tumor has progressed. Squamous cell carcinoma usually begins as an actinic keratosis, from which it progresses into a localized proliferation within epidermis, called SCC *in situ* (Bowen disease). *In situ* carcinoma may present as scaly, hyperkeratotic plaques or a small nodule. As it develops into an invasive phenotype, the lesion may enlarge, become ulcerative, or develop more red or white keratotic nodules (Fig. 6.4). Sometimes these ulcers and plaques develop a raised border although tumor may spread beyond the crater border. The histology displays malignant keratinocytes with varying degrees of nuclear pleomorphism, intracellular abnormal keratinization (dyskeratosis), and extracellular keratin horn pearls (Fig. 6.5). Verrucous, spindle, desmoplastic, acantholytic, and adenosquamous are all histologic SCC variants that have slightly different metastatic disease profiles. For details regarding staging, please refer to the eighth edition of the American Joint Committee on Cancer (AJCC).

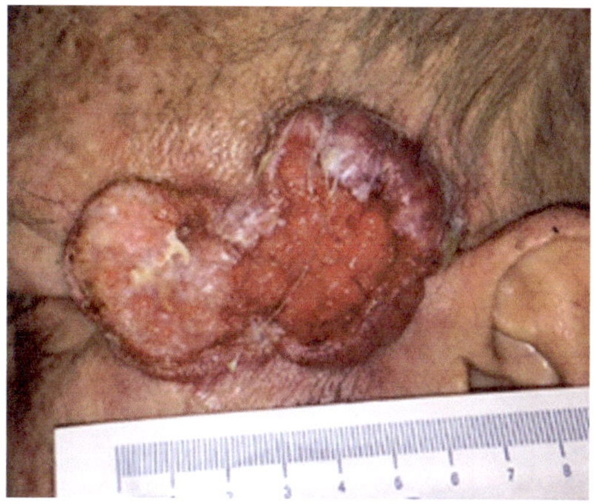

Fig. 6.4 Squamous cell carcinoma. Photograph shows an erythematous, scaly, fungating mass in the temporal scalp with skin erosion

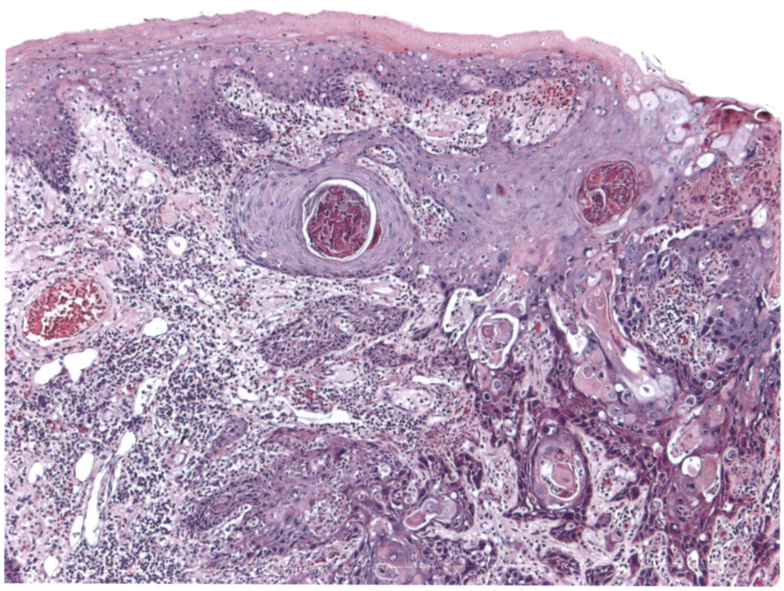

Fig. 6.5 Invasive keratinizing squamous cell carcinoma. Hematoxylin and eosin stained photomicrograph shows invasion of large and small tumor nests into the dermis with associated inflammation

Imaging Findings

Cutaneous squamous cell carcinomas have variable imaging features, ranging from bulky exophytic masses to subtle infiltrative lesions. The role of diagnostic imaging for tumors in the head and neck is to evaluate the depth of invasion, including skull invasion (Fig. 6.6). In addition, approximately 85% of metastases from cutaneous squamous cell carcinoma involve regional lymph nodes, followed by distant metastases to the lungs, liver, brain, and bones (Fig. 6.7). While ultrasound can be used for the initial assessment of cutaneous squamous cell carcinoma and associated lymphadenopathy in the head and neck region, CT or PET/CT is typically performed for

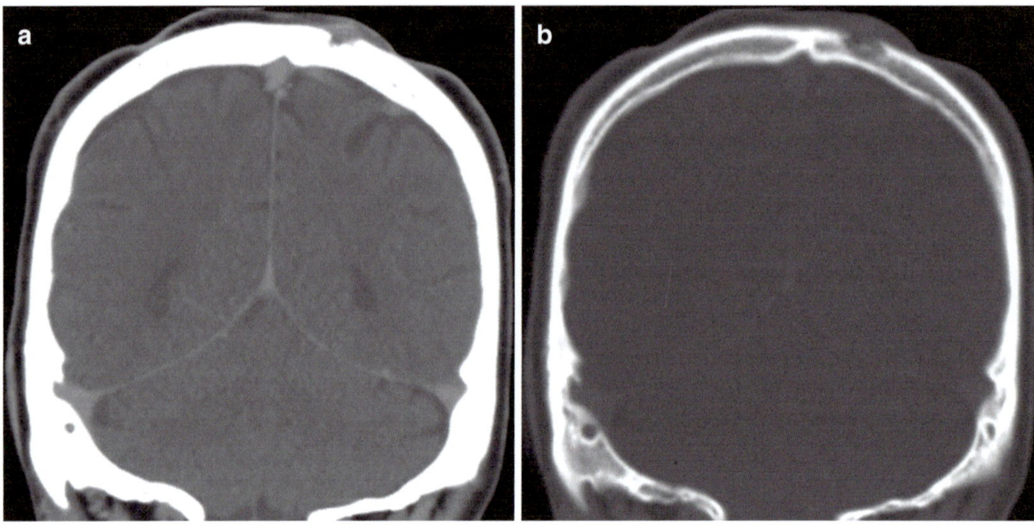

Fig. 6.6 Cutaneous squamous cell carcinoma with bone invasion. Coronal soft tissue (**a**) and bone window (**b**) CT images show a plaque-like, infiltrative lesion in the left scalp, which invades the underlying parietal bone

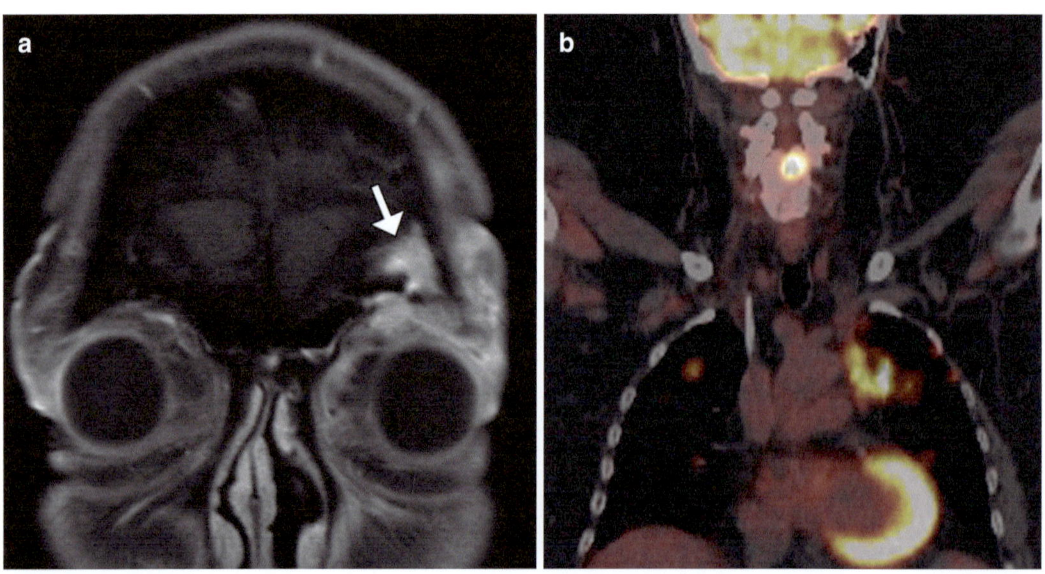

Fig. 6.7 Squamous cell carcinoma. Coronal post-contrast fat-suppressed T1-werighted MRI (**a**) shows a left supraorbital skin tumor with orbital and intracranial extension (*arrow*). Coronal [18]FDG-PET/CT image (**b**) shows hypermetabolic metastases in the cervical spine, lungs, and thoracic lymph nodes

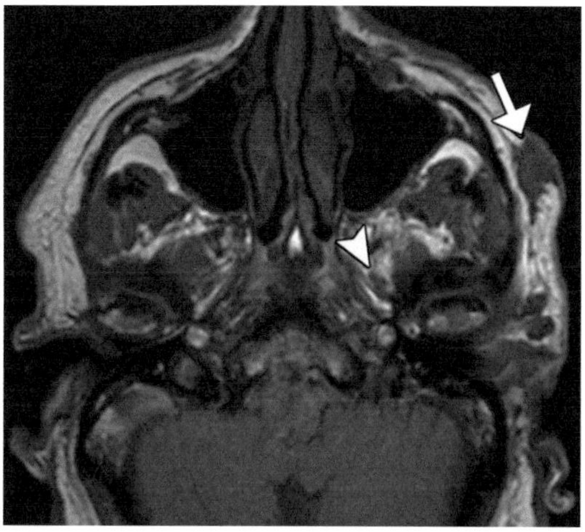

Fig. 6.8 Squamous cell carcinoma with perineural spread. Axial T1-weighted MR image shows an infiltrative left cheek mass (*arrow*) and enhancement of an enlarged left trigeminal nerve (*arrowhead*), indicating perineural spread

more accurate staging. Furthermore, MRI is well suited for evaluating the presence of perineural tumor spread, which can appear as thickening and abnormal enhancement of the nerve involved, most commonly the trigeminal and facial nerves in the head and neck. Of note, the perineural involvement can appear as "skip lesions," with apparent areas of discontinuity in the gross tumor (Fig. 6.8).

Melanoma

Overview

Cutaneous melanoma can be encountered as a primary head and neck skin lesion or as metastasis from elsewhere. Melanoma has a characteristic growth pattern that is divided into two phases: an initial radial growth phase that can last for several months during which it spread only across the epidermis and has low metastatic potential, followed by a vertical growth phase where it penetrates the dermis and often becomes metastatic. There are histologic criteria necessary to classify the tumor in the vertical growth phase, but often the transformation has occurred by the time the dermis is invaded. There are three major classifications of melanoma: superficial spreading melanoma, nodular melanoma, and lentiginous melanoma. Superficial spreading is the most common of all melanomas. Most of them are thin and curable with complete resection. Nodular melanoma is the second most common and has an abnormal growth pattern where it begins in the vertical growth phase and has little to no radial spreading outside of the central nodule. Lentiginous melanoma is the rarest variant that is found in sun damaged areas or on the palms, plantar surface of the foot, and under the nails. There has been a fivefold increased incidence over the past three decades in melanoma. Risk factors include long-term exposure to ultraviolet radiation, frequent tanning, and fair skin. Melanoma has a tendency to spread to lymph nodes, bone, brain, as well as undergo perineural spread. The likelihood of metastasis is correlated with depth of vertical spread. Indeed, tumor staging uses thickness cutoffs of less than 1 mm, 1–2 mm, 2–4 mm, and greater than 4 mm. Each step indicates an incremental decrease in 10 year survival of over 10%. Vascularization, ulceration, perineural invasion, and regression also predispose metastases and auger a worse prognosis. In the head and neck, the brain is the most likely site of metastasis.

Clinicopathological Findings

The acronym ABCDE is often used to identify potential melanoma: Asymmetry, Border irregularity, Color variegation, Diameter greater than or equal 6 mm, and Evolution. Evolution, which refers to changes in size, appearance, and sensation of the lesion, has been shown to have the highest individual specificity for melanoma compared to the other four criteria. Classically, melanoma appears as jet black nodules (Fig. 6.9).

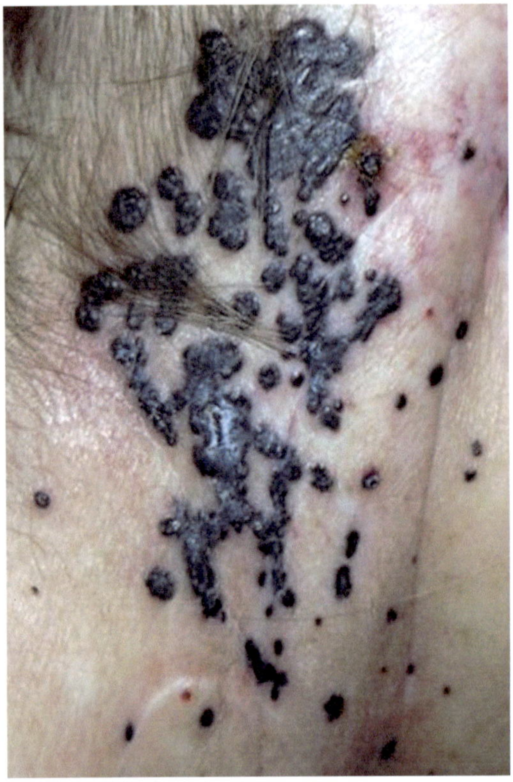

Fig. 6.9 Melanoma. Photograph shows multiple hyperpigmented nodules in the posterior neck

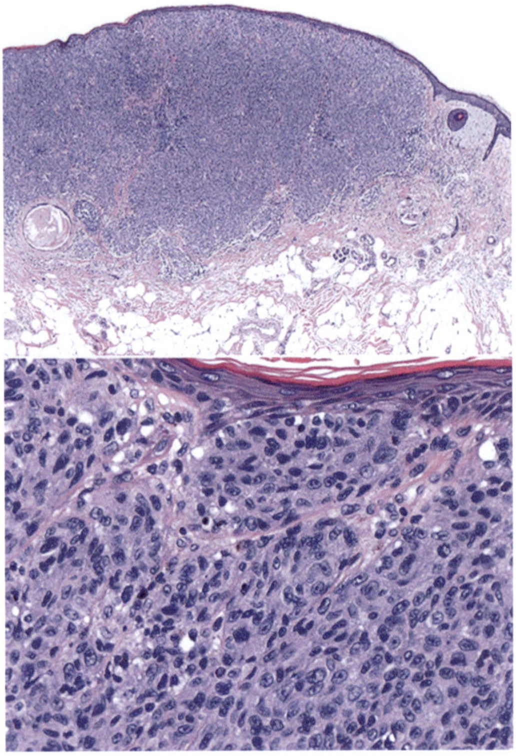

Fig. 6.10 Melanoma. Low (top) and high (bottom) power hematoxylin and eosin stained histological section images show predominantly intradermal nests of cells with large oval nucleoli, prominent nucleoli, mitotic figures, and indistinct cell borders

However, melanoma can have protean features and should be considered in the differential diagnosis of many cutaneous lesions. Amelanotic melanomas are especially difficult to differentiate from other primary neoplasms. Histologically, benign or atypical nevi must be differentiated from malignant melanomas. Asymmetry of the mass, poorly defined borders, infiltration into the superficial layers of the epidermis (Pagetoid spread), confluence of growth at the epidermal base, more than 10 melanocytes per clonal nest in the dermoepidermal junction, abnormal mitoses, and cytoplasmic irregularity may indicate melanoma instead of a nevus (Fig. 6.10). Clinical evaluation of superficial spreading melanoma shows a thin pigmented macule or plaque with irregular borders. It can be red, blue, black, grey, or white. As the neoplasm enters the vertical growth phase, it can become raised. Immunohistochemical stains for S100, SOX10, Melan-A (Mart-1), or HMB45 can be used to differentiate in situ melanoma from Paget disease and pagetoid squamous carcinoma. Nodular melanoma is often a darkly pigmented, polypoid nodule. Lentiginous melanoma forms light brown macules with asymmetric foci. There may be color change and raised areas as the melanoma transitions into a vertical growth phase. Any of the subtypes can be amelanotic melanomas. The amelanotic variety lacks the dark pigmentation and thus is often misidentified. One common melanoma variant is desmoplastic melanoma, which is an amelanotic outgrowth from superficial spreading or more commonly lentiginous melanoma. For details regarding staging, please refer to the eighth edition of the American Joint Committee on Cancer (AJCC).

Imaging Findings

Melanoma is typically very hypermetabolic on ^{18}FDG-PET, which is useful for staging (Fig. 6.11). Otherwise, MRI is the modality of

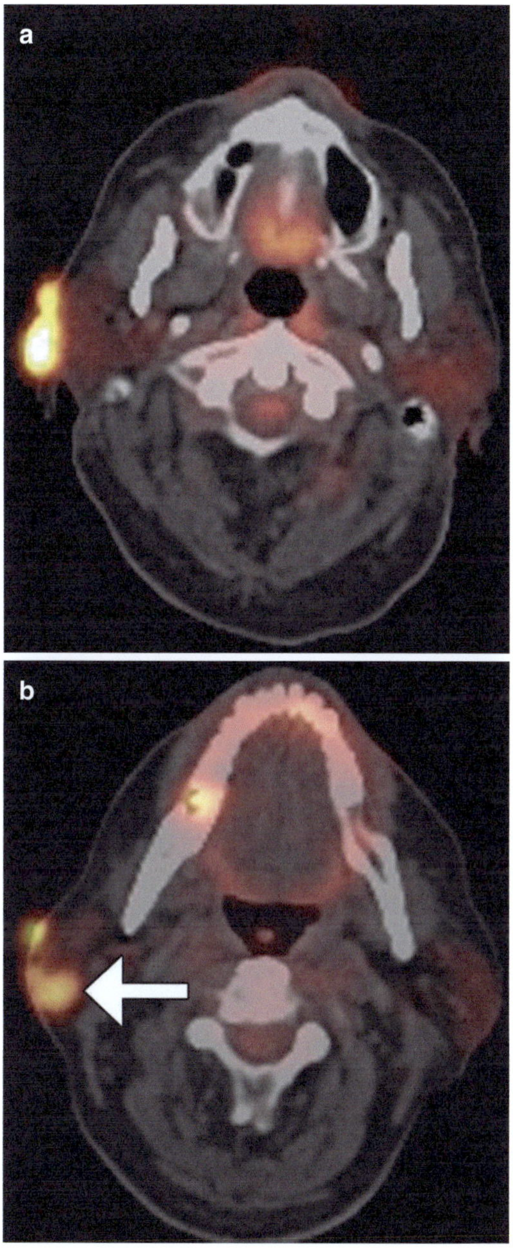

Fig. 6.11 Melanoma with lymph node metastases. Fused ^{18}FDG-PET/CT images show a hypermetabolic right periauricular skin lesion and a subjacent metastatic parotid lymph node (*arrow*)

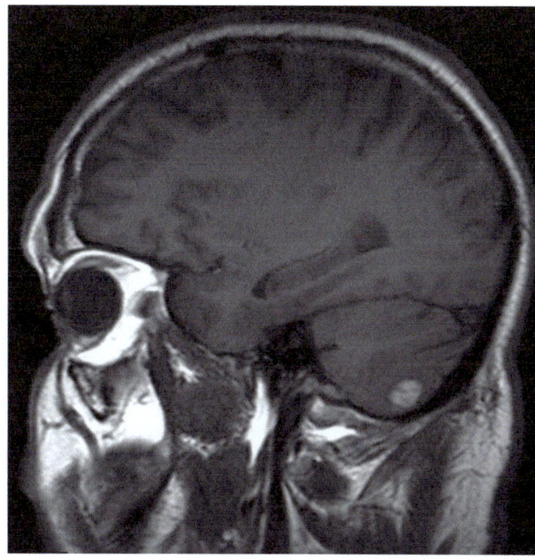

Fig. 6.12 Melanoma brain metastasis. Sagittal T1-weighted MR image shows a high signal intensity lesion in the cerebellum (*arrow*)

choice for evaluating brain metastasis. Melanotic and amelanotic melanomas can have different MRI appearances. Melanotic melanomas typically have intrinsic high signal on T1-weighted imaging and low signal on T2-weighted imaging (Fig. 6.12), due to associated melanin and/or hemorrhage. On the other hand, amelanotic melanomas tend to display lower signal intensity on T1-weighted sequences. SWI or T2*-weighted images can improve lesion detection in either case. Small lesions tend to have homogeneous enhancement, but larger tumors can enhance heterogeneously.

Cutaneous Lymphoma

Overview

Cutaneous lymphoma is composed of a diverse set of diseases with different manifestations and treatments. After the gastrointestinal tract, the skin is the next most common location of extranodal non-Hodgkin lymphoma involvement. Both B-cell and T-cell lymphomas can involve the skin. The majority of cutaneous lymphomas are T-cell lymphomas (65–75%), while B-cell lymphomas make up 25–35%. Hodgkin's lymphoma can also involve the skin, but it is very uncommon.

Symptoms may range in appearance from diffusely infiltrative processes to discrete mass lesions. The most common forms of lymphoma that characteristically involve the skin are mycosis fungoides/Sezary syndrome and CD30+ lymphoproliferative disorders. Together, they make up over 95% of primary cutaneous T-cell lymphomas.

Primary cutaneous T-cell lymphomas proposed by WHO and EORTC include the following:

- Mycosis fungoides (folliculotropic mycosis fungoides, hypopigmented/vitiligenous mycosis fungoides, Pagetoid reticulosis, and granulomatous slack skin)
- Subcutaneous panniculitis-like T-cell lymphoma
- Primary cutaneous CD4+ small/medium pleomorphic T-cell lymphoma
- Sezary syndrome
- Primary cutaneous CD8+ aggressive epidermotropic T-cell lymphoma
- Primary cutaneous gamma/delta T-cell lymphoma
- Extranodal natural killer/T-cell lymphoma, nasal type
- Primary cutaneous peripheral T-cell lymphoma, unspecified

Primary cutaneous B-cell lymphomas proposed by WHO and EORTC include the following:

- Primary cutaneous marginal zone lymphomas
- Primary cutaneous follicle center cell lymphomas
- Primary cutaneous large B-cell lymphomas:
  - Primary cutaneous large B-cell lymphomas, leg type
  - Primary cutaneous large B-cell lymphomas, other (intravascular large B-cell lymphomas and other primary cutaneous large B-cell lymphomas)

Clinicopathological Findings

Cutaneous lymphoma can initially present as scaly erythematous patches, which later become plaque-like in nature and then progress to papules, nodules, or tumors (Figs. 6.13 and 6.14). Ulceration can occur in the later stages. Most types show slow growth and are commonly seen to wax and wane. Alopecia and pruritus are com-

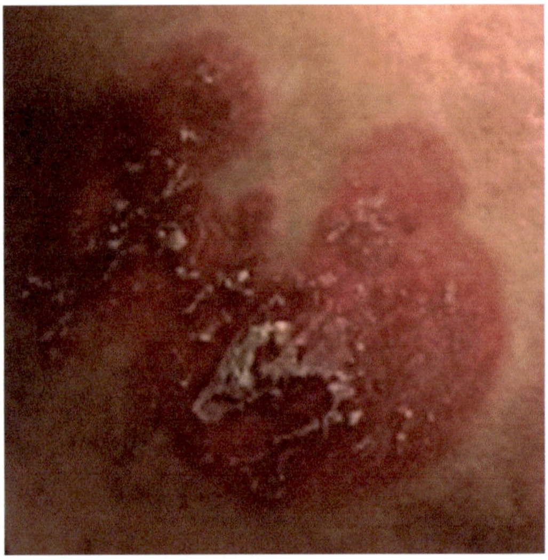

Fig. 6.13 Mycosis fungoides. Photograph shows an erythematous and scaling rash

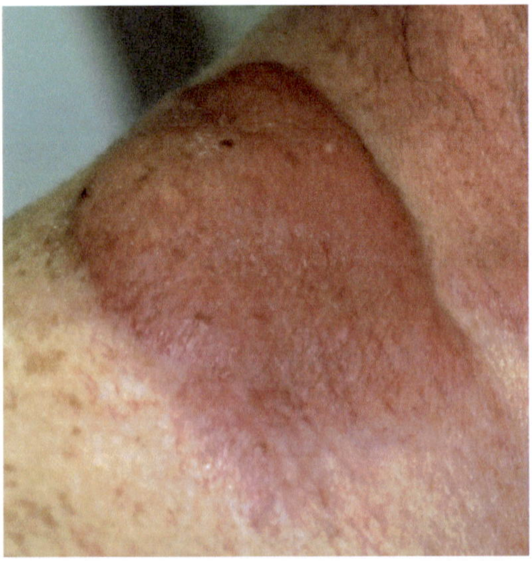

Fig. 6.14 Cutaneous B-cell lymphoma. Photograph shows an erythematous mass in the lower neck

mon. Close histologic examination is imperative in suspected primary cutaneous lymphoma cases to rule out inflammation, other lymphoproliferative disorders, or secondary neoplasms. Each type of cutaneous lymphoma is histologically distinct, reflecting its developmental lineage. The most common cutaneous T-cell lymphoma is mycosis fungoides, which consists of small T-helper cells with cerebriform nuclei and frequent perinuclear halos (Fig. 6.15). Pautrier's microabscesses, which are accumulations of mononuclear cells in the epidermis, may form during the later stages of the disease. There are occasionally band-like lymphocyte infiltrates in the dermis and along the epidermal border. The T-helper cells are CD4 and CD45RO positive but CD26 and CD8 negative. Primary cutaneous CD30 lymphoproliferative disorders are CD30 positive and usually present as sheets of large T cells mixed with granulocytes. Primary B-cell lymphomas show a proliferation of B lymphocytes; however, the morphology can vary between subtypes. For example, marginal zone lymphoma contains small B cells and plasma cells, while follicle center cell lymphoma is composed of centrocytes and centroblasts (Fig. 6.16). For details regarding staging, please refer to the eighth edition of the American Joint Committee on Cancer (AJCC).

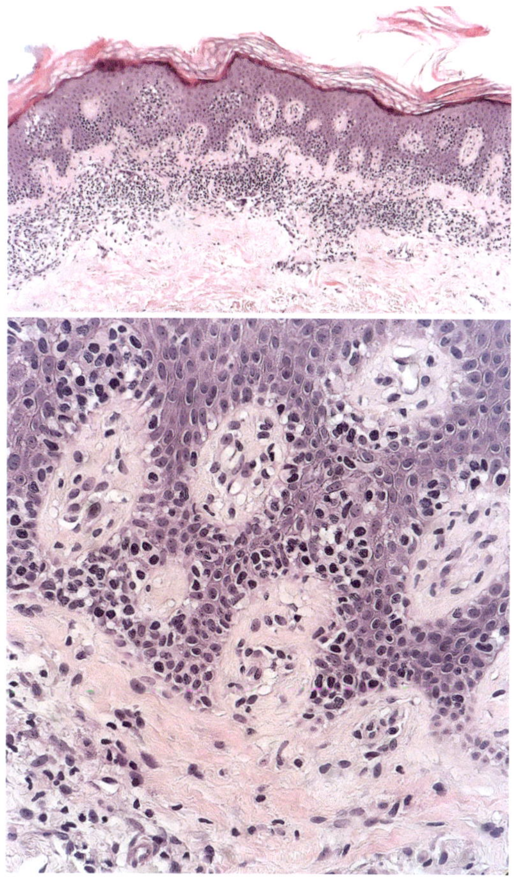

Fig. 6.15 Mycosis fungoides. Low (top) and high (bottom) power hematoxylin and eosin stained photomicrograph show band-like subepidermal infiltrates and intraepithelial neoplastic T cells

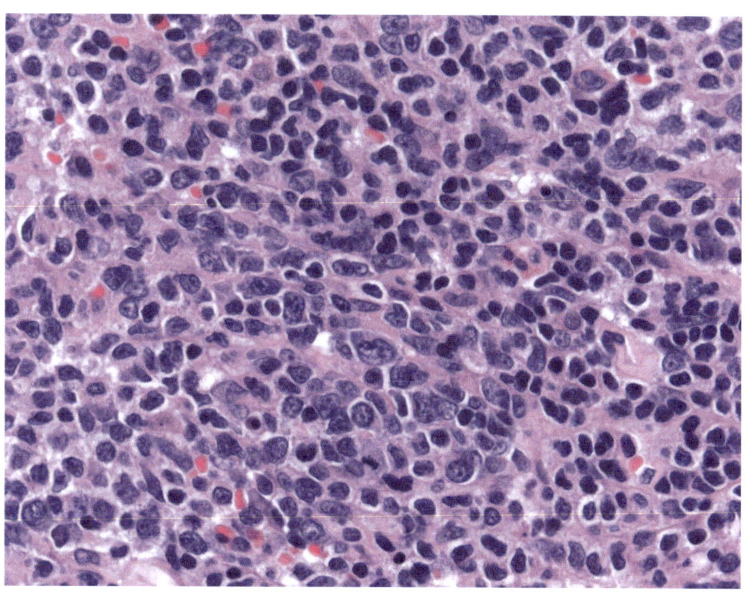

Fig. 6.16 Cutaneous B-cell lymphoma. Hematoxylin and eosin stained photomicrograph shows sheets of cells with variably large nuclei, wrinkled nuclear contours, and occasional nucleoli

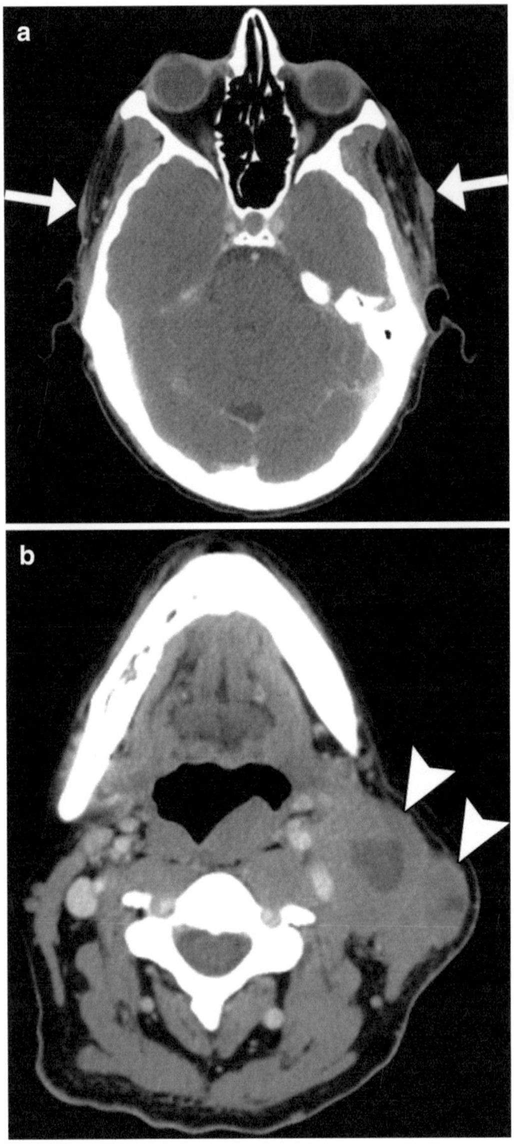

Fig. 6.17 Sezary syndrome. Axial CT images (**a**, **b**) show nodular skin thickening (*arrows*) and lymphadenopathy (*arrowheads*)

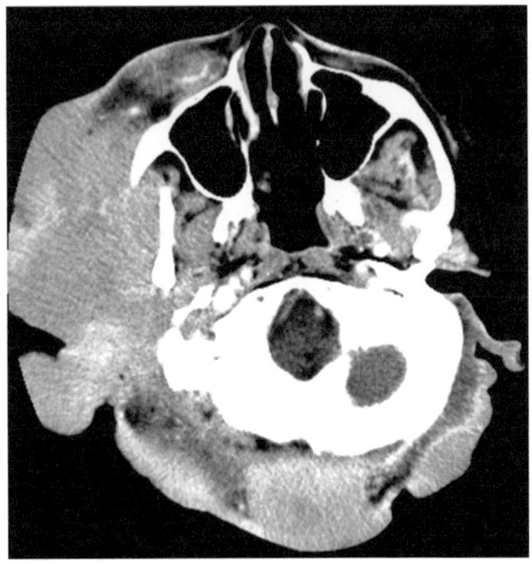

Fig. 6.18 Mycosis fungoides. Axial CT shows multiple, bulky, infiltrative, enhancing tumors in the face and scalp

Imaging Findings

CT, MRI, and ^{18}FDG-PET/CT can all be used to assess tumor thickness, size, local extent, and lymph node involvement. In particular, PET/CT is more accurate than CT in the staging and assessment of treatment response of cutaneous lymphoma and also in guiding biopsy to the most metabolically active component. However, since the primary cutaneous lesions are clinically apparent, PET/CT has limited role during the early stage of disease, but rather is useful in assessing local skin recurrence and distant spread. The presence of restricted diffusion in lymphoproliferative lesions can be exploited by whole-body MRI with diffusion weighted imaging for providing both morphologic and functional information of the disease status.

There can be a wide range of imaging features of cutaneous lymphoma in the head and neck region. For example, the imaging findings for Sezary syndrome and mycosis fungoides can range from barely discernible skin thickening to bulky, infiltrative, enhancing tumors (Figs. 6.17 and 6.18).With cutaneous type anaplastic large cell lymphoma, there can be more discrete tumors with ulceration and necrosis (Fig. 6.19). Panniculitis-like T-cell lymphoma often appears as small nodules with stranding of the subcutaneous fat on imaging (Fig. 6.20),

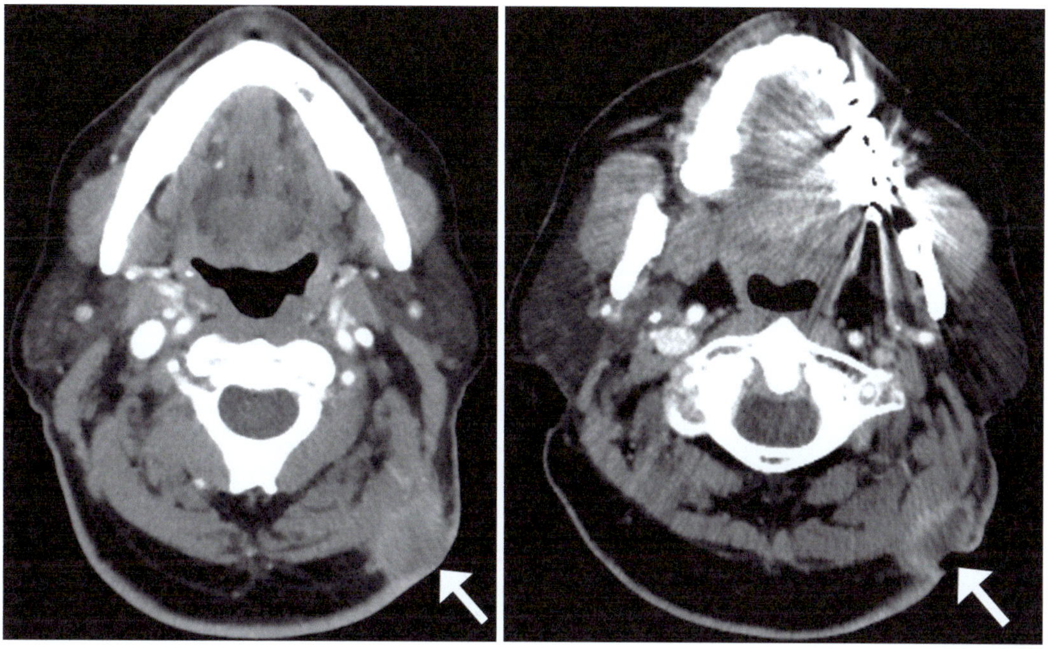

Fig. 6.19 Anaplastic large T-cell lymphoma. Axial contrast-enhanced CT shows a necrotic mass with skin ulceration in the posterior left neck (*arrow*)

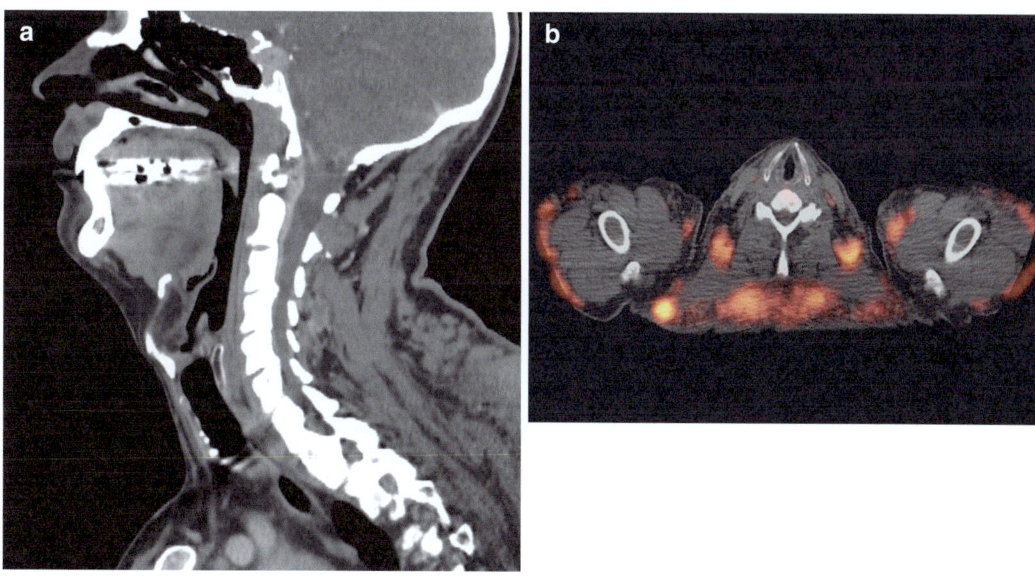

Fig. 6.20 Panniculitis-like T-cell lymphoma. Sagittal CT (**a**) and fused ^{18}FDG-PET/CT (**b**) images show diffuse areas of nodular subcutaneous fat stranding with corresponding hypermetabolism in the posterior neck. There is also posterior bilateral cervical lymphadenopathy

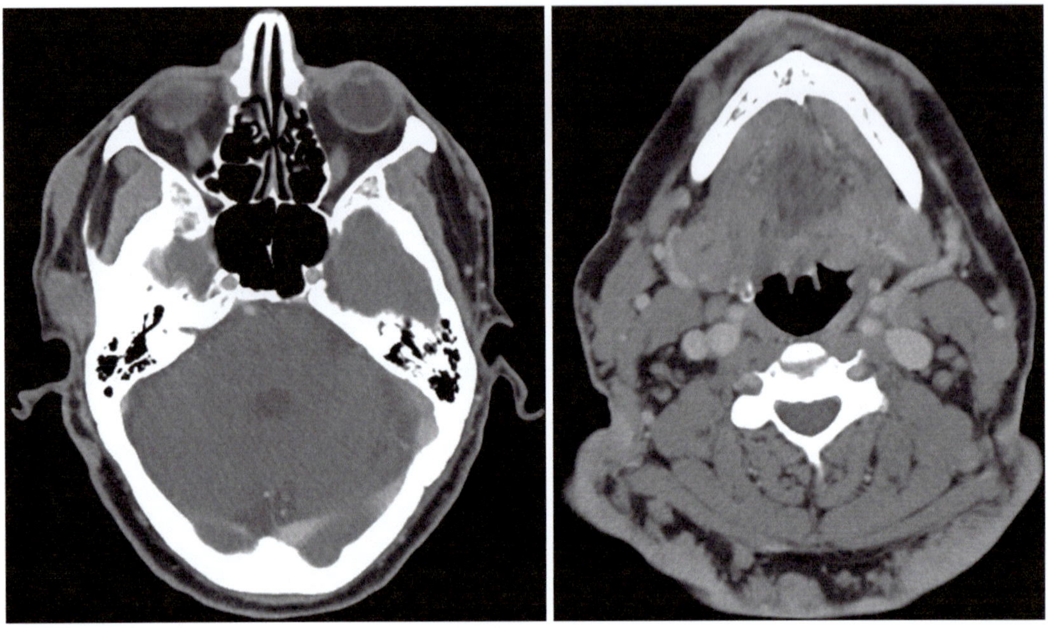

Fig. 6.21 Cutaneous B-cell lymphoma. Axial CT images show numerous skin and subcutaneous nodules

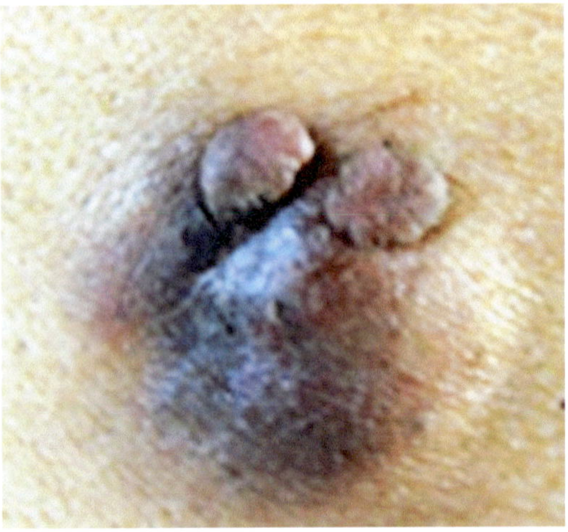

Fig. 6.22 Dermatofibrosarcoma protuberans. Photograph shows a multinodular mass with hyperpigmentation of the overlying skin

which can mimic an infectious process. Cutaneous B-cell lymphomas can appear as a "shower of lesions" in the skin and subcutaneous tissues on imaging, without or with associated systemic involvement, such as lymphadenopathy (Figs. 6.21 and 6.22).

Dermatofibrosarcoma Protuberans

Overview

Dermatofibrosarcoma protuberans (DFSP) is a fibrohistiocytic tumor that can be locally invasive, but nodal metastasis, perineural spread, and bone destruction are uncommon. Approximately 50% of the lesions are located in the midline. Fibrosarcomatous transformation of DFSP (DFSP-FS) is classified as high grade and has a greater propensity for metastasis. Low-grade DFSP and DFSP-FS are clinically indistinguishable and require histologic diagnosis. Bednar tumors are rare variants that comprise less than 5% of DFSPs and contain melanin-producing dendritic cells. The prognosis is generally very good unless there are metastases.

Clinicopathological Findings

DFSP often presents as a pigmented multinodular mass arising from the dermis with subcutaneous infiltration (Fig. 6.22). Approximately half of the lesions demonstrate bulging of the skin. It is typically a slow-growing reddish-brown tumor with multiple nodules. Clinical subtypes include morphea-like white or brown indurated plaques, atrophoderma-like soft depressed white or brown plaques, and angioma-like soft red plaques. Bednar tumors are a dark brown color and often have an irregular surface. The presence of tumor fixation and nodularity indicate locally advenced disease. Histologically, DFSP is composed of spindle cells in a short fasciculated to storiform growth pattern (Fig. 6.23). There is infiltration into subcutaneous tissue that tends to follow septa. A honeycomb pattern of invasion is often seen within adipose tissue. Mitotic activity is generally low. If the lesion has at least 5–10% fibrosarcomatous content manifesting as long, hypercellular "herringbone" fascicles of neoplastic cells with increased mitoses, then it is considered fibrosarcomatous transformation of DFSP (DFSP-FS). There is usually no epidermal involvement although the overlying epidermis can show thinning or atrophy. Most DFSPs are CD34 positive although DFSP-FS is often CD34 negative. A characteristic translocation between COL1A1 and PDGFB is present in most cases.

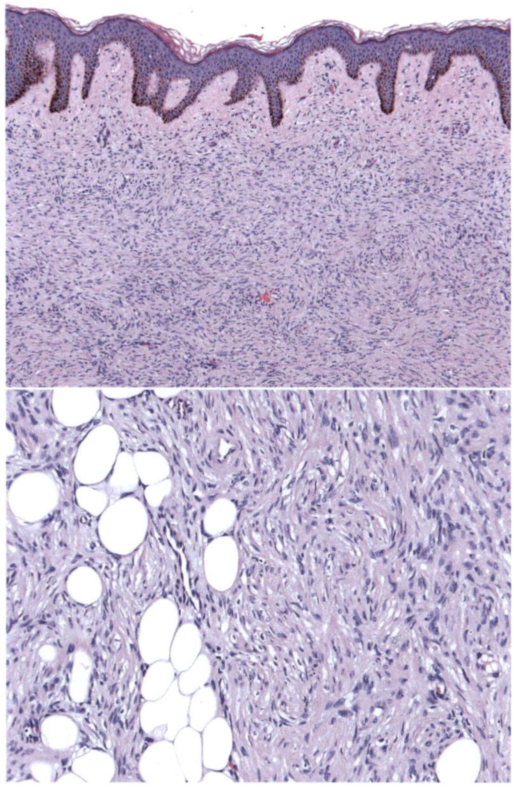

Fig. 6.23 Dermatofibrosarcoma protuberans. Low (top) and high (bottom) power hematoxylin and eosin stained photomicrographs show dermal involvement by a bland, fasciculated spindle cell neoplasm with honeycomb invasion into subcutaneous fat

Imaging Findings

Most cases of dermatofibrosarcoma protuberans are superficial and well defined and bone invasion, perineural spread, and metastases are atypical. Both CT and MRI are helpful for delineating the size and extent of the tumor. On imaging, dermatofibrosarcoma protuberans typically appears as a fairly well-defined lobulated or nodular mass with bulging of the skin surface and avid, but heterogeneous enhancement, as well as hyperintensity on T2-weighted MRI

(Figs. 6.24 and 6.25). There is usually no associated bone invasion, perineural spread, or nodal/distant metastasis.

Kaposi Sarcoma

Overview

Kaposi sarcoma (KS) is a low-grade vascular tumor that is caused by human herpes virus 8 infection. There are four variants of this disease: classic KS, endemic (African) KS, iatrogenic (organ transplant-related) KS, or acquired immunodeficiency syndrome (AIDS)-related KS. Several clinical and epidemiologic differences have been noted among the four KS variants. For example, classic KS has the lowest rate of metastasis, a slow growth rate, and represents the majority of cases in patient above the age of 65. Endemic and iatrogenic KS are more aggressive than classic KS, and AIDS-related KS is the most aggressive. Cutaneous involvement in the head and neck is present in 66% of cases, while enlarged lymph nodes are present in up to 13% of cases. KS that originates in the skin is often indolent, with a 5-year survival rate of over 75%.

Clinicopathological Findings

The skin and mucosa are the most common areas of involvement. Kaposi sarcoma often presents as red, purple, or brown nodules, papules, macules, or less commonly plaques (Fig. 6.26). The disease can present in a wide range of sizes, and lesions are generally not painful. The lesions can appear cystic due to local lymphatic swelling surrounded by lymphedema resulting from regional lymphatic obstruction. All four KS variants are indistinguishable histologically, and manifest as sheets of spindle cells in vague fascicles with abundant extravasated red blood cells (Fig. 6.27). The tumor is often accompanied an accumulation of monocytes, plasma cells, and T cells, which is more pronounced in early KS. Spindle cells stain for immunohistochemical markers of vascular endothelium (such as CD31 and ERG) and the viral protein latent nuclear antigen-1 (HHV8).

Imaging Findings

Imaging can be used to quantitatively assess the extent of head and neck cutaneous Kaposi sarcoma, which often appear as multiple irreg-

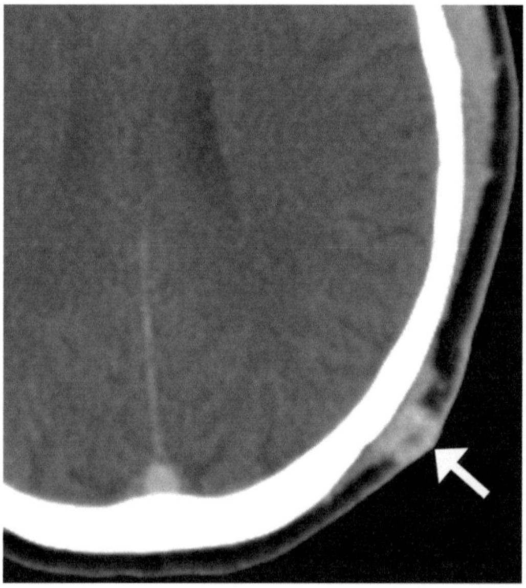

Fig. 6.24 Dermatofibrosarcoma protuberans. Axial CT image shows a heterogeneous nodule in the left scalp (*arrow*) with extension to the periosteum of the calvarium, but no bone erosions

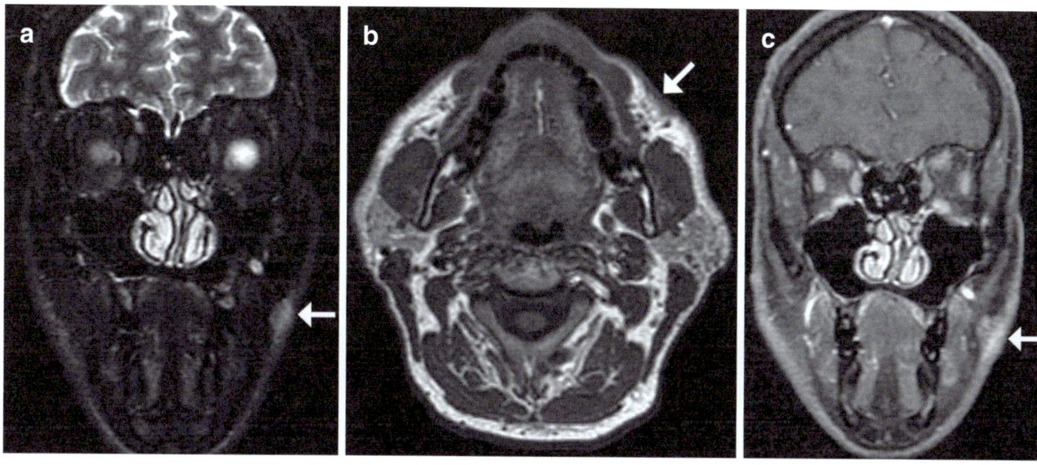

Fig. 6.25 Dermatofibrosarcoma protuberans. Coronal fat-suppressed T2-weighted (**a**), axial T1-weighted (**b**), and coronal fat-suppressed post-contrast T1-weighted (**c**) MR images show a nodular lesion in the left cheek (*arrows*)

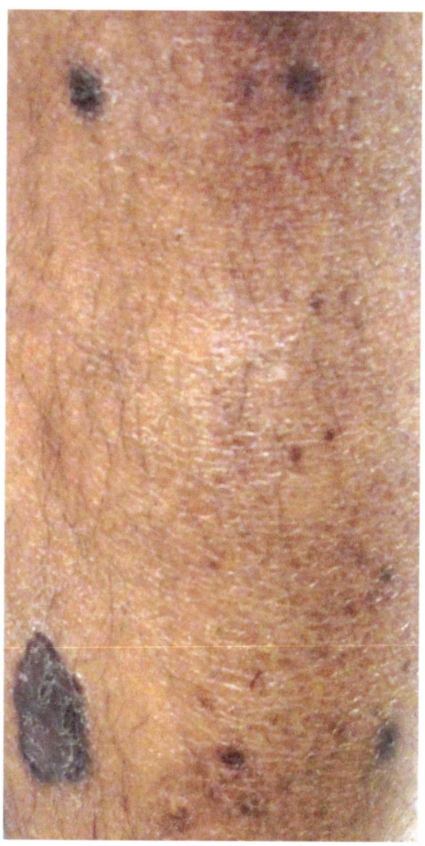

Fig. 6.26 Kaposi sarcoma. Photograph shows multiple hyperpigmented macules and plaques on the skin of the lower extremity. Courtesy of Ashley Jenkins MD

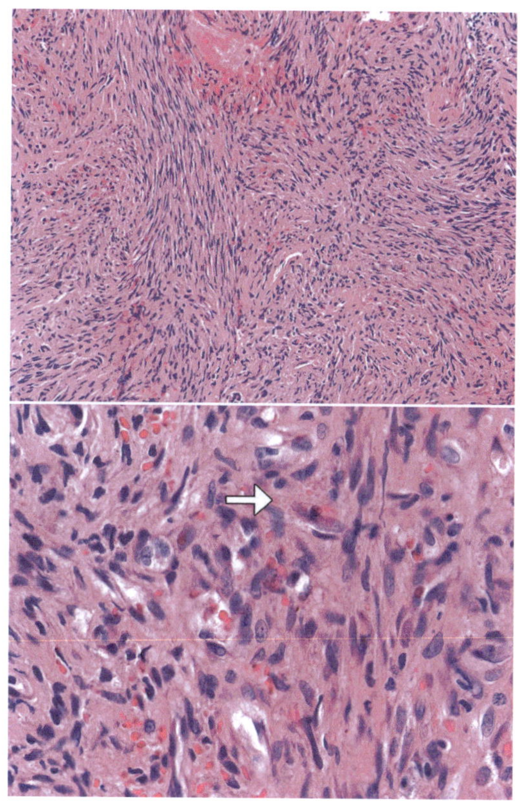

Fig. 6.27 Kaposi sarcoma. Low (top) and high (bottom) hematoxylin and eosin stained photomicrographs show spindle cells in long intersecting fascicles with extravasated red blood cells and eosinophilic globules (*arrow*)

ularly shaped nodules (Fig. 6.28). Otherwise, diagnostic imaging is mainly performed to assess the extent of visceral and lymphatic involvement by Kaposi sarcoma, which can be performed using CT, MRI, ^{18}FDG-PET, or ^{99m}Tc-Tetrofosmin scintigraphy. Pharyngeal involvement can manifest as polypoid lesions and the lymphadenopathy can be necrotic, particularly when large (Fig. 6.29).

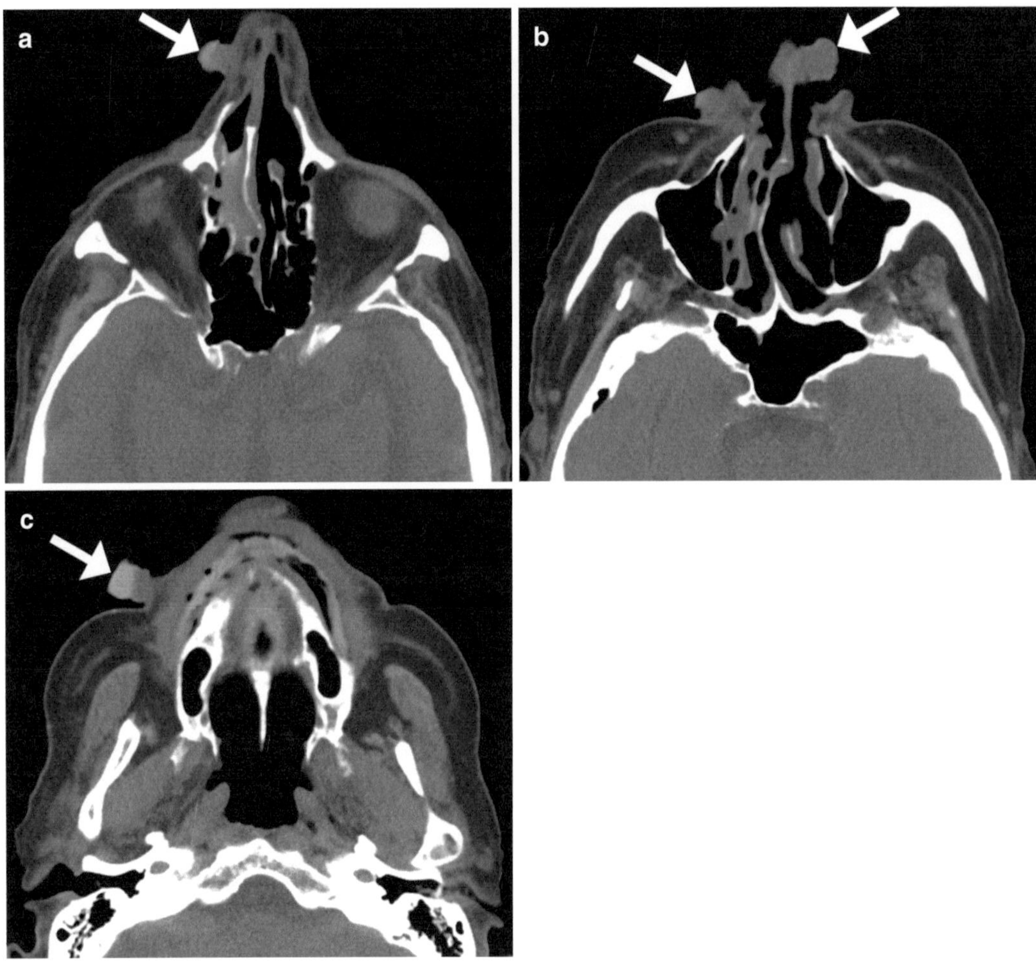

Fig. 6.28 Kaposi sarcoma. Axial CT images (**a** through **c**) show multiple exophytic skin lesions involving the face (*arrows*)

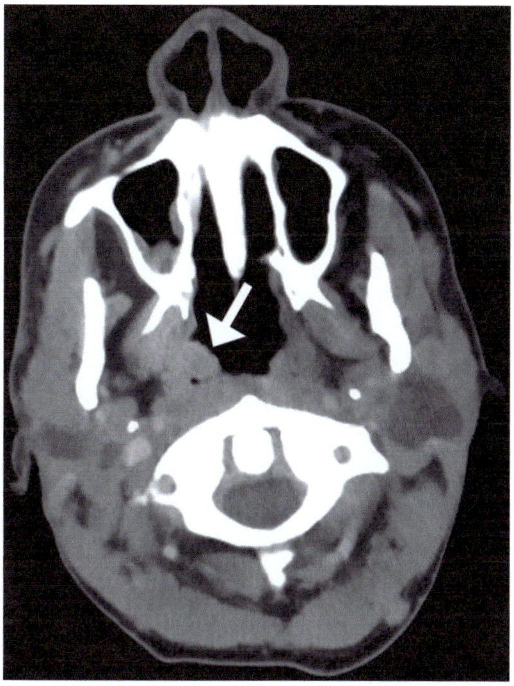

Fig. 6.29 Kaposi sarcoma. Axial CT image shows bilateral centrally hypoattenuating lymphadenopathy and a polypoid lesion in the right nasopharynx (*arrow*). The lesions regressed with treatment in this HIV-positive patient

Merkel Cell Carcinoma

Overview
Merkel cell carcinoma is a rare, aggressive cutaneous neoplasm that mainly occurs in the head and neck. This tumor is predisposed by exposure to ultraviolet light and therefore tends to affect elderly individuals with fair skin. Immunosuppression and Merkel cell polyomavirus have also been linked to the development of Merkel cell carcinoma. There is a high prevalence of second neoplasms, such as squamous cell carcinoma, and the prognosis is generally poor.

Clinicopathological Findings

Merkel cell carcinoma is believed to arise from stem cells in the epidermis. Upon clinical examination, Merkel cell carcinomas often appear as nontender, dome-shaped red, violaceous, or purple nodules (Fig. 6.30). There may also be associated ulcerative, acneiform, or telangiectatic features. These tumors can grow rapidly and there are distant metastases in approximately one-third of patients. A combination of light microscopy and immunohistochemistry is often used to make a definitive diagnosis. It usually presents as a mixture of three morphologies: trabecular, intermediate, and small cell. The trabecular type demonstrates chords of cells with abundant cytoplasm, round nuclei, and inconspicuous nucleoli. The intermediate and small cell carcinomas are more densely cellular and composed of intermediate to small cells with minimal cytoplasm, round to oval nuclei, and inconspicuous to prominent nucleoli, respectively (Fig. 6.31). Merkel cell carcinoma is positive for neuroendocrine markers, including synaptophysin, chromogranin, as well as cytokeratin 20, usually in a perinuclear dot-like distri-

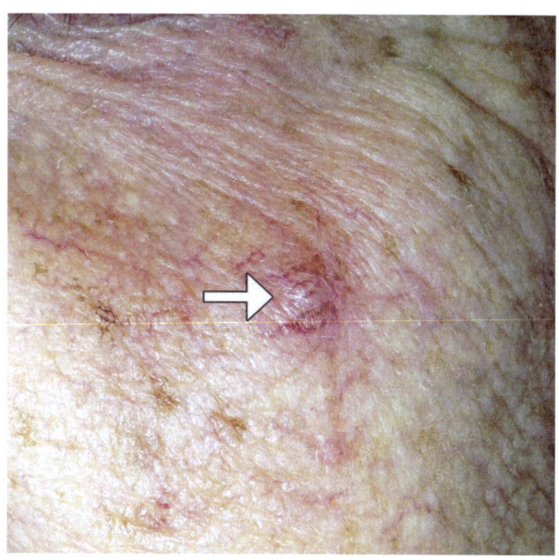

Fig. 6.30 Merkel cell carcinoma. Photograph shows a dome-shaped, red cutaneous nodule in the cheek (*arrow*)

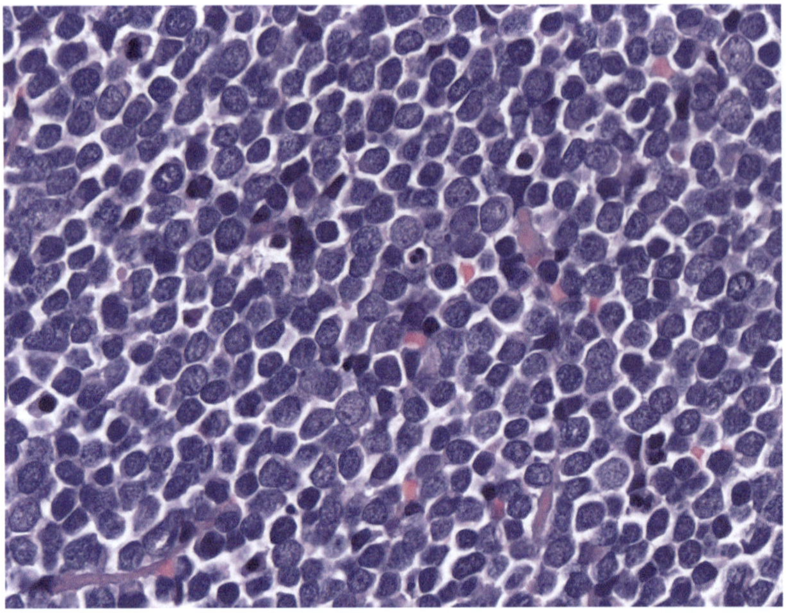

Fig. 6.31 Merkel cell carcinoma Hematoxylin and eosin stained photomicrograph shows intermediate-sized cells with minimal cytoplasm, round to oval nuclei, finely stipple chromatin, and absent to inconspicuous nucleoli. Apoptotic and mitotic figures are also present

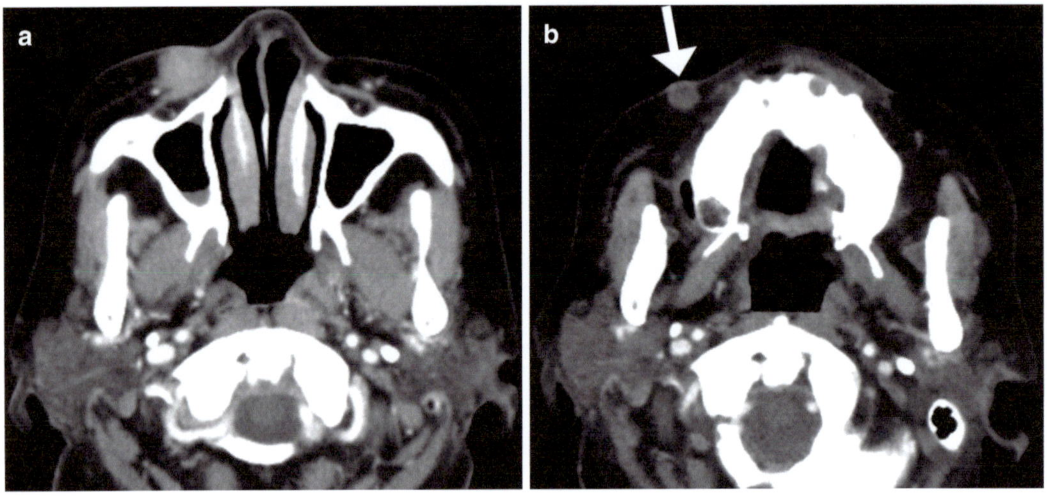

Fig. 6.32 Merkel cell carcinoma. Axial post-contrast CT image (**a**) at initial presentation of a patient with Merkel cell carcinoma shows a mildly infiltrative tumor in the right cheek. Axial post-contrast CT image after surgery (**b**) shows a small subcutaneous nodule at the surgical margin (*arrow*), which proved to be recurrent tumor

bution. For details regarding staging, please refer to the eighth edition of the American Joint Committee on Cancer (AJCC).

Imaging Findings

CT or MRI can be used to characterize the extent of the Merkel cell carcinoma. On CT and MRI, the tumor appears as a nonspecific soft tissue nodule, but there can be cutaneous fat stranding adjacent to the tumor, which suggests lymphedema (Figs. 6.32 and 6.33). CT is useful for evaluating lymph node metastases, which appear as high-attenuation. MRI is useful for evaluating brain, spine, and bone metastases. ^{18}FDG-PET/CT and sentinel lymph node biopsy may also play a role in staging.

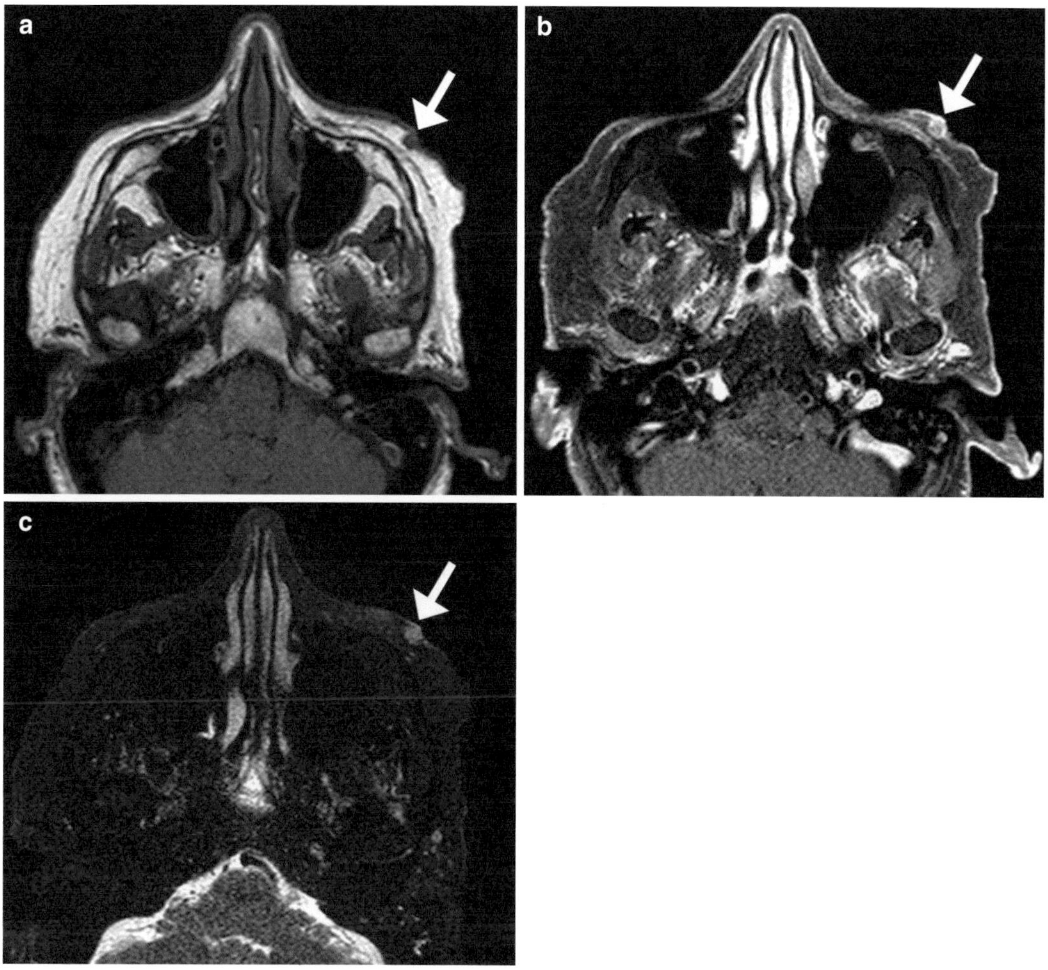

Fig. 6.33 Merkel cell carcinoma. Axial T1-weighted (**a**), fat-suppressed post-contrast T1-weighted (**b**), and fat-suppressed T2-weighted (**c**) MR images show an enhancing subcutaneous nodule in the left cheek (*arrows*)

Microcystic Adnexal Carcinoma

Overview
Microcystic adnexal carcinoma is a locally aggressive skin adnexal carcinoma that most commonly involves the head and neck region. It has been proposed that microcystic adnexal carcinoma is an apocrine tumor. The tumor is characterized by slow, but locally aggressive growth with infiltration of subcutaneous fat, muscles, perichondrium, periosteum, and/or perineurium. As a result, surgical treatment often leads to ablation defects, which are many times the size of the clinical lesion. The local recurrence rate by standard excision is about 50%, but there may be more favorable cure rates with Mohs micrographic surgery.

Clinicopathological Findings

Microcystic adnexal carcinoma is a rare tumor of the skin that grows indolently over the course of years. Clinically, the neoplasm often masquerades

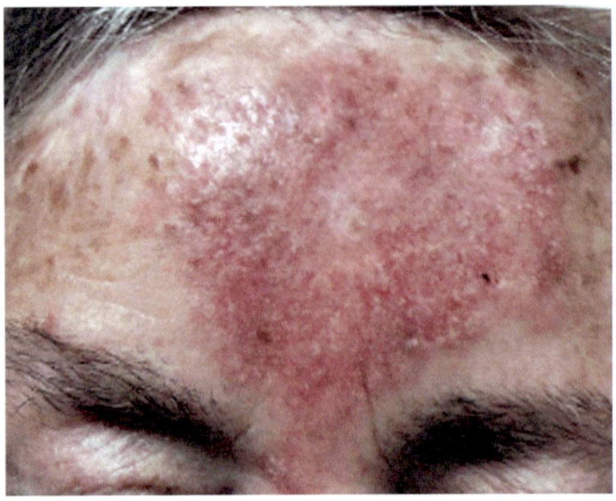

Fig. 6.34 Microcystic adnexal carcinoma. Photograph shows a geographic erythematous patch in the forehead

as a flesh-colored, yellow, or erythematous, indurated papule or plaque, with a predilection for the central portion of the face (Fig. 6.34). Histologically, the neoplasm is characterized by a combination of small keratocysts in the upper dermis, islands, strands, and ducts of small basaloid or squamoid cells, and deep infiltration by very small nests and strands of cells with densely eosinophilic hyalinized stroma (Fig. 6.35). Microcystic adnexal carcinomas are CK15 positive, similar to desmoplastic trichoepithelioma and different from SCC and BCC.

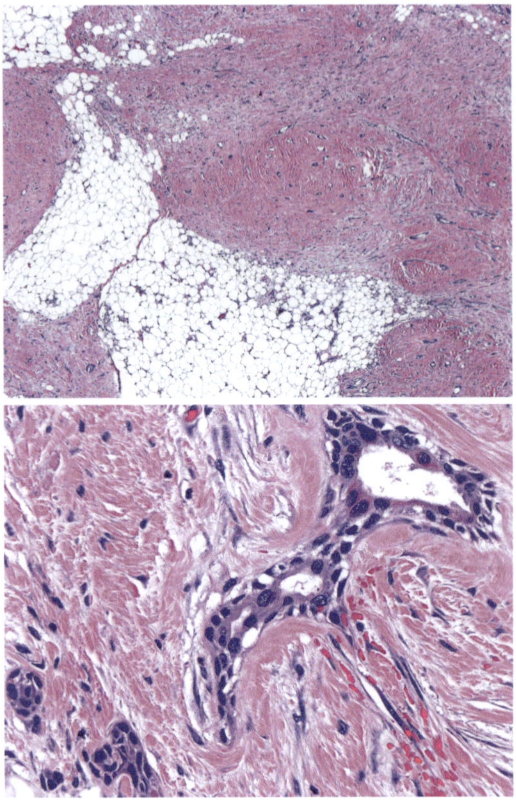

Fig. 6.35 Microcystic adnexal carcinoma. Low (top) and high (bottom) power hematoxylin and eosin stained photomicrographs show deep invasion into adipose tissue by small bilayered ducts and nests composed of atypical epithelial and myoepithelial cells surrounded by abundant hyalinized stroma

Imaging Findings

MRI is a suitable imaging modality for evaluating the extent and depth of the microcystic adnexal carcinoma. The neoplasm can manifest as an enhancing nodule with low T2 signal, whereby it can mimic a fibrous tumor. Alternatively, microcystic adnexal carcinoma can appear as a diffuse, infiltrative, enhancing lesion rather than a discrete mass (Fig. 6.36), whereby it can mimic an inflammatory process.

Sebaceous Carcinoma

Overview

Sebaceous carcinoma is a rare malignant epithelial adnexal neoplasm with a predilection for the periocular region, arising from Meibomian or Zeiss glands of the eyelids, but represents the third most common malignancy in this region after squamous cell carcinoma and basal cell carcinoma. Other favored extra-ocular sites in the head and neck include the parotid area, followed by nose, scalp, neck, external auditory canal, retro-auricular, and submandibular region. The diagnosis can be challenging to make at initial presentation since sebaceous carcinoma can clinically and histopathologically mimic other malignant and benign conditions.

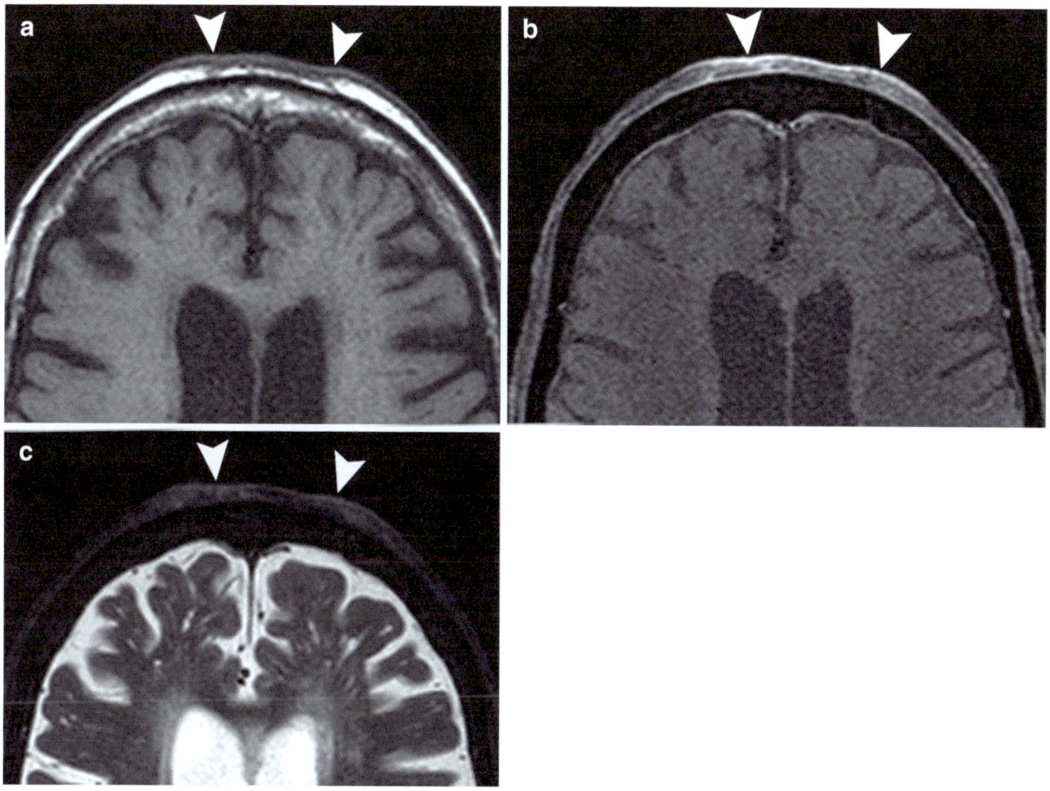

Fig. 6.36 Microcystic adnexal carcinoma. Axial T1-weighted (**a**), fat-suppressed post-contrast T1-weighted (**b**), and fat-suppressed T2-weighted (**c**) MR images show an infiltrative enhancing lesion in the frontal scalp (*arrowheads*)

Clinicopathological Findings

Sebaceous carcinomas can appear as variably colored masses that may be ulcerated on clinical exam (Fig. 6.37). Indeed, the clinical appearance is not pathognomonic and can also mimic benign conditions, such as keratoacanthomas. Histologic evaluation demonstrates a high-grade carcinoma with nested growth, central necrosis, and brisk mitotic activity. Cytoplasm usually demonstrates variably sized optically clear vacuoles (Fig. 6.38). Definite identification of intracytoplasmic fat droplets using fat stains such as Oil-Red-O or Sudan Black IV on frozen tissue, or lipid-associated proteins, such as adipophilin on formalin-fixed tissue can help differentiate sebaceous carcinoma from glycogenated SCC or BCC. The presence of intra-conjunctival pagetoid spread presents a surgical challenge and

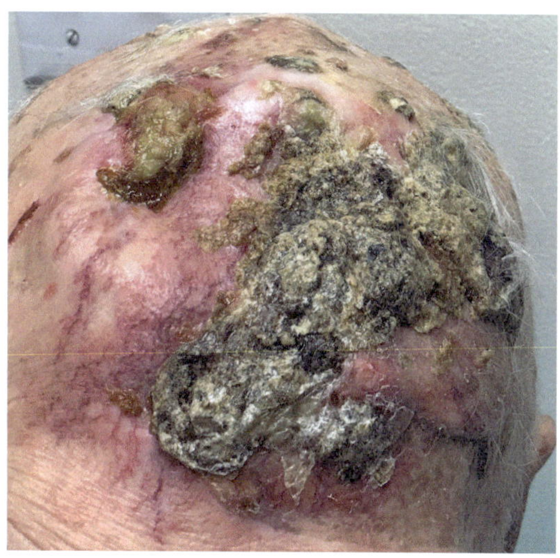

Fig. 6.37 Sebaceous carcinoma. Photograph shows multiple scaly, irregular, pigmented exophytic tumors in the scalp

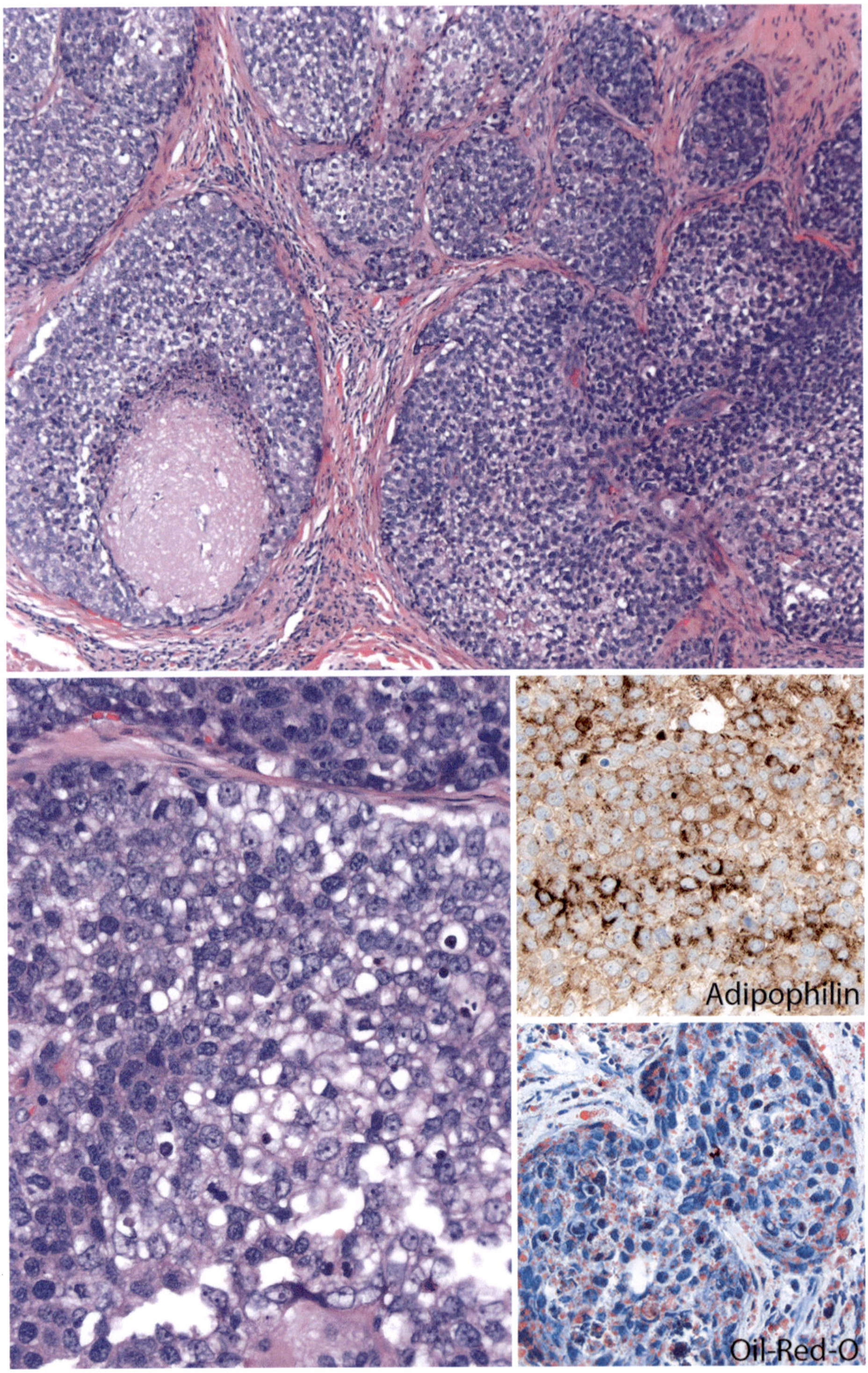

Fig. 6.38 Sebaceous carcinoma. Low power hematoxylin and eosin stained photomicrograph (top) of conjunctival sebaceous carcinoma growing in large nests with central necrosis. Higher power hematoxylin and eosin stained photomicrograph (bottom left) demonstrates clear cytoplasmic vacuoles, mitoses, and apoptoses. Immunostain for adipophilin (granular, cytoplasmic) and histochemical stain for fat (Oil- Red-O) are relatively specific for sebaceous carcinoma

more frequently requires orbital exenteration. The risk of tumor-related metastases does not change with pagetoid spread.

Imaging Findings

CT and MRI are useful for evaluating the extent of the sebaceous carcinoma in the head and neck. The periocular tumors may appear as irregular thickening of the eyelid (Fig. 6.39), but attenuation should be made to the orbital fat for infiltration and to the orbital walls for bone erosions. Extra-ocular tumors may appear infiltrative, enhancing masses that may protrude from the skin and extend into the deep structures (Fig. 6.40). The tumors may be multiple, particularly in the setting of recurrent disease.

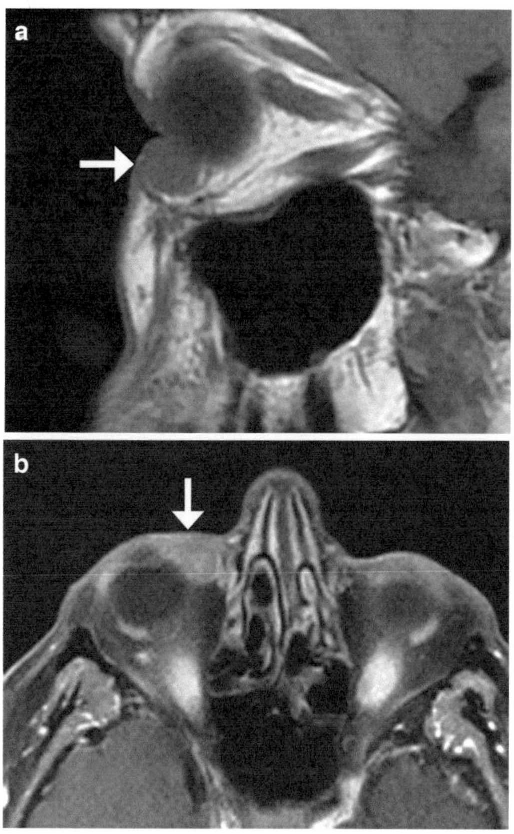

Fig. 6.39 Sebaceous carcinoma. Sagittal T1-weighted (**a**) and axial fat-suppressed T1-weighted (**b**) MR images show an enhancing mass in the inferior right eyelid (*arrows*)

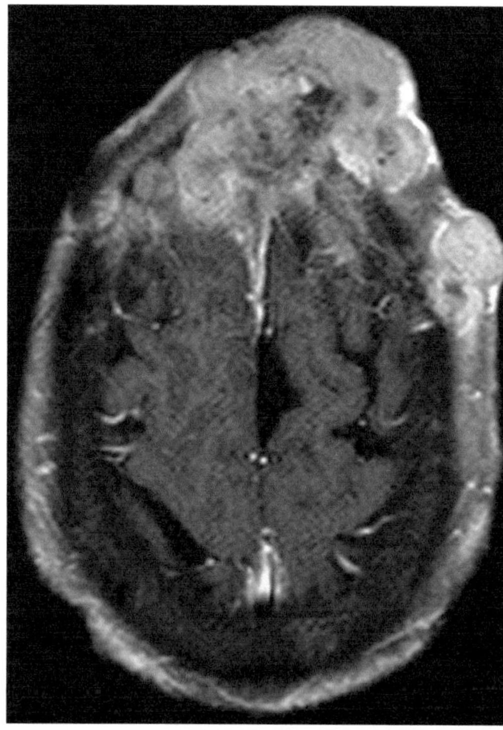

Fig. 6.40 Sebaceous carcinoma. Axial fat-suppressed post-contrast T1-weighted MRI shows multiple invasive enhancing scalp nodules

Cutaneous Adenoid Cystic Carcinoma

Overview

Cutaneous adenoid cystic carcinoma arises from sweat glands, ectopic salivary glands, or ceruminous glands, which are specialized sudoriferous glands located mainly in the lateral external auditory canal. External auditory canal adenoid cystic carcinoma has a more indolent clinical course than its salivary gland counterparts.

Clinicopathological Findings

Adenoid cystic carcinoma of the external auditory canal is much less common than squamous cell carcinoma and basal cell carcinoma. Patients may present with discharge from the ear,

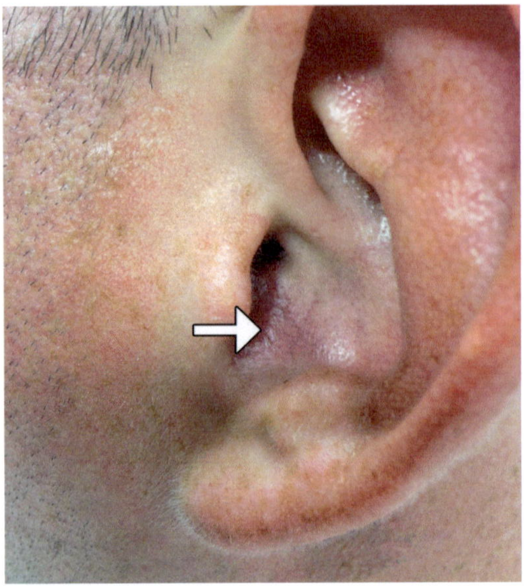

Fig. 6.41 Adenoid cystic carcinoma. Clinical photograph shows a reddish nodular lesion raising the skin of the lateral external auditory canal (*arrow*)

progressive hearing loss, and the presence of swelling, discoloration, and induration of the lateral third of the external auditory canal (Fig. 6.41). Histologically, adenoid cystic carcinoma is composed of basaloid cells with dual epithelial and myoepithelial cell differentiation and can have cribriform, tubular, or solid growth patterns (Fig. 6.42). Myoepithelial cells produce basement membrane matrix material, resulting in characteristic eosinophilic to pale blue-grey myxoid stromal globules. Higher percentages of solid growth portend worse prognosis. Immunohistochemically, epithelial cells are positive for CD117 and myoepithelial cells for high molecular weight keratin and p63/p40. Radical resection and radiation is recommended in order to minimize the risk of local recurrence, which can manifest many years after treatment. Adenoid cyst carcinoma rarely undergoes lymphatic spread to the lymph nodes, but commonly spreads hematogenously, particularly to the lungs. In addition, adenoid cystic carcinoma has a propensity for perineural spread.

Imaging Findings

CT and MRI are complementary for the evaluation of external auditory canal adenoid cystic carcinoma, which appears as an enhancing soft tissue mass that can erode bone (Fig. 6.43). Adenoid cystic carcinoma is often not very hypermetabolic on ^{18}FDG-PET.

Angiosarcoma

Overview

Cutaneous angiosarcomas are vascular malignancies that can derive from the endothelium of the blood vessels (hemangiosarcomas) or lymphatic vessels (lymphangiosarcomas). Approximately 60% of angiosarcomas occur in the head and neck. Angiosarcomas tend to spread rapidly, with the highest rate of lymph node metastasis among all soft tissue sarcomas of the head and neck. Consequently, angiosarcomas tend to have a poor prognosis, with a 5-year survival rate of less than 40% overall. The most effective treatment is resection with preoperative or postoperative radiation therapy.

Clinicopathological Findings

The clinical types of cutaneous angiosarcoma include angiosarcoma of the head and neck of the elderly, angiosarcoma associated with chronic lymphedema, and post-irradiation angiosarcoma. Cutaneous angiosarcomas can have a variety of appearances on physical examination, including erythematic lesions, violaceous nodules and plaques, and flat infiltrating hemorrhagic areas (Fig. 6.44). The neoplasm can also mimic benign conditions such as rosacea, xanthelasma, cellulitis, and facial angioedema, or other malignant neoplasms. Histologically, angiosarcoma can manifest a variety of histologic appearances, from vasoformative to epithelioid to spindled. Nuclei are usually highy atypical with hyperchromasia, prominent nucleoli, and abundant mitoses (Fig. 6.45). In a poorly differentiated tumor, search for a malignant vasoformative component and extravasated red blood cells may aid in diagnosis. Helpful immunomarkers include CD31, CD34, ERG, FLI-1, and Factor VIII antigen.

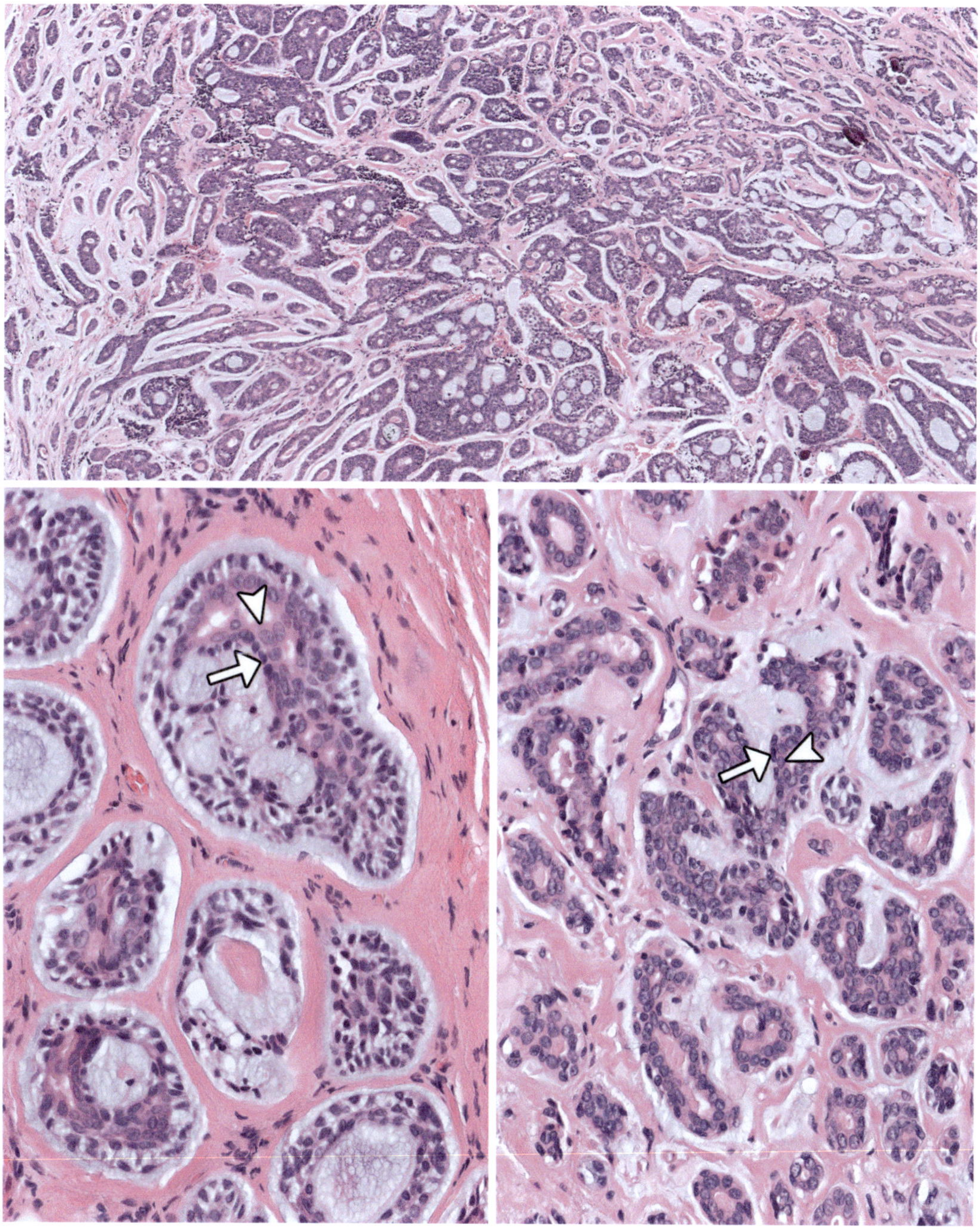

Fig. 6.42 Adenoid cystic carcinoma. Hematoxylin and eosin stained photomicrographs show cribriform and tubular growth patterns composed of myoepithelial cells with dark nuclei and clear cytoplasm (*arrows*), as well as epithelial cells with vesicular nuclei and eosinophilic cytoplasm (*arrowheads*). The stroma is variably collagenous and eosinophilic to bluish and myxoid

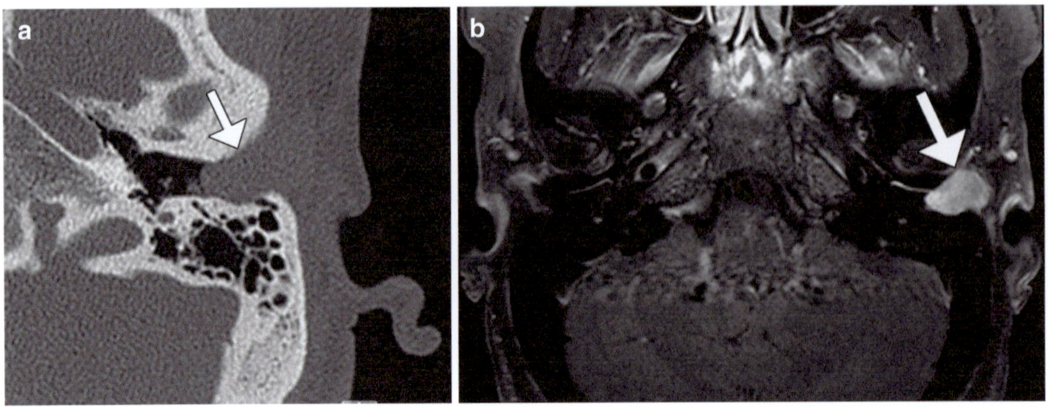

Fig. 6.43 Adenoid cystic carcinoma. Axial CT image (**a**) shows a mass (*arrow*) within the left external auditory canal with perhaps mild bony erosions (*arrow*). The mass (*arrow*) demonstrates avid enhancement of the corresponding fat-suppressed post-contrast T1-weighted MRI (**b**)

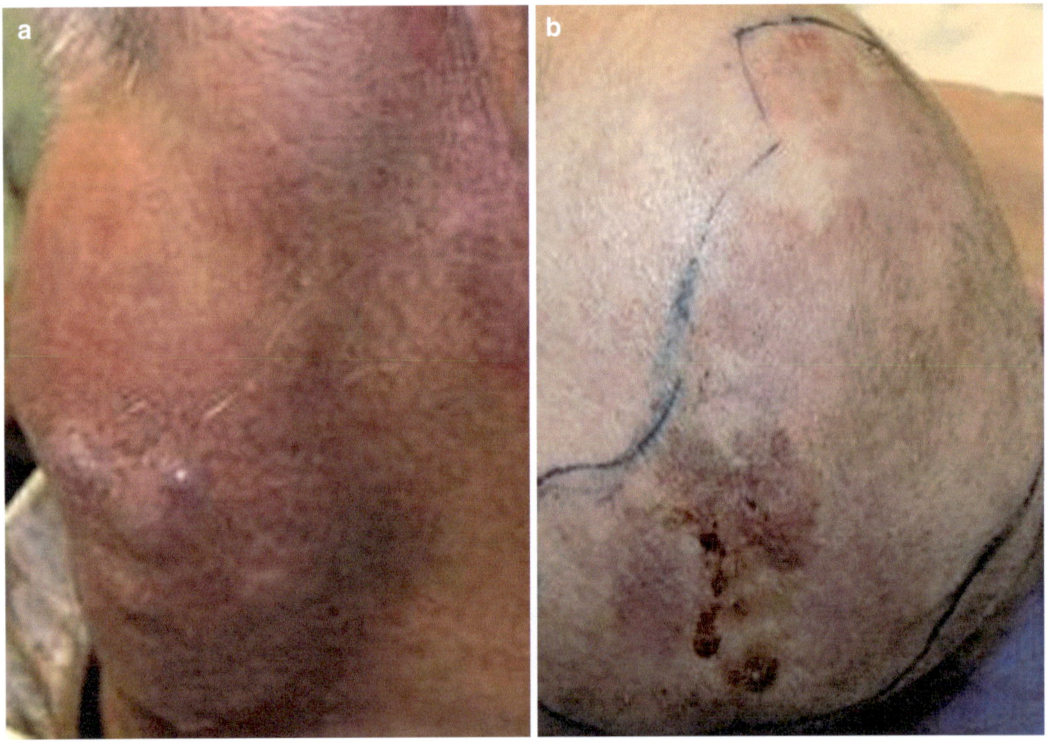

Fig. 6.44 Angiosarcoma. Photograph (**a**) shows an erythematous hematoma-like mass in the posterior neck. Photograph in a different patient (**b**) shows geographic areas of violaceous discoloration in the scalp. The lesion was outlined with blue ink for surgical planning

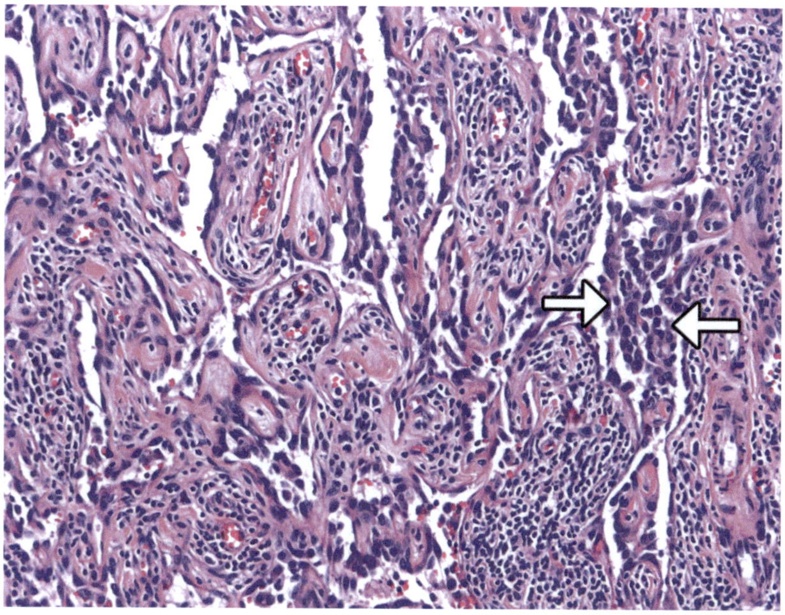

Fig. 6.45 Angiosarcoma. Hematoxylin and eosin stained photomicrograph shows vascular channels with complex branching architecture, highly atypical endothelial cells, intraluminal endothelial proliferation (*arrows*), and associated inflammatory cells

Imaging Findings

Angiosarcomas tend to appear as high T2 and intermediate T1 signal intensity tumors, with occasional areas of T1 hyperintensity due to hemorrhage. In addition, the tumors often contain flow voids and display avid enhancement although areas that do not enhance may be apparent due to necrosis. Cross-sectional imaging is useful for evaluating the extent of tumor, which can be infiltrative and associated with head and neck lymph node metastases (Fig. 6.46).

Cutaneous Metastases

Overview

Cutaneous metastases occur in 0.7–9% of cancers overall and can be the initial clinical manifestation of underlying malignancy. Lung cancer is the most common source of cutaneous metastases in men, while breast cancer is the most common cause in women.

The scalp and face are common locations for distant metastases. Alternatively, primary cancers in the head and neck can involve the skin by direct extension. Ultimately, metastasis to the skin is often a pre-terminal event that heralds poor outcome.

Clinicopathological Findings

The clinical presentation of skin metastases can be variable, including erythema, rash, nodules, and mass (Figs. 6.47 and 6.48). Distant metastases usually deposit in the dermis and less commonly the epidermis (Fig. 6.49). Most metastatic lesions maintain a similar histology appearance to the primary tumor, but some metastases cannot be easily distinguished under light microscopy, such as small cell lung cancer, small cell melanoma, and Merkel cell carcinoma, so immunohistochemical staining helps to identify primary lesions from metastases. It is common to observe inflammatory responses and angiogenesis within the cutaneous lesions.

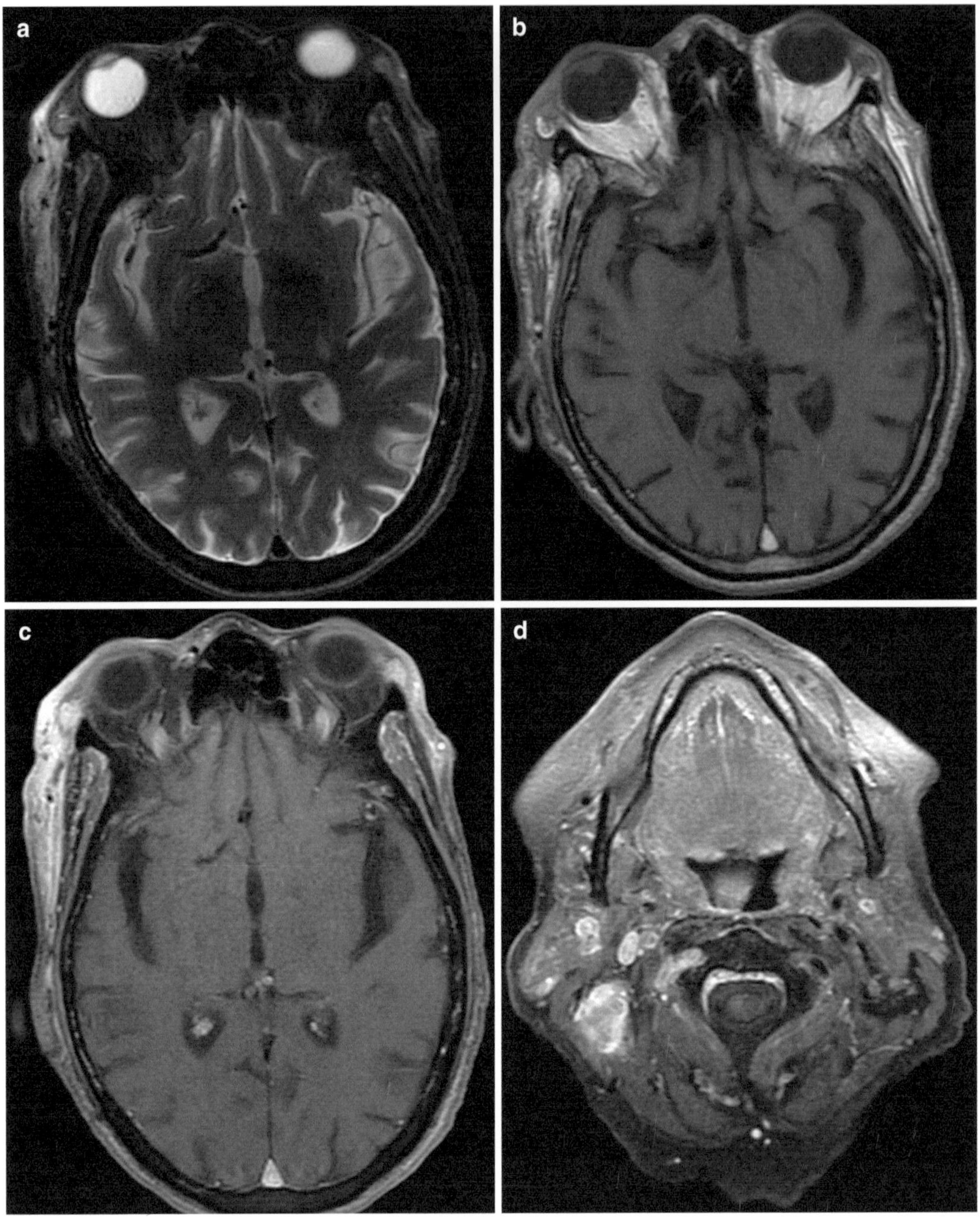

Fig. 6.46 Angiosarcoma. Axial fat-suppressed T2-weighted (**a**), T1-weighted (**b**), post-contrast fat-suppressed T1-weighted (**c**, **d**) MR images show an infiltrative mass with prominent flow voids in the right scalp and ipsilateral metastatic lymphadenopathy

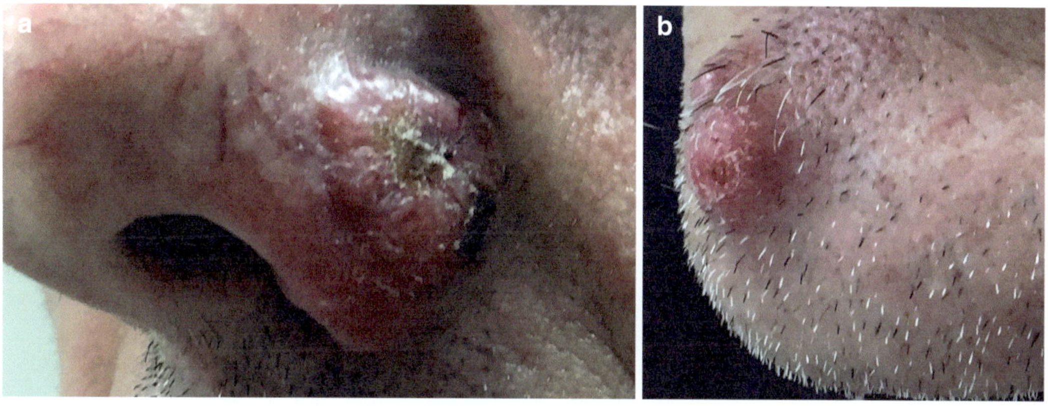

Fig. 6.47 Distant metastases. Photographs (**a**, **b**) show nasal ala and chin erythematous nodular lesions with skin ulceration in a patient with metastatic oropharyngeal squamous cell carcinoma

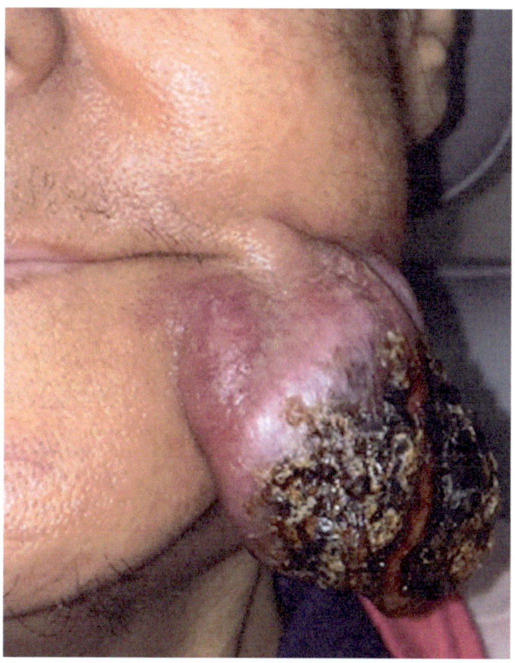

Fig. 6.48 Direct tumor invasion of the skin, Photograph shows a bulky exophytic mass with skin erythema and crusting from extension of a buccal squamous cell carcinoma

Imaging Findings

Cutaneous metastases may be encountered incidentally on staging imaging examinations or may undergo imaging specifically to image the extent of the lesions. Most distant metastases involving the skin and subcutaneous tissues appear as small enhancing nodules (Fig. 6.50). Although these may initially appear innocuous and nonspecific, growth on follow-up examinations suggest the true malignant nature of the lesions. Depending on the type of primary tumor, skin metastases may be hypermetabolic on ^{18}FDG-PET, which may be used for staging (Fig. 6.51). Involvement of the skin and subcutaneous tissues from direct extension is a criterion in the staging of certain head and neck tumors and can be recognized on imaging as effacement of the subcutaneous fat and contour deformity of the overlying skin (Fig. 6.52).

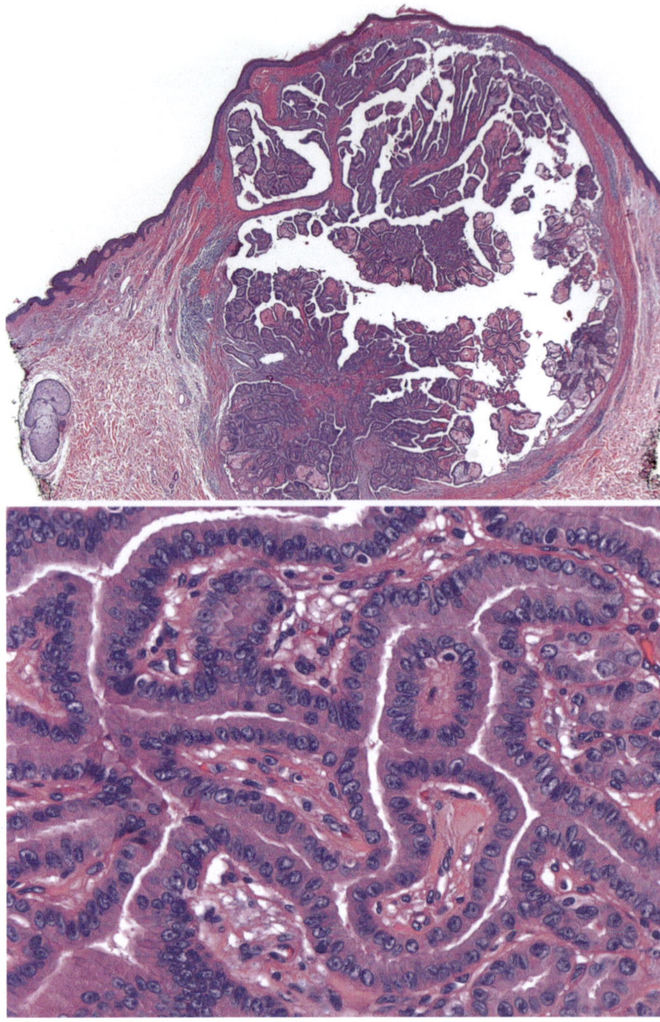

Fig. 6.49 Cutaneous metastasis. Low (top) and high (bottom) power hematoxylin and eosin stained photomicrographs show a nodular, circumscribed dermal proliferation of neoplastic cells with papillary architecture, eosinophilic cytoplasm, and enlarged, elongated, and grooved nuclei of papillary thyroid carcinoma

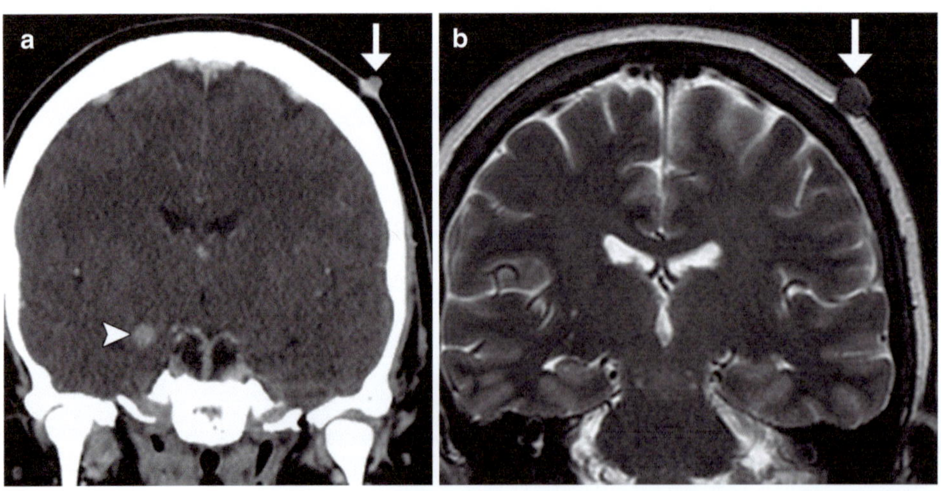

Fig. 6.50 Cutaneous metastatic disease. Coronal contrast-enhanced CT (**a**) and T2-weighted MR (**b**) images show a nodule left scalp metastasis that grew on follow-up 2 months later (*arrows*) in a patient with esophageal carcinoma. There is also a right medial temporal lobe metastasis shown on the CT image (*arrowhead*)

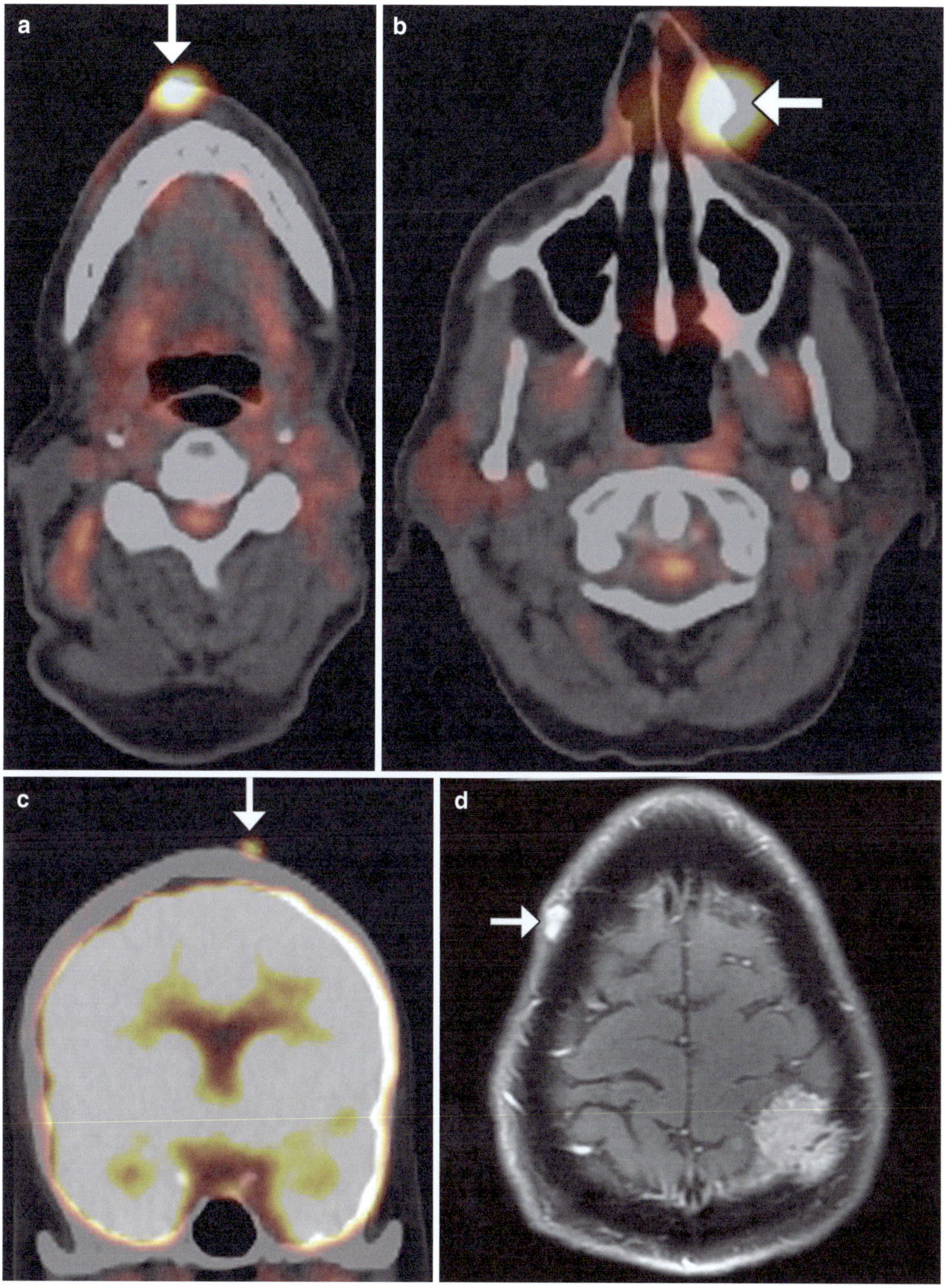

Fig. 6.51 Cutaneous metastatic disease. Axial (**a**, **b**) and coronal (**c**) ^{18}FDG-PET/CT images show multiple hypermetabolic head and neck skin metastases in the same patient as shown in Fig. 6.47. Axial fat-suppressed post-contrast T1-weighted MRI (**d**) shows an enhancing right scalp nodule (*arrow*)

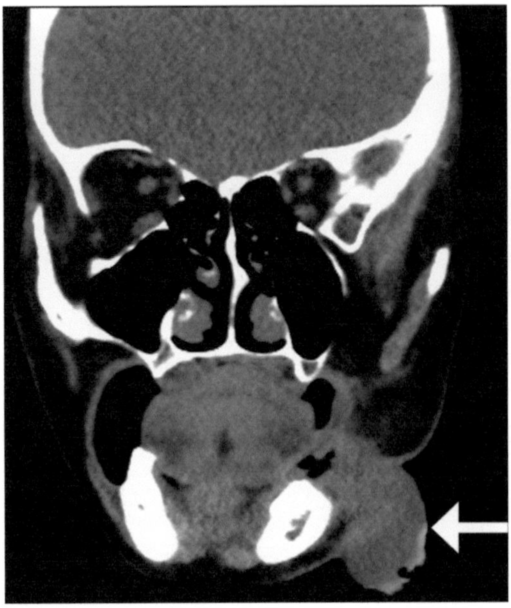

Fig. 6.52 Direct tumor extension into the skin. Coronal CT Image shows a buccal squamous cell carcinoma that extends from the oral cavity to the skin (*arrow*). This is the same patient as shown in Fig. 6.48

Suggested Reading

Ambujam S, Audhya M, Reddy A, Roy S. Cutaneous angiosarcoma of the head, neck, and face of the elderly in type 5 skin. J Cutan Aestheth Surg. 2013;6(1):45–7.

Anderson SE, Beer KT, Banic A, Steinbach LS, Martin M, Friedrich EE, Stauffer E, Vock P, Greiner RH. MRI of merkel cell carcinoma: histologic correlation and review of the literature. AJR AM J Rotentgenol. 2005;185(6):1441–8.

Baheti AD, Tirumani SH, Giardino A, Rosenthal MH, Tirumani H, Krajewski K, Ramaiya NH. Basal cell carcinoma: a comprehensive review for the radiologist. Am J Roentgenol. 2015;204(2):W132–40.

Balamucki CJ, DeJesus R, Galloway TJ, Mancuso AA, Amdur RJ, Morris CG, Kirwan JM, Mendenhall WM. Impact of radiographic findings on for prognosis skin cancer with perineural invasion. Am J Clin Oncol. 2015;38(3):248–51.

Belkin DA, Wysong A. Radiographic imaging for skin cancer. Semin Cutan Med Surg. 2016;35(1):42–8.

Bolm I, Babaryka G, Moergel M, Al-Nawas B, Kämmerer PW. Multifocal metastasizing extra-ocular facial sebaceous carcinoma as diagnostic challenge: case report and systematic review. J Maxillofac Oral Surg. 2015;14(Suppl 1):331–7.

Cassarino DS, DeRienzo DP, Barr RJ. Cutaneous squamous cell carcinoma: a comprehensive clinicopathologic classification. J Cutan Pathol. 2006;33(4):261–79.

Chao AN, Shields CL, Krema H, Shields JA. Outcome of patients with periocular sebaceous gland carcinoma with and without conjunctival intraepithelial invasion. Ophthalmology. 2001;108(10):1877–83.

Crowson AN. Basal cell carcinoma: biology, morphology and clinical implications. Mod Pathol. 2006;19:S127–47.

D'Ambrosio N, Lyo JK, Young RJ, Haque SS, Karimi S. Imaging of metastatic CNS neuroblastoma. AJR Am J Roentgenol. 2010;194(5):1223–9.

Dammann F, Horger M, Mueller-Berg M, et al. Rational diagnosis of squamous cell carcinoma of the head and neck region: comparative evaluation of CT, MRI and 18-FDG PET. Am J Roentgenol. 2005;184:1326–31.

Dong F, Gidley PW, Ho T, Luna MA, Ginsberg LE, Sturgis EM. Adenoid cystic carcinoma of the external auditory canal. Laryngoscope. 2008;118(9):1591–6.

Escott EJ. A variety of appearances of malignant melanoma in the head: a review. Radiographics. 2001;21(3):625–39.

Fischer S, Breuninger H, Metzler G, Hoffmann J. Microcystic adnexal carcinoma: an often misdiagnosed, locally aggressive growing skin tumor. J Craniofac Surg. 2005;16(1):53–8.

Fliss DM, Kraus M, Tovi F. Adenoid cystic carcinoma of the external auditory canal. Ear Nose Throat J. 1990;69(9):635, 638–9, 642 passim.

Gaballah AH, Jensen CT, Palmquist S, Pickhardt PJ, Duran A, Broering G, Elsayes KM. Angiosarcoma: clinical and imaging features from head to toe. Br J Radiol. 2017;90(1075):20170039.

Gaviani P, Mullins ME, Braga TA, Hedley-Whyte ET, Halpern EF, Schaefer PS, Henson JW. Improved detection of metastatic melanoma by T2*-weighted imaging. AJNR Am J Neuroradiol. 2006;27(3):605–8.

Gershenwald JE, Scolyer RA, Hess KR, Sondak VK, Long GV, Ross MI, Lazar AJ, Faries MB, Kirkwood JM, McArthur GA, Haydu LE, Eggermont AMM, Flaherty KT, Balch CM, Thompson JF, for members of the American Joint Committee on Cancer Melanoma Expert Panel and the International Melanoma Database and Discovery Platform. Melanoma staging: evidence-based changes in the American Joint Committee on Cancer eighth edition cancer staging manual. CA Cancer J Clin. 2017;67(6):472–92.

Glastonbury CM, Mukherji SK, O'Sullivan B, Lydiatt WM. Setting the stage for 2018: how the changes in the American Joint Committee on Cancer/Union for International Cancer Control Cancer Staging Manual Eighth Edition Impact Radiologists. AJNR Am J Neuroradiol. 2017;38(12):2231–7.

Godden D, Brennan P, Milne J. Update on melanoma: the present position. Br J Oral Maxillofac Surg. 2010;48:575–8.

Goessling W, McKee PH, Mayer RJ. Merkel cell carcinoma. J Clin Oncol. 2002;20(2):588–98.

Gomez-Maestra MJ, España-Gregori E, Aviñó-Martinez JA, et al. Brainstem and cavernous sinus metastases arising from a microcystic adnexal carcinoma of the eyebrow by perineural spreading. Can J Ophthalmol. 2009;44(3):17.

Gramolelli S, Schulz TF. The role of Kaposi sarcoma-associated herpesvirus in the pathogenesis of Kaposi sarcoma. J Pathol. 2015;235(2):368–80.

Gufler H, Franke FE, Rau WS. High-resolution MRI of basal cell carcinomas of the face using a microscopy coil. Am J Roentgenol. 2007;188:W480–4.

Hoang MP, Dresser KA, Kapur P, High WA, Mahalingam M. Microcystic adnexal carcinoma: an immunohistochemical reappraisal. Mod Pathol. 2008;21(2):178–85.

Juan YH, Saboo SS, Tirumani SH, Khandelwal A, Shinagare AB, Ramaiya N, Krajewski KM. Malignant skin and subcutaneous neoplasms in adults: multimodality imaging with CT, MRI, and 18F-FDG PET/CT. AJR Am J Roentgenol. 2014;202(5):W422–38.

Kapoor PG, Chabbra R. Neuroblastoma presenting as raccoon eyes. Cancer. 2003;98:155–65.

Kim EY, Kim SS, Ryoo JW, Na DG, Roh HG, Byun HS, Ko YH. Primary peripheral T-cell lymphoma of the face other than mycosis fungoides. Computed tomography and magnetic resonance findings. J Comput Assist Tomogr. 2004;28(5):670–5.

Kransdorf MJ, Meis-Kindblom JM. Dermatofibrosarcoma protuberans: radiologic appearance. AJR Am J Roentgenol. 1994;163(2):391–4.

Kreimer A, Clifford G, Boyle P. Human papillomavirus types in head and neck squamous cell carcinomas worldwide: a systematic review. Cancer Epidemiol Biomarkers Prev. 2005;14:467–75.

Lee HJ, Im JG, Goo JM, Kim KW, Choi BI, Chang KH, Han JK, Han MH. Peripheral T-cell lymphoma: spectrum of imaging findings with clinical and pathologic features. Radiographics. 2003;23(1):7–26, discussion 26–8.

Lee F, King A, Ma B, Yeung D. Dynamic contrast enhancement magnetic resonance imaging for differential diagnosis in head and neck cancers. Eur J Radiol. 2012;81:784–8.

Lemm D, Mügge LO, Mentzel T, Höffken K. Current treatment options in dermatofibrosarcoma protuberans. J Cancer Res Clin Oncol. 2009;135(5):653.

Li X, Zhang W, Xiao L, Zeng Q, Wu X, Qin J, Shen Y. Computed tomographic and pathological findings of dermatofibrosarcoma protuberans. J Comput Assist Tomogr. 2012;36(4):462–8. https://doi.org/10.1097/RCT.0b013e31825d5a24.

Liapakis IE, Korkolis DP, Koutsoumbi A, Kokkalis G, Gherardini G, Vassilopoulos PP. Merkel cell carcinoma: clinicopathological aspects of an unusual neoplasm. J BUON. 2007;12(2):173–9.

Lomas A, Leonardi-Bee J, Btth-Hextall F. A systematic review of worldwide incidence of nonmelanoma skin cancer. Br J Dermatol. 2012;166:1069–80.

Miketic LM, Chambers TP, Lembersky BC. Cutaneous T-cell lymphoma: value of CT in staging and determining prognosis. AJR Am J Roentgenol. 1993;160(5):1129–32.

Millare GG, Guha-Thakurta N, Sturgis EM, El-Naggar AK, Debnam JM. Imaging findings of head and neck dermatofibrosarcoma protuberans. AJNR Am J Neuroradiol. 2014;35(2):373–8.

Morrison WH, Byers RM, Garden AS, Evans HL, Ang KK, Peters LJ. Cutaneous angiosarcoma of the head and neck. A therapeutic dilemma. Cancer. 1995;76(2):319.

Nguyen BD, McCullough AE. Imaging of Merkel cell carcinoma. Radiographics. 2002;22(2):367–76.

O'Mahony D, Gandjbakhche AH, Hassan M, Vogel A, Yarchoan R. Imaging techniques for Kaposi Sarcoma (KS). J HIV Ther. 2008;13(3):65–71.

O'Rorke M, Ellison M, Murray L, Moran M, James J, Anderson A. Human papillomavirus related head and neck cancer survival: a systematic review and meta-analysis. Oral Oncol. 2012;48:1191–201.

Otero HJ, Jagannathan JP, Prevedello LM, Johnston CJ, Ramaiya NH, Van den Abbeele AD, DiPiro PJ. CT and PET/CT findings of T-cell lymphoma. Am J Roentgenol. 2009;193:349–58.

Petter G, Haustein UF. Histologic subtyping and malignancy assessment of cutaneous squamous cell carcinoma. Dermatol Surg. 2000;26(6):521–30.

Plaza JA, Mackinnon A, Carrillo L, Prieto VG, Sangueza M, Suster S. Role of immunohistochemistry in the diagnosis of sebaceous carcinoma: a clinicopathologic and immunohistochemical study. Am J Dermatopathol. 2015;37(11):809–21.

Ramakrishnan R, Chaudhry IH, Ramdial P, Lazar AJ, McMenamin ME, Kazakov D, Brenn T, Calonje E. Primary cutaneous adenoid cystic carcinoma: a clinicopathologic and immunohistochemical study of 27 cases. Am J Surg Pathol. 2013;37(10):1603–11.

Rao P, Lahat G, Arnold C, Gavino AC, Lahat S, Hornick JL, Lev D, Lazar AJ. Angiosarcoma: a tissue microarray study with diagnostic implications. Am J Dermatopathol. 2013;35(4):432–7.

Restrepo CS, Ocazionez D. Kaposi's sarcoma: imaging overview. Semin Ultrasound CT MR. 2011;32(5):456–69.

Restrepo CS, Martínez S, Lemos JA, Carrillo JA, Lemos DF, Ojeda P, Koshy P. Imaging manifestations of Kaposi sarcoma. Radiographics. 2006;26(4):1169–85.

Rippey JJ. Why classify basal cell carcinomas? Histopathology. 1998;32(5):393–8.

Rohren EM. PET/computed tomography and patient outcomes in melanoma. PET Clin. 2015;10(2):243–54.

Rubin AI, Chen EH, Ratner D. Basal-cell carcinoma. N Engl J Med. 2005;353:2262–9.

Saeed S, Keehn CA, Morgan MB. Cutaneous metastasis: a clinical, pathological, and immunohistochemical appraisal. J Cutan Pathol. 2004;31(6):419–30.

Sanderson R, Ironside J. Squamous cell carcinomas of the head and neck. BMJ. 2002;325:822–7.

Sariya D, Ruth K, Adams-McDonnell R, et al. Clinicopathologic correlation of cutaneous metastases: experience from a cancer center. Arch Dermatol. 2007;143(5):613–20.

Sidiropoulos KG, Martinez-Escala ME, Yelamos O, Guitart J, Sidiropoulos M. Primary cutaneous T-cell lymphomas: a review. J Clin Pathol. 2015;68:1003–10.

Smith V, Walton S. Treatment of facial basal cell carcinoma: a review. J Skin Cancer. 2011;2011:Article ID 380371.

Snow S, Madjar DD, Hardy S, Bentz M, Lucarelli MJ, Bechard R, Aughenbaugh W, McFadden T, Sharata H, Dudley C, Landeck A. Microcystic adnexal carcinoma: report of 13 cases and review of the literature. Dermatol Surg. 2001;27(4):401–8.

Stiller CA, Trama A, Brewster DH, Verne J, Bouchardy C, Navarro C, Chirlaque MD, Marcos-Gragera R, Visser O, Serraino D, Weiderpass E, Dei Tos AP, Ascoli V, RARECARE Working Group. Descriptive epidemiology of Kaposi sarcoma in Europe. Report from the RARECARE project. Cancer Epidemiol. 2014;38(6):670–8.

Stratigos A, Garbe C, Lebbe C, Malvehy J, del Marmol V, Pehamberger H, Peris K, Becker JC, Zalaudek I, Saiag P, Middleton MR, Bastholt L, Testori A, Grob JJ, European Dermatology Forum (EDF); European Association of Dermato-Oncology (EADO); European Organization for Research and Treatment of Cancer (EORTC). Diagnosis and treatment of invasive squamous cell carcinoma of the skin: European consensus-based interdisciplinary guideline. Eur J Cancer. 2015;51(14):1989–2007.

Suárez AL, Pulitzer M, Horwitz S, Moskowitz A, Querfeld C, Myskowski PL. Primary cutaneous B-cell lymphomas: part I Clinical features, diagnosis, and classification. J Am Acad Dermatol. 2013;69(3):329.e1–13.

Swann MH, Yoon J. Merkel cell carcinoma. Semin Oncol. 2007;34(1):51–6.

Tawfik AM, Kreft A, Wagner W, Vogl TJ. MRI of a microcystic adnexal carcinoma of the skin mimicking a fibrous tumour: case report and literature review. Br J Radiol. 2011;84(1002):e114–7.

Timmerman R. Images in clinical medicine. Raccoon eyes and neuroblastoma. J Pediatr. 2014;164(6):1495.

Torreggiani W, Al-Ismail K, Munk P, Nicolaou S, O'Connell J, Knowling M. Dermatofibrosarcomapr otuberans: MR imaging features. Am J Roentgenol. 2001;178:989–93.

Vikey A, Vikey D. Primary malignant melanoma, of head and neck: a comprehensive review of literature. Oral Oncol. 2012;48:399–403.

Wick MR. Cutaneous melanoma: a current overview. Semin Diagn Pathol. 2016;33(4):225–41.

Zhang L, Liu QY, Cao Y, Zhong JS, Zhang WD. Dermatofibrosarcoma protuberans: computed tomography and magnetic resonance imaging findings. Medicine (Baltimore). 2015;94(24):e1001.

Neuroimaging of Vascular Skin Lesions and Related Conditions

7

Daniel Thomas Ginat, Sarah L. Stein, Stephanie McCann, and Gregory Christoforidis

Contents

Abstract

Vascular lesions that may have skin manifestations can be classified as tumors, malformations, and miscellaneous according to the ISSVA. Vascular tumors can be benign, such as congenital and infantile hemangiomas, or aggressive and malignant, such as Kaposi sarcoma and angiosarcoma (refer to Chap. 6). Vascular malformations can be classified as simple, such as capillary malformations, lymphatic malformations, and venous malformations, combined, such as arteriovenous malformations and lymphatic-venous malformation, and associated with other anomalies, such as Klippel-Trenaunay syndrome, Sturge-Weber syndrome (also refer to Chap. 3), and Maffucci syndrome. Furthermore, coagulation abnormalities such as disseminated intravascular coagulopathy and hemoglobinopathies, such as sickle cell disease can have both skin and neuroimaging findings. Certain examples of these different types of vascular lesions with skin involvement and associated neuroimaging findings are reviewed in this chapter.

D. T. Ginat (✉) · S. McCann · G. Christoforidis
Department of Radiology, University of Chicago, Pritzker School of Medicine, Chicago, IL, USA
e-mail: dtg1@uchicago.edu

S. L. Stein
Section of Dermatology, Departments of Medicine and Pediatrics, University of Chicago, Chicago, IL, USA

D. T. Ginat (ed.), *Neuroradiological Imaging of Skin Diseases and Related Conditions*,
https://doi.org/10.1007/978-3-319-90931-8_7

Vascular Tumors

Infantile Hemangiomas

Overview

Infantile hemangioma is the most common vascular tumor in infancy. Hemangiomas may be focal and localized or segmental in distribution. Associated anomalies are occasionally present, such as PHACES syndrome, which is composed of posterior fossa malformations, segmental hemangiomas of the head and neck, intracranial arterial anomalies, cardiac defects or coarctation of the aorta, eye and endocrine anomalies, and sternal defects.

Clinical Findings

Infantile hemangiomas are often not noted at birth, but grow rapidly during the first weeks to months of life. The tumor occurs as a superficial, deep, or mixed lesion within the skin and subcutaneous tissues. Visually, the lesion may initially appear as a blanched patch, telangiectasia, bluish discoloration, or as a bright red spot, followed by progressive enlargement of the mass. Those that are most superficial will demonstrate a deep red to purple surface color, while deeper lesions may impart a bluish hue to the overlying skin or remain mostly flesh-colored (Fig. 7.1). Focal hemangiomas are most common, generally appearing as spongy nodules ranging in size from a few millimeters to several centimeters. Segmental lesions are plaques or masses following embryologic development patterns or other

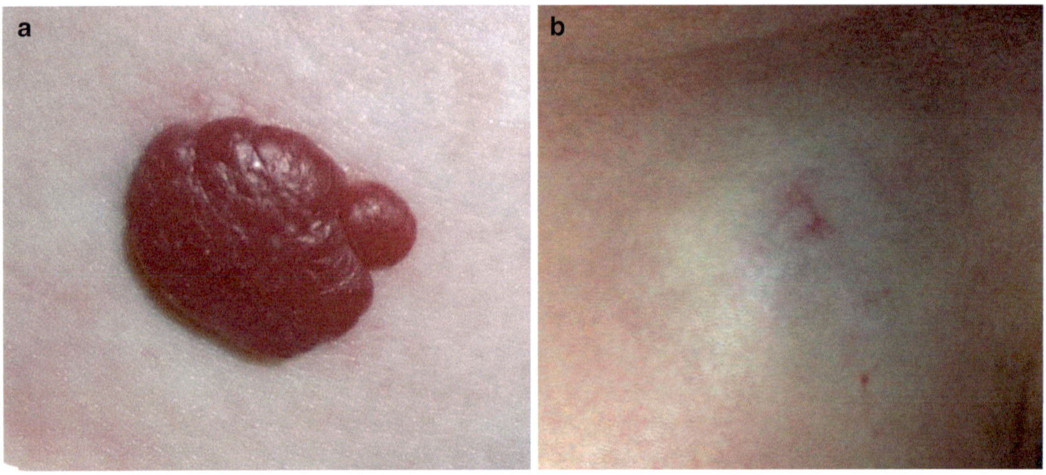

Fig. 7.1 Infantile hemangioma. Photograph shows a focal, superficial, bright red nodule (**a**). Photograph in a different patient shows a deep mass with overlying purple hue (**b**)

Fig. 7.2 Infantile hemangioma. Photograph shows segmental distribution of bright red papules that coalesce into a plaque

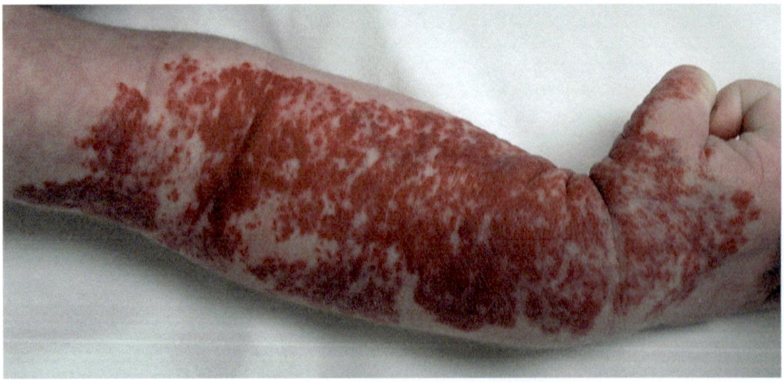

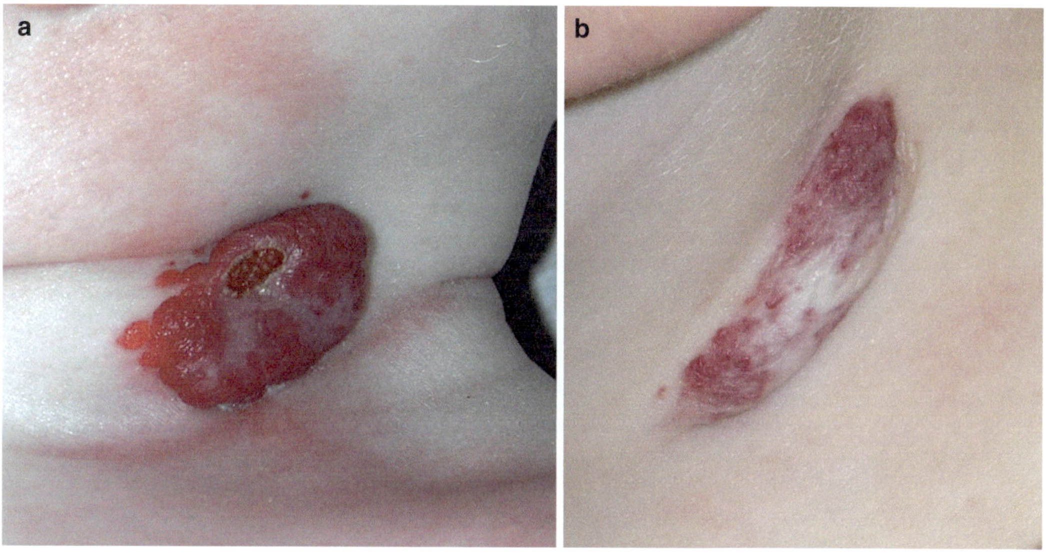

Fig. 7.3 Infantile hemangioma. Photograph shows a bright red nodule in the neck crease at 4 months of age with overlying erosion (**a**). Photograph at 3 years of age shows that nodule has flattened to a soft baggy texture and the red coloration has become lighter with areas clear of vascular markings (**b**)

anatomic distributions (Fig. 7.2). The hemangioma growth phase hits a plateau at approximately 8–10 months of age. After 1 year of life, the hemangioma enters the involution phase, during which it slowly regresses over the subsequent 4–6 years of life. During involution, the hemangioma becomes more dusky red to gray, softer and more compressible. Ultimately, most of the vascular markings dissipate and the site may be left with minimal remnants of the preceding tumor, though if the mass was significantly exophytic, then a fibrofatty residua or redundant loose skin may be left at the site (Fig. 7.3). Histologically, hemangiomas are comprised of hyperplastic proliferating masses of endothelial cells with increased numbers of mast cells. Positive endothelial cell staining with erythrocyte-type glucose transporter (Glut)-1 protein helps to differentiate infantile hemangiomas from other congenital vascular neoplasms.

The hemangiomas associated with PHACES syndrome are typically large, often segmental, plaque-type hemangiomas most commonly located on the head and neck (Fig. 7.4). Hemangiomas located on the head and neck and measuring larger than 5 cm in diameter should prompt consideration of this syndrome. Further evaluation for PHACES includes complete MRI of the brain and MR angiography, cardiac assessment with echocardiogram, and ophthalmologic examination.

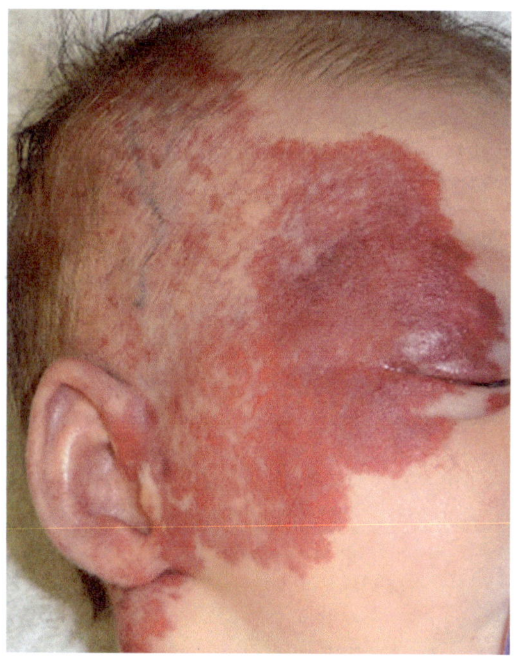

Fig. 7.4 PHACES syndrome. Photograph shows a segmental plaque-type facial hemangioma in the right V1 and V2 distributions

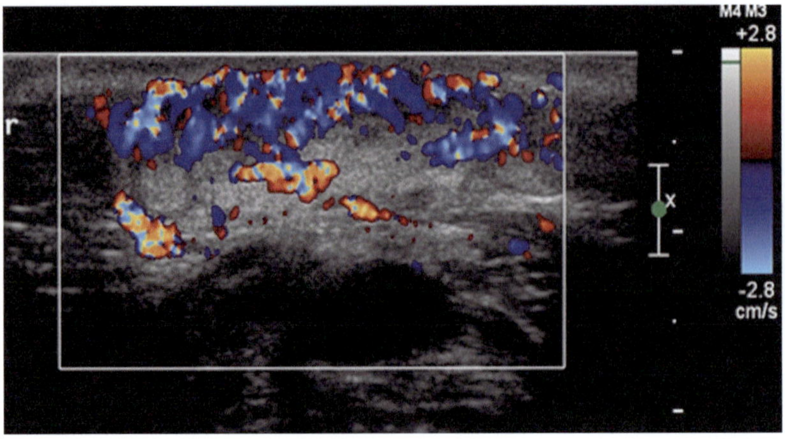

Fig. 7.5 Infantile hemangioma. Doppler ultrasound image shows a hypervascular superficial lesion

Treatment is often not necessary for small, focal hemangiomas that do not compromise functional structures, are not ulcerated, and are not likely to cause critical cosmetic deficits. When intervention is indicated for complicated hemangiomas, medical management with propranolol may be considered. Propranolol has been shown to reliably interrupt the growth phase of infantile hemangiomas and in some cases may accelerate involution.

Imaging Findings

MRI is useful for evaluating the full extent of a hemangioma. The MRI findings differ depending on the biological stage of the lesion. Proliferative stage lesions appear as well-defined, lobulated, high T2 and intermediate T1 signal masses with prominent flow voids and avid early enhancement. Involuting hemangiomas may demonstrate fat signal characteristics. Ultrasonography is also useful for the evaluation of superficial hemangiomas. The lesions tend to be hypervascular on Doppler ultrasound (Fig. 7.5).

MRI and MRA of the head and neck is recommended to evaluate for PHACES syndrome (Fig. 7.6). Cerebral arterial anomalies are present in approximately 90% of patients with PHACES syndrome, including stenoses or occlusions, aneurysms, and anomalous vessels ipsilateral to the facial hemangioma. Prominence of the posterior fossa cerebrospinal fluid space and incidental intracranial hemangiomas may be noted. Ophthalmologic abnormalities observed on imaging include intraorbital hemangiomas, microphthalmia, and coloboma. Other head and neck imaging findings rarely include ectopic lingual thyroid, which can be associated with congenital hypothyroidism.

Congenital Hemangiomas

Overview

Congenital hemangiomas differ from infantile hemangiomas in that they are fully formed at birth and have characteristic clinical features and evolution. In addition, immunohistochemical staining of the tissue demonstrates that these tumors are Glut1 negative. Congenital hemangiomas are sub-classified based on how they evolve over time as rapidly involuting congenital hemangioma (RICH) or non-involuting congenital hemangioma (NICH).

Clinical Findings

Non-involuting congenital hemangiomas tend to be pink to purple in color, round to ovoid

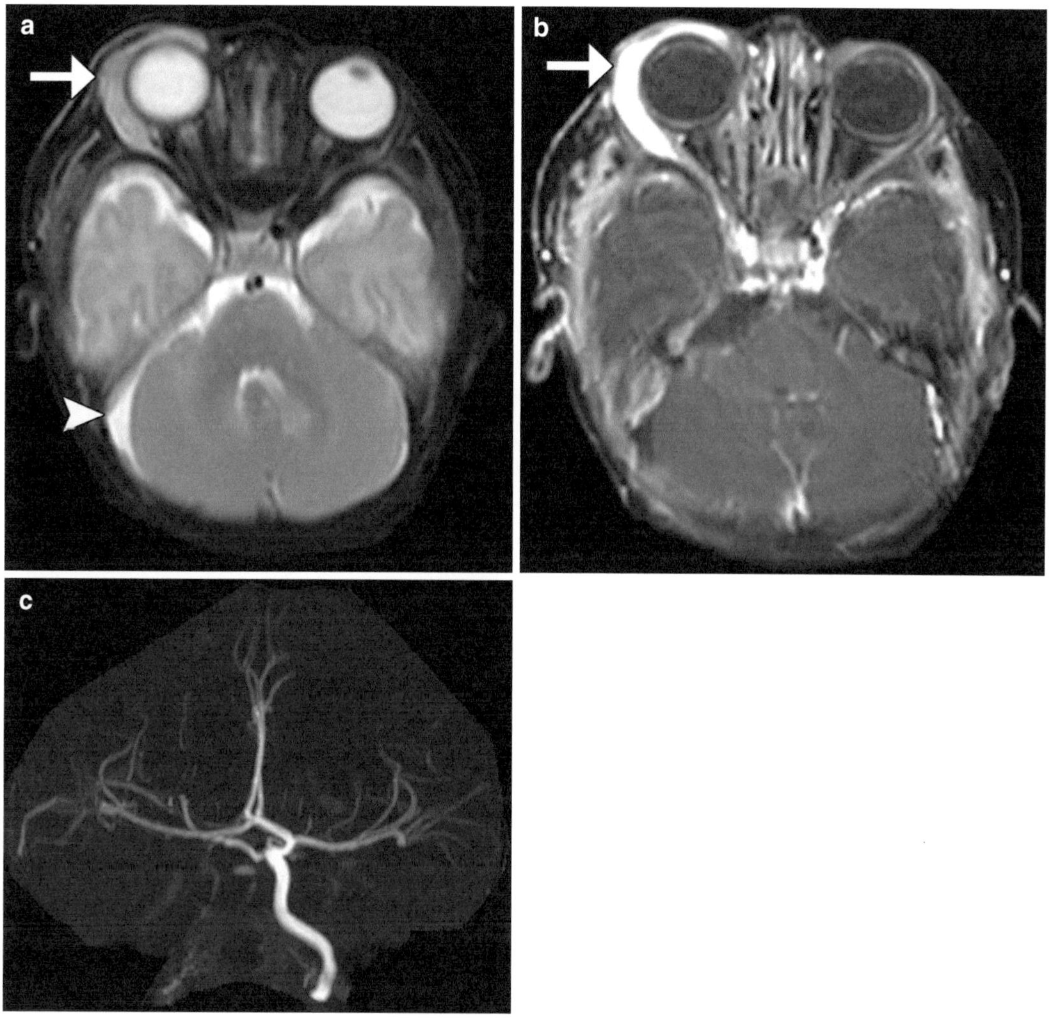

Fig. 7.6 PHACES syndrome. Axial T2-weighted (**a**) and fat-suppressed post-contrast T1-weighted (**b**) MR images demonstrate an enhancing right extraconal hemangioma (arrows). There is also asymmetric prominence of the extra-axial cerebrospinal fluid space along the right cerebellar convexity (arrowhead). In addition, there is diffuse right face skin thickening and enhancement. The 3D MIP MRA (**c**) demonstrates a hypoplastic right internal carotid artery

in shape, and demonstrate prominent overlying telangiectasias with a peripheral blanched pale halo. Rapidly involuting congenital hemangiomas may present similarly to a NICH, or more like that of a typical infantile hemangioma. RICH that undergo rapid involution become softer, flatter, and smaller over weeks to months, with complete involution generally by 12–15 months of age, often leaving residual dermal and subcutaneous atrophy (Fig. 7.7).

Radiology Findings

Sonographic and MR imaging features are similar to that of infantile hemangiomas (Fig. 7.8). Characteristics that favor congenital hemangiomas include intravascular thrombi, ill-defined margins, aneurysms, increased venous component, and areas of arteriovenous shunting. Rapidly involuting congenital hemangiomas tend to appear heterogeneous and have larger flow voids. Fat stranding is found to be slightly more common in non-involuting congenital hemangiomas.

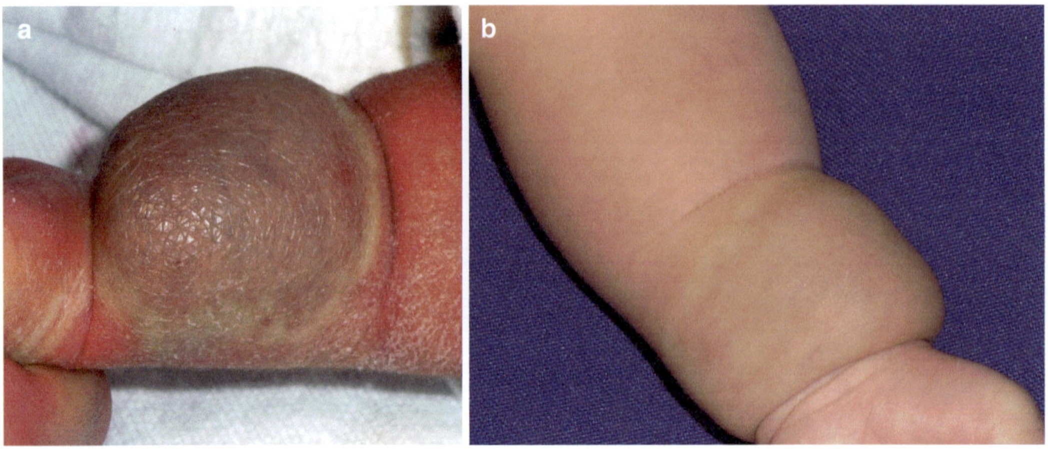

Fig. 7.7 Rapidly involuting congenital hemangioma (RICH). Photograph at 5 days of age shows an exophytic bluish pink mass with surrounding blanched halo (**a**). Photograph obtained at 3 months of age shows that the mass has flattened considerably and lightened to a pinkish blanched hue (**b**)

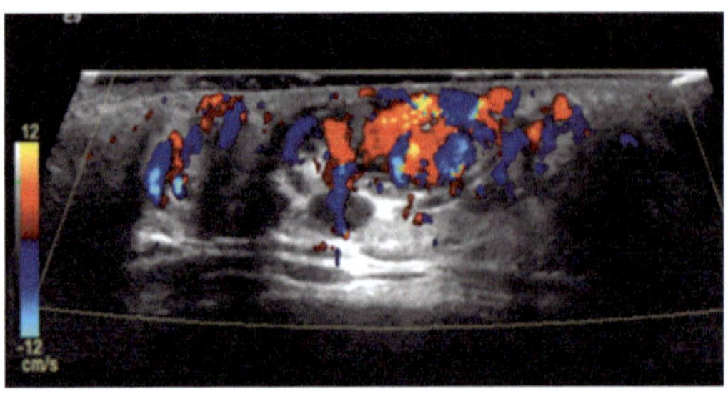

Fig. 7.8 Congenital hemangioma. Doppler ultrasound shows a superficial lesion with prominent low-flow vascularity

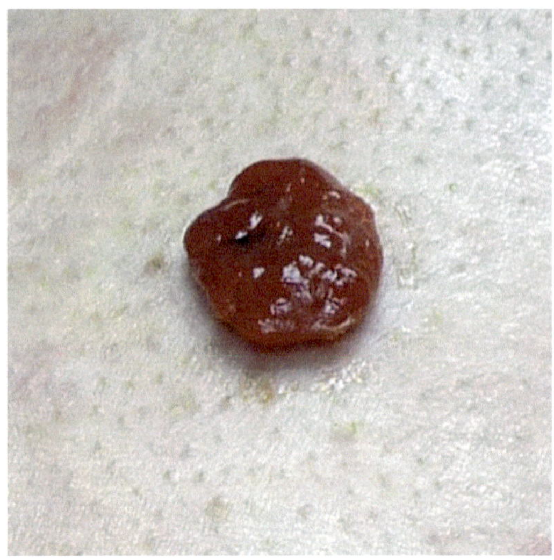

Fig. 7.9 Lobular capillary hemangioma. Photograph shows a bright red exophytic vascular nodule with a shiny, moist, friable surface

Lobular Capillary Hemangioma

> **Overview**
>
> Lobular capillary hemangioma (pyogenic granuloma) is a benign vascular tumor of the skin and mucosa with onset outside of the neonatal period. The tumor consists of a capillary proliferation likely precipitated by minor trauma or possibly the result of hormonal influences.

Clinical Findings

Lobular capillary hemangiomas in the skin appear as localized pedunculated bright red vascular nodules (Fig. 7.9). The lesions frequently bleed as a result of the friable surface. Lobular capillary hemangiomas may occur during pregnancy, with increasing incidence during the third trimester.

Radiology Findings

Lobular capillary hemangiomas appear as sharply marginated tumors with increased echogenicity on ultrasound, with increased blood flow on Doppler images. On MRI, the lesion demonstrates isointense signal to muscle on T1 and increased signal intensity on T2-weighted

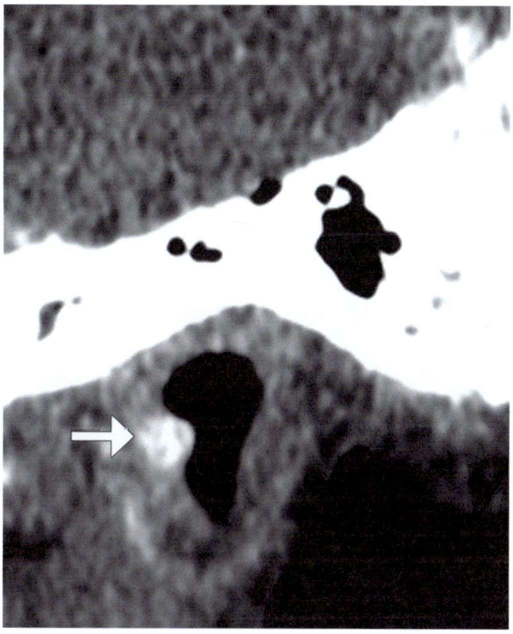

Fig. 7.10 Lobular capillary hemangioma. Sagittal post-contrast CT image demonstrates an avidly enhancing nodular lesion in the anterior external auditory canal (arrow)

images. The lesions display avid enhancement on post-contrast CT and MRI (Fig. 7.10).

Vascular Malformations

Arteriovenous Malformations

Overview
Arteriovenous malformations consist of feeding arteries and draining veins connected by a nidus of tortuous vascular channels without an intervening capillary bed. Complications include high output heart failure, arterial steal phenomenon, cutaneous ischemia and ulceration, osseous overgrowth, and hemorrhage.

Clinical Findings

Arteriovenous malformations in the superficial head and neck soft tissues present as masses with a reddish to bluish hue, and on palpation feel like a collection of vascular channels, or worm-like.

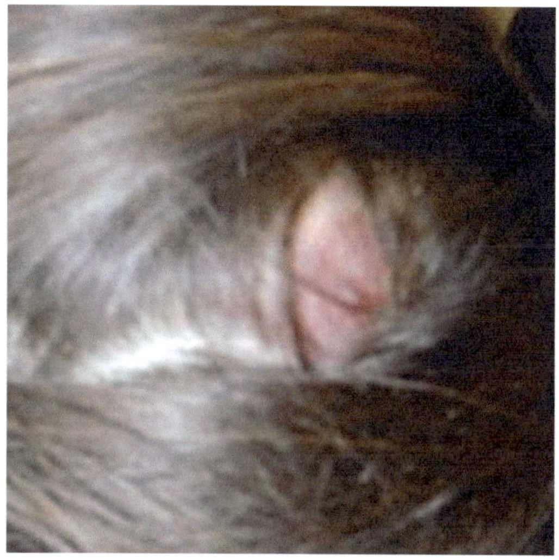

Fig. 7.11 Arteriovenous malformation. Photograph shows a mass in the scalp with reddish skin discoloration

These masses are often pulsatile and may demonstrate a systolic bruit or thrill (Fig. 7.11). Scalp arteriovenous malformations sometimes have a cirsoid aneurysm or varicose configuration and may be prone to hemorrhage.

Imaging Findings

Imaging of arteriovenous malformations is generally performed for treatment planning. CTA or MRA can often effectively delineate the enlarged and tortuous feeding arteries and early-draining veins, which typically have a serpiginous configuration (Fig. 7.12). Ultimately, digital subtraction angiography remains the gold standard modality and allows endovascular embolization, when needed (Fig. 7.13).

Venous Malformations

Overview
Venous malformations are congenital slow-flow vascular malformations that represent a non-proliferative collection of abnormal vessels. Venous malformations can occur in any part of the body, but head and neck region tends to be most commonly involved. These anomalies can be classified as isolated malformations without venous drain-

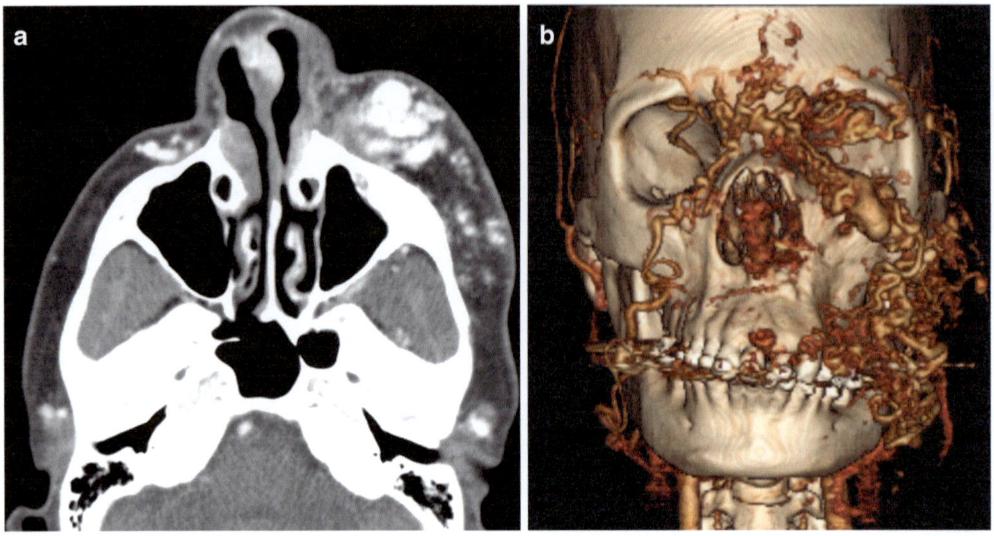

Fig. 7.12 Arteriovenous malformation. Axial (**a**) and 3D (**b**) CTA images demonstrates numerous enlarged serpiginous feeding arteries and draining veins in the face

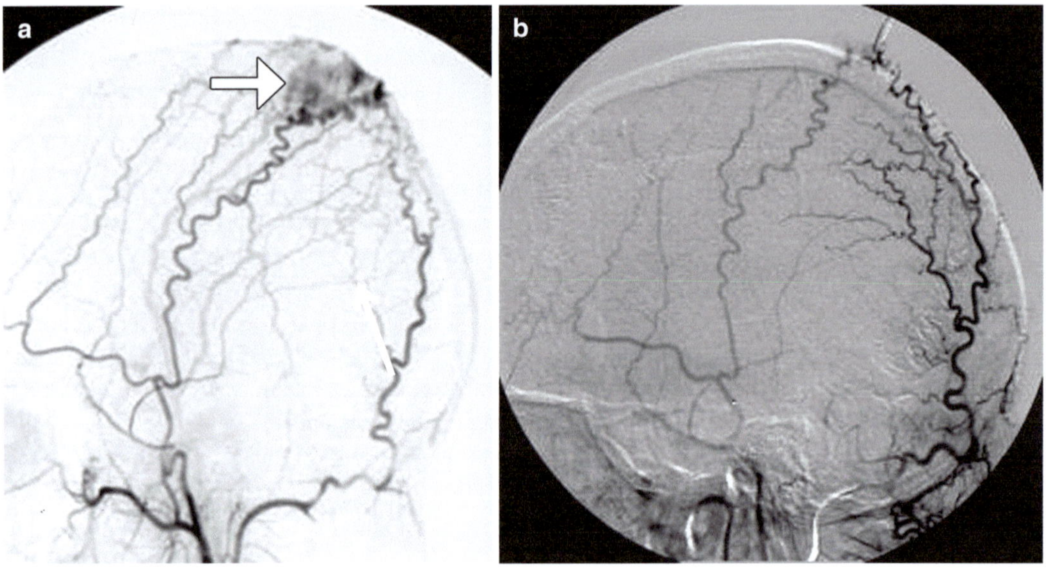

Fig. 7.13 Arteriovenous malformation. Initial digital subtraction angiogram shows a nidus (arrow) supplied by the superficial temporal and occipital artery branches with early venous drainage (**a**). DSA obtained during the late arterial phase after direct injection of glue shows resolution of the arteriovenous malformation without early venous drainage (**b**)

age; malformations that drain into normal veins; malformations that drain into dysplastic veins; and malformations consisting primarily of venous ectasia. These malformations can occur in isolation, but can also be components of various syndromes, including blue rubber bleb syndrome (Bean syndrome) and familial cerebral cavernous malformation syndrome (CCM). Blue rubber bleb syndrome is characterized by multiple venous malformations in the skin and gastrointestinal tract.

Clinical Findings

Superficial venous malformations typically appear as blue to purple, soft, compressible, non-pulsatile nodules, or as a discrete soft-tissue mass with a blue-purple hue (Fig. 7.14), sometimes with prominent surrounding veins. The lesions can be observed to enlarge with Valsalva maneuver or the application of a tourniquet. The malformations may also expand with trauma or thrombosis and during puberty or pregnancy. Approximately 9% of patients with familial CCM demonstrate cutaneous lesions, particularly patients with the CCM1 mutation, which encodes KRIT1 (krev interaction trapped 1).

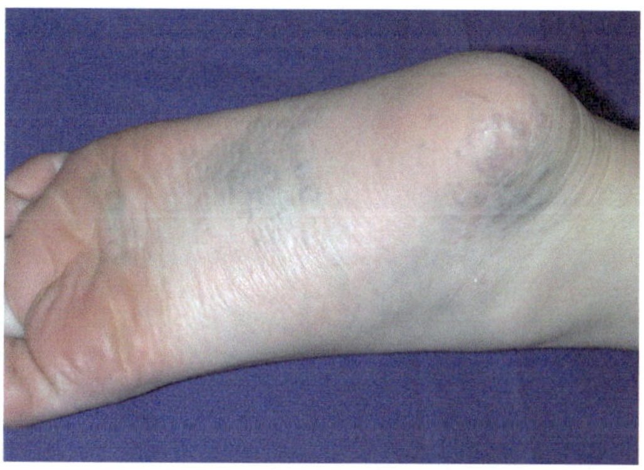

Fig. 7.14 Venous malformations. Photograph shows multiple clusters of deep purple papules on the plantar foot and lateral heel

Imaging Findings

Diagnostic imaging can be useful for confirming the diagnosis of venous malformation and assessing the extent of disease since there can be involvement of deeper tissues than may be apparent on clinical examination. Ultrasound with color Doppler is often the first-line imaging modality for the evaluation of suspected venous malformations. Superficial venous malformations are compressible and generally display heterogeneous echotexture. Deeper venous malformations appear as well-defined, spongiform masses or as infiltrative, tortuous, and beaded vascular channels with typical venous waveforms.

MRI is a particularly useful imaging modality for evaluating the deep lesions in patients with blue rubber bleb syndrome. On MRI, the malformations appear as T2 hyperintense tumors that may contain septations and typically avidly enhance, but flow voids tend to be lacking (Fig. 7.15). Notably, venous malformations may undergo hemorrhage, imparting a heterogeneous appearance on imaging. The lesions can be well-defined or infiltrative. Well-defined lesions tend to have superior outcomes after percutaneous sclerotherapy.

MRI is also the modality of choice to evaluate for cerebral cavernous malformations, which tend to be numerous in patients with KRIT1

Fig. 7.15 Blue rubber bleb syndrome. Axial fat-suppressed T2-weighted MRI shows numerous T2-hyperintense, enhancing subcutaneous, intramuscular, and intrathyroidal venous malformations

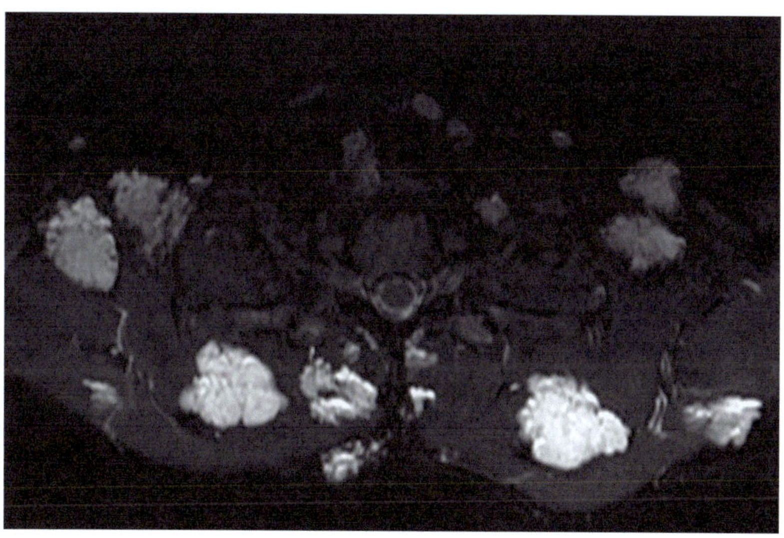

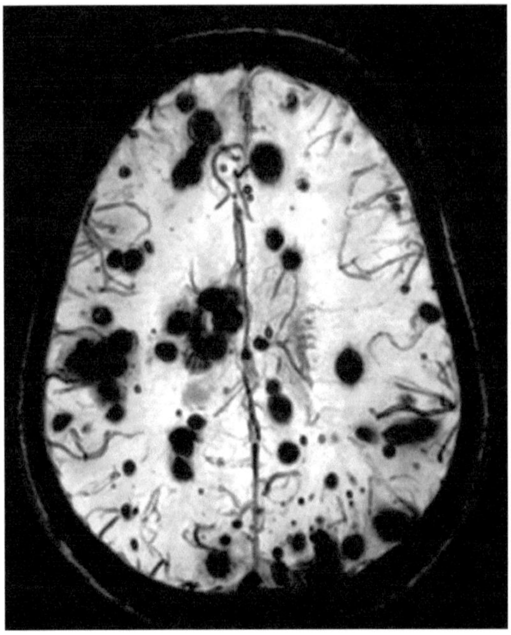

Fig. 7.16 Familial CCM syndrome. Axial SWI MRI shows numerous low signal lesions in the bilateral cerebral hemispheres

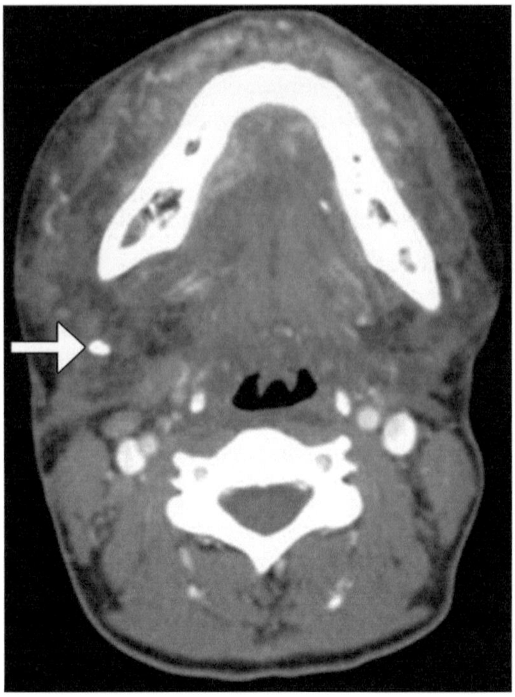

Fig. 7.17 Venous malformation. Axial post-contrast CT image demonstrates an infiltrative lesion involving the skin and underlying soft tissues of the face, with a phlebolith (arrow)

mutations. In particular, the lesions are most conspicuous on T2* gradient echo or susceptibility-weighted sequences due to associated prominent low signal blooming effect (Fig. 7.16). In addition, patients with familial cerebral cavernous malformations tend to have an increased number of white matter lesions.

Although CT plays a relatively limited role in the assessment of venous malformations, this modality can readily depict the presence of phleboliths, which are highly suggestive of the diagnosis (Fig. 7.17).

Percutaneous sclerotherapy with ethanol causes nearly instantaneous endothelial death and thrombosis, followed shortly after by exuberant edema. The lesion will shrink and fibrose over the weeks following treatment. Evaluation of the treatment response with imaging should be performed several months after the therapy to allow for resolution of inflammation, as T2 signal hyperintensity can persist up to 3 months after treatment.

Sinus Pericranii

Overview

Sinus pericranii is a rare abnormal communication between the intracranial dural sinuses and the epicranial venous system, most often through an emissary transosseous vein. Contraindications to treatment include venous drainage of crucial brain area through the malformation, significant amount of blood drainage through the abnormality, and risk of severe bleeding or brain ischemia from venous hypertension. Surgical treatment is reserved for complex cases with other associated anomalies and malformations, cases of intracranial hemorrhage, or cases that have failed endovascular treatment.

Clinical Findings

Skin manifestations of sinus pericranii are variable and may resemble other vascular disorders of the scalp and cranium. Patients can present with a non-pulsatile compressible soft-tissue mass that can enlarge with increased venous pressure. The majority of sinus pericranii are in the midline frontal region. Up to 20% of patients have associated venous malformations elsewhere. Complications include hemorrhage, infection, and thrombosis.

Imaging Findings

Imaging is utilized to confirm the diagnosis of sinus pericranii and evaluate for potential complications. Doppler ultrasound is useful for demonstrating the low-flow character of these lesions and at least a portion of the intracranial connection (Fig. 7.18). However, CT/CTV, MRI/MRA, and digital subtraction can more comprehensively depict the extent of sinus pericranii (Fig. 7.19) Well-defined bone defects in the calvarium through which the anomalous vessels pass may be observed on CT. Areas of non-enhancement in the veins may be apparent and suggest the presence of thrombus. Digital subtraction angiography is useful for assessing flow dynamics, particularly in the case of pretreatment planning. Depending on the amount of blood being drained into the sinus pericranii from particular portions of brain parenchyma, endovascular intervention via coiling or embolization may be an option.

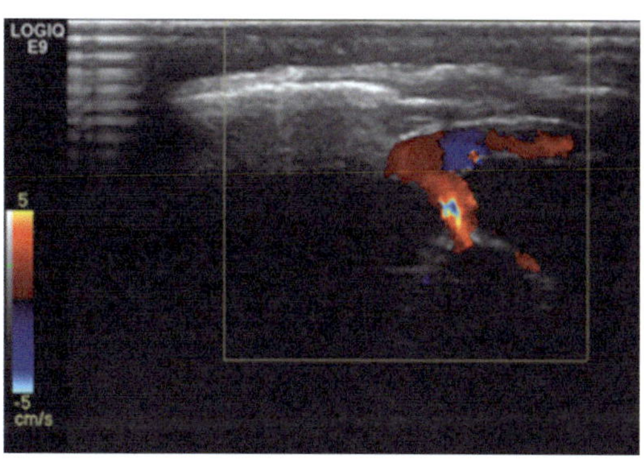

Fig. 7.18 Sinus pericranii. Doppler ultrasound shows communication between a scalp vein and a dural venous sinus

Capillary Malformations

> **Overview**
> Capillary malformations are composed of dilated capillaries and venules. There are several patterns and morphologies of capillary malformation, such as nevus simplex, port-wine stain, reticulated, geographic, capillary malformation–arteriovenous malformation, cutis marmorata telangiectatica congenita, and telangiectasia.

Clinical Findings

The clinical features of capillary malformations depend upon the pattern and morphology as follows:

- Nevus simplex (salmon patch, angel kiss, stork bite) is the most common vascular lesion seen in newborns. These lesions tend to be pink to red flat patches with irregular borders, located in a characteristic midline location at the nape of the neck and posterior scalp, over the glabella, or on the medial aspect of the upper eyelids (Fig. 7.20). These lesions are usually isolated findings without associated abnormalities and likely represent persistence of the fetal circulation rather than a true malformation.
- Port-wine stain (nevus flammeus) appears as a well-demarcated flat confluent pink to dark red patch that may be an isolated finding or associated with a variety of syndromes, such as Sturge-Weber syndrome (Fig. 7.21).
- Reticulated capillary malformations are often diffuse or multifocal with indistinct borders and are composed of a fine network of vascular markings (Fig. 7.22). They may be an isolated finding or associated with bone or soft-tissue overgrowth.
- Geographic capillary malformations are well-demarcated, dark red, confluent patches in the shape of a continent or landmass on a map (Fig. 7.23). There is an increased incidence of associated lymphatic-venous malformations

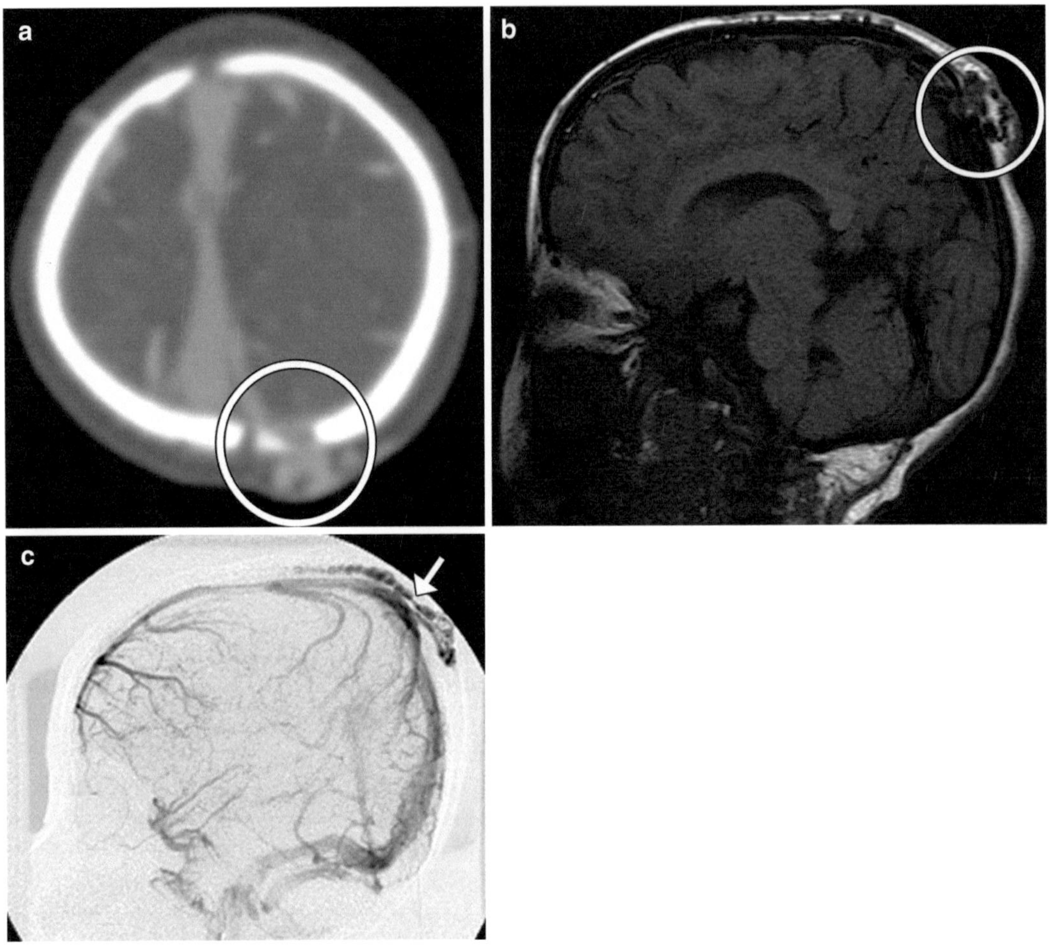

Fig. 7.19 Sinus pericranii. Axial CTV (**a**), sagittal MRI (**b**), and digital subtraction angiogram (**c**) show enlarged veins in the left scalp (encircled) that communicate with the intracerebral veins. An associated calvarial defect is apparent on the CT

and other anomalies, as seen in syndromes such as CLOVES and Klippel-Trenaunay.

- Capillary malformation–arteriovenous malformation syndrome describes a familial condition associated with mutations of the RASA1 gene. The cutaneous capillary malformations of this disorder are typically multiple, in a scattered distribution, and are a rusty red-brown in color, occasionally with a surrounding pale halo (Fig. 7.24). AVMs are also a part of this syndrome and may be cutaneous, subcutaneous, intramuscular, intraosseous, or cerebral, and are often not associated with the cutaneous capillary malformations.
- Cutis marmorata telangiectatica congenita describes a localized mottling of the skin that resembles physiologic cutis marmorata of the newborn, but doesn't resolve with rewarming. The lesions are red to violaceous, stellate, or marble-like patches, sometimes with associated prominent veins, telangiectasia, and atrophy (Fig. 7.25). Overlying ulceration may also be present.
- Telangiectasias are small flat clusters of thin, branching, pink to red vessels visible on the skin surface (Fig. 7.26). The vessels will blanch with pressure. Telangiectasias are common and most often insignificant, but rarely can be the

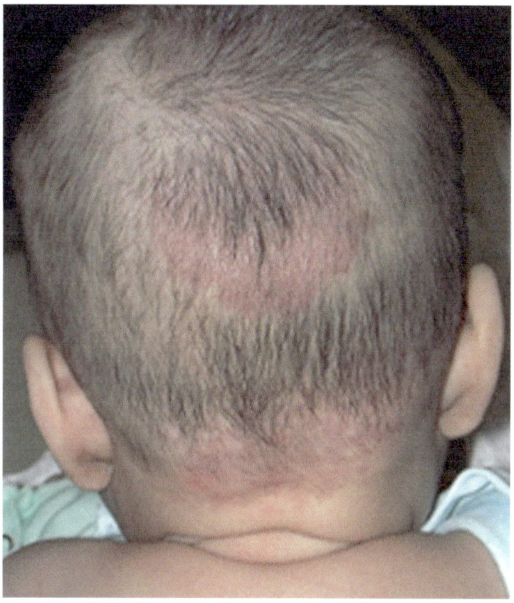

Fig. 7.20 Nevus simplex. Photograph shows pink vascular patches overlying the posterior scalp and at the nape of the neck

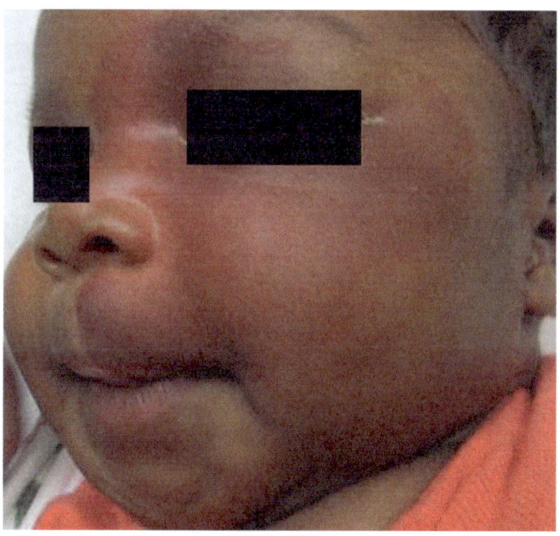

Fig. 7.21 Port-wine stain. Photograph shows a well-demarcated confluent red purple patch on the left face in a patient with Sturge-Weber syndrome

result of co-existing cutaneous atrophy (such as corticosteroid-induced atrophy or solar damage) or metabolic derangements, or may occur in the setting of genetic conditions such as hereditary benign telangiectasia, unilateral nevoid telangiectasia, hereditary hemorrhagic telangiectasia (Osler-Weber-Rendu syndrome), and ataxia telangiectasia.

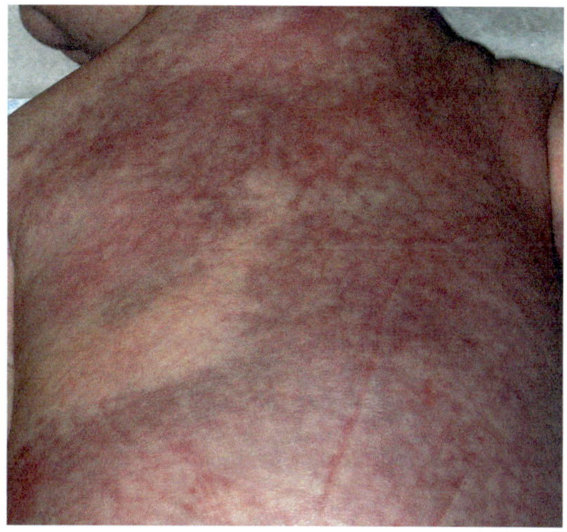

Fig. 7.22 Reticulated capillary malformation. Photograph shows a network of reddish vascular markings over the back with skip areas

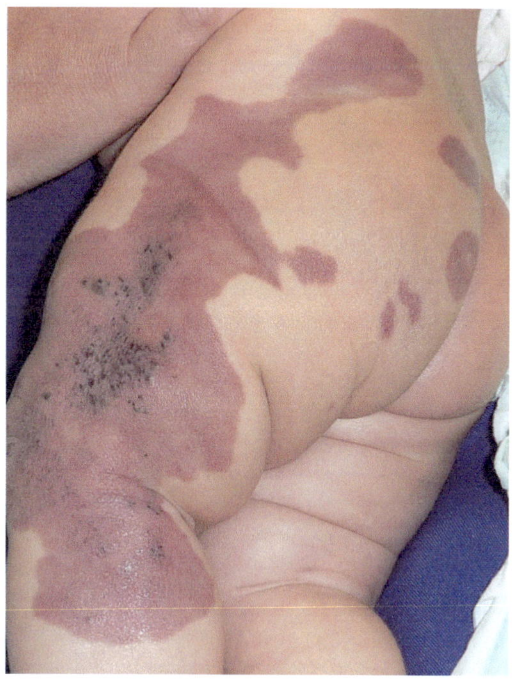

Fig. 7.23 Geographic capillary malformation. Photograph shows well-demarcated purple-red confluent figurate patches with dark purple overlying papules indicating a lymphatic component within the malformation

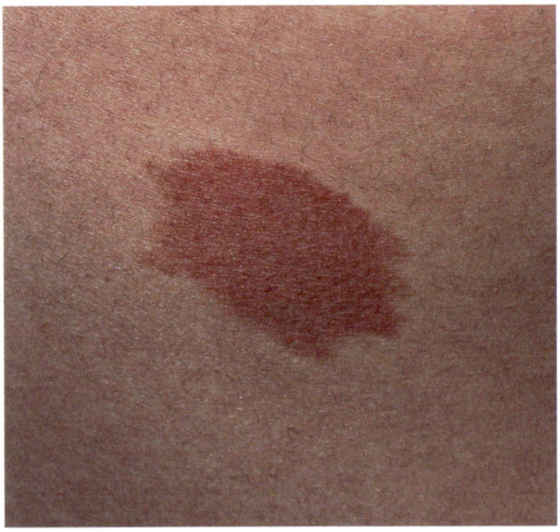

Fig. 7.24 Capillary malformation–arteriovenous malformation syndrome. Photograph shows a rusty brown well-demarcated macule in a patient with RASA1 mutation

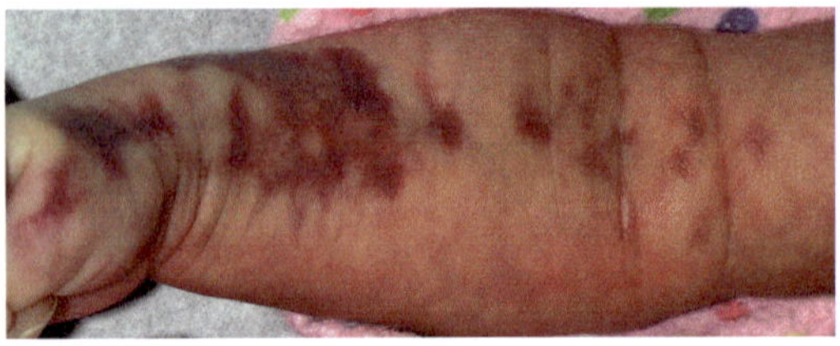

Fig. 7.25 Cutis marmorata telangiectatica congenita. Photograph shows violaceous stellate and reticulated vascular markings resembling accentuated mottling

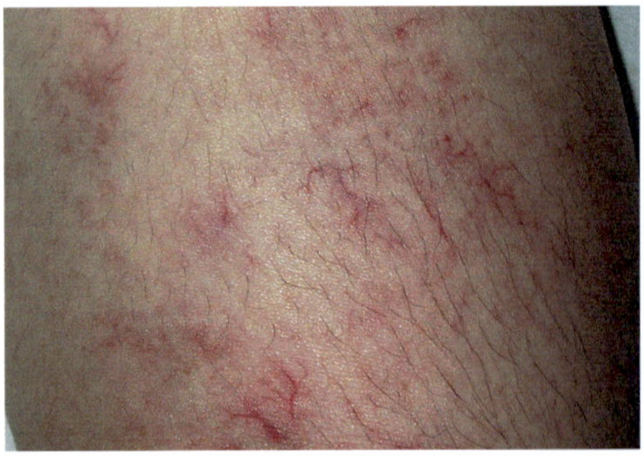

Fig. 7.26 Telangiectasia. Photograph shows scattered fine, red, branching, superficial vascular markings

Imaging Findings

Cutaneous capillary malformations do not necessarily have discernible imaging correlates. However, associated abnormalities can have manifestations on neuroimaging. For example, pulmonary arteriovenous malformations are common in patients with hereditary hemorrhagic telangiectasia and can predispose to cerebral infarction and intracranial abscesses (Fig. 7.27). In addition, 10–20% of patients have a vascular malformation in the brain, including high flow pial fistulas, nidus type brain arteriovenous malformations, often associated with aneurysms (Fig. 7.28), and microarteriovenous malformations, which are capillary malformations and do not demonstrate shunting. Other conditions associated with capillary malformations are described in the "Vascular Malformations Associated with Other Anomalies" section.

Lymphatic Malformations

Overview

Lymphatic malformations are low-flow simple vascular malformations that most commonly involve the subcutaneous tissues, with up to 80% occurring in the head and neck region. These malformations are classically transspatial, whereby multiple tissue planes can be involved. Lymphatic malformations can be macrocystic with cystic compartments measuring greater than 1 cm, microcystic, or a combination. In some cases, lymphatic malformations cause mass effect on adjacent structures, which can lead to soft-tissue and osseous hypertrophy. Alternatively, lymphatic malformations can induce osteolysis, such as in the case of Gorham-Stout syndrome.

Clinical Findings

Lymphatic malformations are typically evident during early childhood and may expand, particularly when hemorrhage into the malformation occurs. There is a wide range of clinical presentations associated with lymphatic malformations. Some lesions present as clusters of skin-colored to purple red papules and translucent vesicle-like structures, which are typically soft, but not necessarily compressible

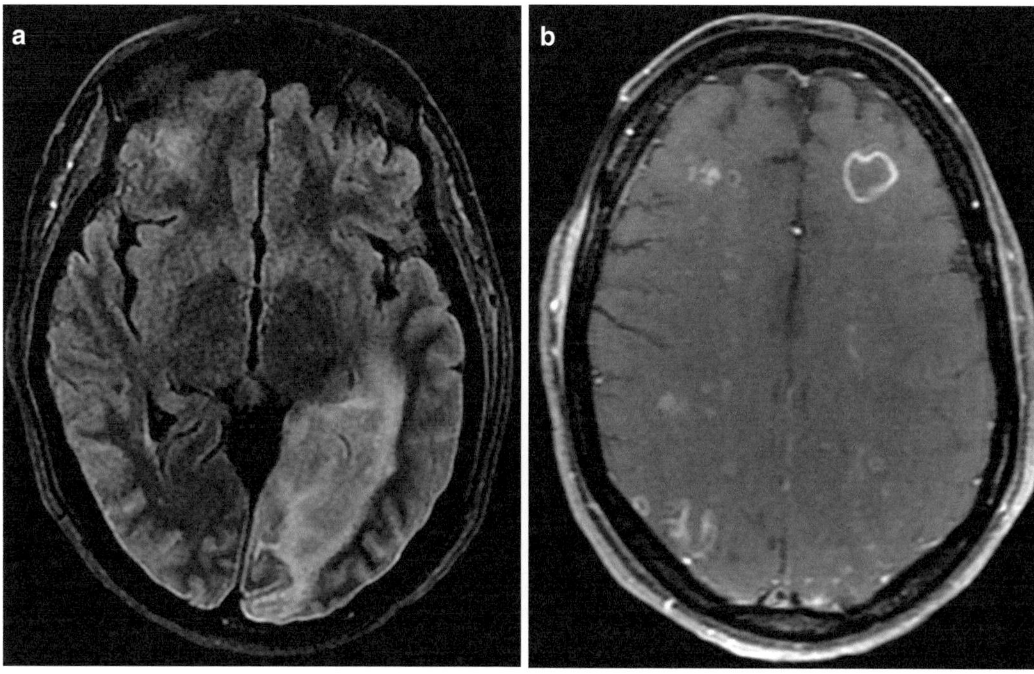

Fig. 7.27 Hereditary hemorrhagic telangiectasia. Axial T2-weighted FLAIR MRI (**a**) shows a large subacute infarct in the left posterior cerebral artery territory. Axial post-contrast T1-weighted MRI in the same patient (**b**) shows multiple ring-enhancing lesions in the bilateral cerebral hemispheres that represent septic embolic with abscess formation

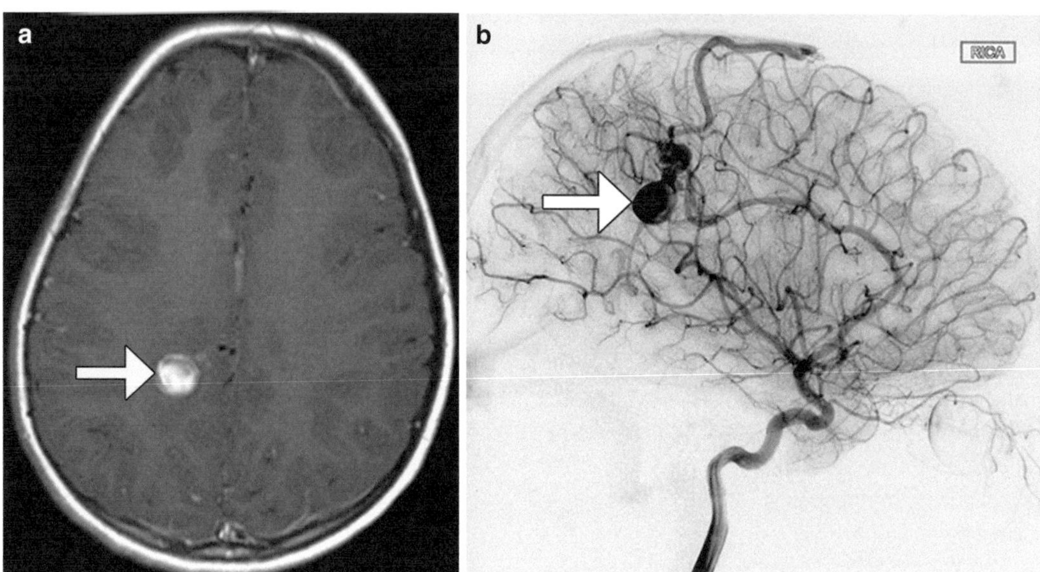

Fig. 7.28 Hereditary hemorrhagic telangiectasia. Axial post-contrast T1-weighted MRI (**a**) shows an enhancing lesion in the right paracentral lobule, which represents an aneurysm (arrow). Catheter digital subtraction angiography image (**b**) shows an atypical arteriovenous malformation with an associated aneurysm (arrow)

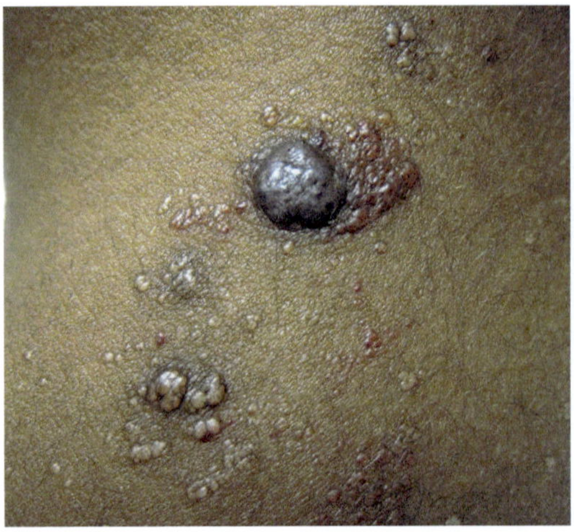

Fig. 7.29 Lymphatic malformation. Photograph shows scattered and clustered, shiny, translucent papules and vesicles with intermixed red to purple papules and nodules

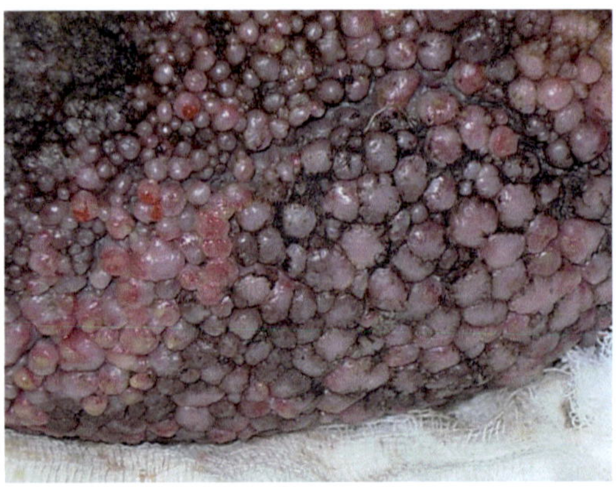

Fig. 7.30 Lymphatic malformation. Photograph shows extensive coalescing pink and flesh-colored shiny and translucent papules and nodules in the scalp

(Fig. 7.29). Alternatively, tumorous soft-tissue masses, or regions of apparent extensive cutaneous swelling are present (Fig. 7.30). The lesions typically transilluminate and are not pulsatile. Lymphatic malformations are prone to developing secondary infection.

Imaging Findings

Although lymphatic malformations may be suspected clinically based on history and physical examination, imaging is usually necessary to confirm the diagnosis, evaluate the extent of the lesion, and for treatment planning, which may entail percutaneous sclerotherapy. Ultrasound is often the first-line imaging modality in the workup of suspected superficial lymphatic malformations. MRI is necessary to investigate deep and extensive lesions, particularly including multiplanar STIR or T2-weighted sequences with fat suppression and pre- and post-contrast T1-weighted sequences.

On ultrasound, lymphatic malformations most commonly appear as multiloculated cystic masses with imperceptible walls and anechoic contents, unless there has been superimposed infection or hemorrhage. Similarly on MRI, lymphatic malformations typically appear as septated with fluid signal and no flow voids, although fluid levels may be present secondary to hemorrhage (Fig. 7.31). There may be fine enhancement of the capsule and septations. The enhancement may be more pronounced when infected and may be accompanied by fat stranding.

CT is useful for delineating the degree of osteolysis in patients with Gorham-Stout syndrome (Fig. 7.32). The degree of bone resorption can be vast and associated with pathological fractures. MRI may reveal associated edema and enhancement in the areas surrounding the osteolysis.

Vascular Malformations Associated with Other Anomalies

Overview

Many conditions can feature at least one type of vascular malformation associated with non-vascular lesions. Some such syndromes include the following:

- *Klippel-Trenaunay syndrome*: capillary, venous, and/or lymphatic malformations with limb overgrowth.
- *Beckwith-Wiedemann syndrome*: capillary malformation with limb overgrowth, abdominal wall defect, temporal bone anomalies, renal anomalies, and increased risk for embryonal tumors.

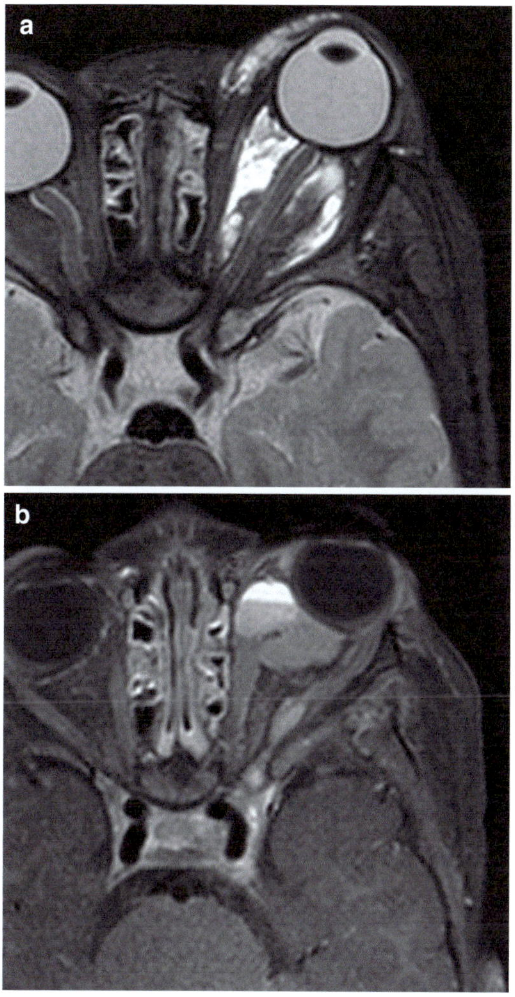

Fig. 7.31 Lymphatic malformation. Axial fat-suppressed T2-weighted (**a**) and fat-suppressed post-contrast T1-weighted (**b**) MR images show a transparatial loculated mass with fluid-fluid levels that involves the left periorbital and orbital soft tissues with associated proptosis

- *Sturge-Weber syndrome*: cutaneous facial and leptomeningeal capillary malformations with eye anomalies and/or bone and soft-tissue overgrowth (refer to Chap. 3).
- *Maffucci syndrome*: venous malformations with or without spindle-cell hemangioendothelioma and enchondromas, with heightened risk for chondrosarcoma.

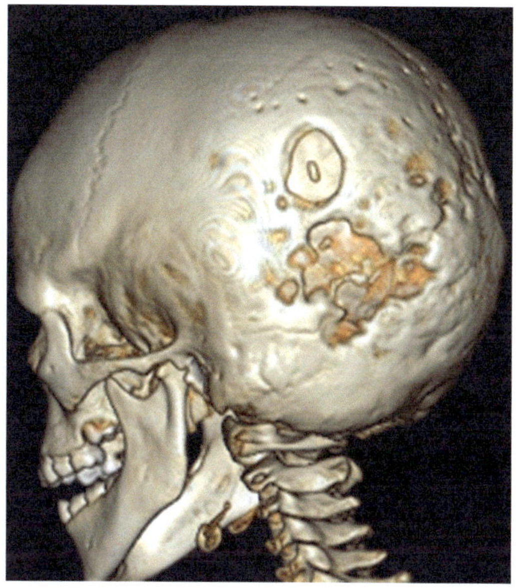

Fig. 7.32 Gorham-Stout syndrome. 3D CT image shows multiple lytic lesions in the skull

- *CLOVES syndrome*: capillary, venous, and lymphatic malformations and/or arteriovenous malformation with lipomatous overgrowth and spinal and skeletal anomalies.
- *Proteus syndrome*: capillary, venous, and/or lymphatic malformations with asymmetric overgrowth, connective tissue hamartomas of the palms and soles, and lipomas.

Clinical Findings

- *Klippel-Trenaunay syndrome*: Comprises the triad of vascular malformations, varicose veins, and bone and soft-tissue hyperplasia. The vascular malformation is most often a capillary malformation present from birth and ranging from light pink to dark red or purple in color which may be fairly localized to extensive in distribution. Geographic vascular stains are associated with a higher risk of complications and associated lymphatic malformations. These geographic stains appear red to deep purple, often with superficial vascular blebs and pseudoverrucous papules. Prominent superficial veins may be present, with varicosities developing with age. Hypertrophy of the affected body part presents with increased limb girth and length due to soft-tissue and fat overgrowth, as well as sometimes even bony hypertrophy. Soft tissue and vascular overgrowth can also affect the head and neck region in an asymmetric manner and can be complicated by stroke, intracranial hemorrhage, and headaches, for example.

- *Beckwith-Wiedemann syndrome*: An overgrowth syndrome characterized by macrosomia and macroglossia, persistent mid-facial nevus simplex, abdominal wall defects, neonatal hypoglycemia, visceromegaly, and renal anomalies. In addition, these patients have predisposition for several types of neoplasms, including Wilms tumor, rhabdomyosarcoma, hepatoblastoma, and adrenal tumors. The clinical diagnosis is based on clinical and imaging identification of the constellation of findings. The facial capillary malformations appear similar to nevus simplex and tend to involve the midforehead, glabella, and upper eyelids with occasional extension to the nose and upper lip.
- *Maffucci syndrome*: Rare sporadic genetic disorder characterized by enchondromatosis and multiple venous malformations. In the neck, the cricoid cartilage is the most common location for enchondromas, while in the skull, enchondromas most commonly involve the sphenoid bone. Enchondromas undergo malignant transformation into chondrosarcomas in approximately 15–20% of patients. Other neoplasms in the head and neck region associated with Maffuci syndrome include pituitary adenoma, olfactory neuroblastoma, malignant chordoma, and spindle-cell hemangioendothelioma.
- *CLOVES syndrome*: Associated with PIK3CA mutation and consists of congenital lipomatous asymmetric overgrowth of the trunk with lymphatic, capillary, venous, and combined-type vascular malformations, epidermal nevi, and skeletal anomalies. Patients with this syndrome can present with neurological deficits and are also susceptible to thromboembolism.
- *Proteus syndrome*: Associated with AKT1 mutations and characterized by postnatal segmental overgrowth of multiple tissues, including skin, subcutis, connective tissues, CNS, and viscera. The disproportionate overgrowth may involve the extremities, skull, vertebrae, and external auditory meatus and are associated with dysmorphic facial features. Lipomas and fatty hyperplasia can be extensive. Cutaneous manifestations include connective tissue hamartomas primarily of the palms and soles, resulting in characteristic cerebriform hyperplasia. Epidermal nevi are frequently present. A variety of vascular malformations may occur, including capillary, venous, and lymphatic.

Imaging Findings

- *Klippel-Trenaunay syndrome*: Neuroimaging may reveal asymmetry of the cerebral and cerebellar hemispheres and associated vasculature (Fig. 7.33). In particular, the thickness of the gray matter is normal and there are no sulcation abnormalities, but the amount of the white matter is increased and there may be slightly reduced size of the ipsilateral lateral ventricle. Limb hypertrophy and cutaneous stigmata tend to be on the same side as the brain abnormality.
- *Beckwith-Wiedemann syndrome*: An enlarged tongue (glossomegaly) can be evident on head and neck imaging, which can be used to characterize the degree of airway narrowing (Fig. 7.34). Patients with conductive hearing loss may undergo temporal bone CT, which can reveal congenital stapedial fixation (Fig. 7.35). Stapedial fixation may be related to malformation of the second branchial arch. Imaging may also be used to evaluate for metastases from the various malignancies associated with Beckwith-Wiedemann syndrome.
- *Maffucci syndrome*: Besides assessing the venous malformations themselves, diagnostic imaging can also be useful for evaluating associated abnormalities, such as enchondromas and malignancies (Fig. 7.36).
- *CLOVES syndrome*: MRI is a suitable screening modality for patients with this syndrome. In particular, MRI (Fig. 7.37) can help define the type and extent of vascular malformations, scoliosis, tethered cord and spinal lipomas,

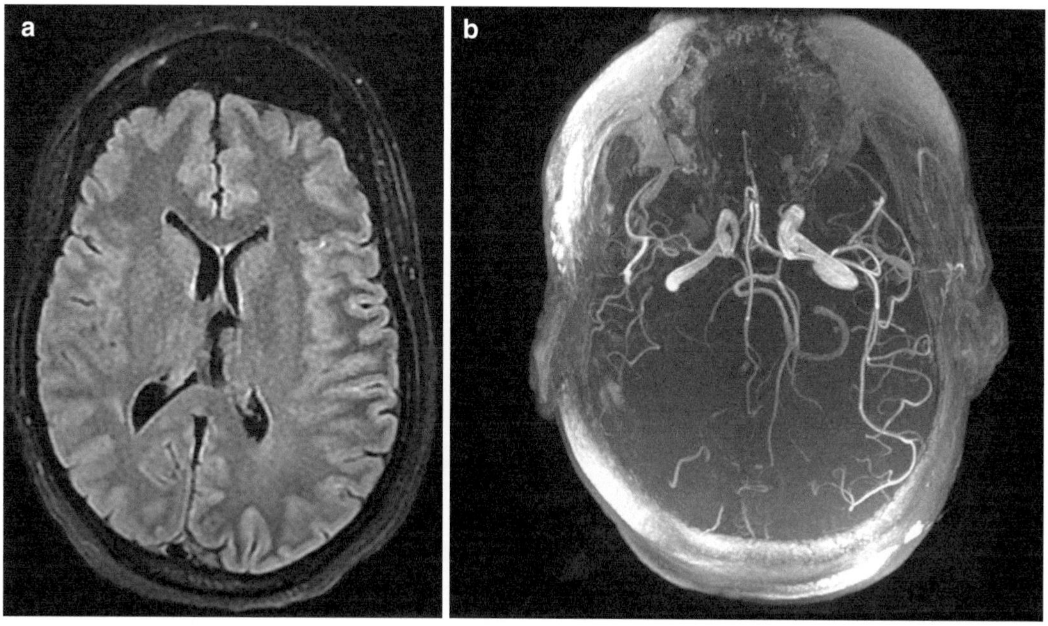

Fig. 7.33 Klippel-Trenaunay syndrome. Axial T2-weighted FLAIR MRI (**a**) and MIP MRA (**b**) show asymmetric enlargement of the left cerebral hemisphere due to increased white matter bulk diffusely and associated prominence of the ipsilateral cerebral arteries

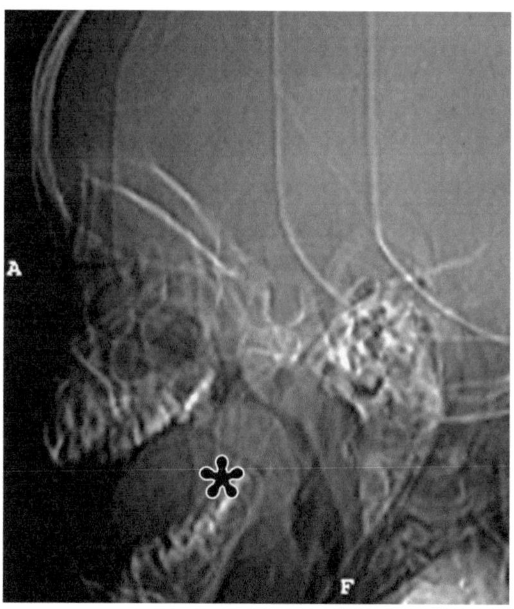

Fig. 7.34 Beckwith-Wiedemann syndrome. CT scout image shows glossomegaly (*) with narrowing of the oropharyngeal airway

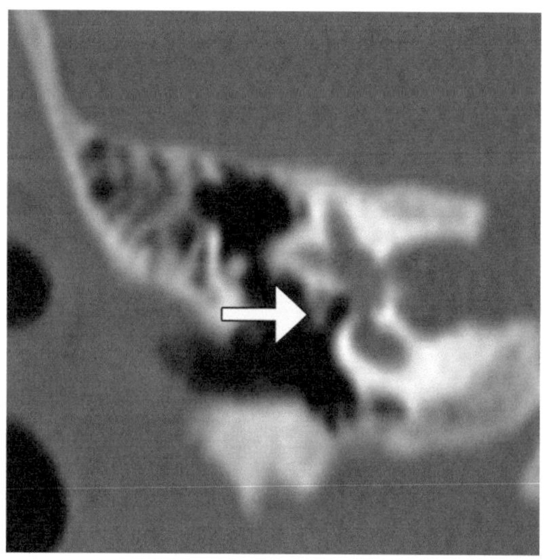

Fig. 7.35 Beckwith-Wiedemann syndrome. Coronal right temporal bone CT image shows that the stapes (arrow) abuts the tympanic segment of the facial nerve, causing conductive hearing loss

megalencephaly/hemimegalencephaly, Chiari malformation, and polymicrogyria.

- *Proteus syndrome*: Although the diagnosis is largely clinical, imaging can demonstrate skull enlargement (Fig. 7.38), asymmetric overgrowth of soft tissue, bones, or internal organs, fat hypertrophy, cystic lung disease, and thickening of the gastrointestinal walls.

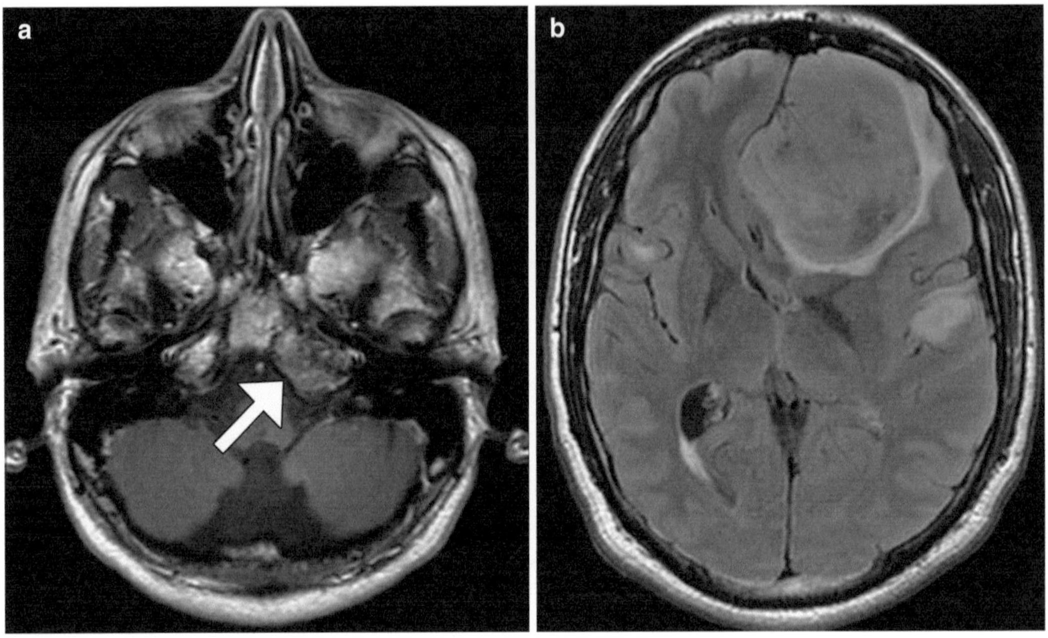

Fig. 7.36 Maffuci syndrome. Axial post-contrast T1-weighted MRI (**a**) demonstrates a mildly enhancing left skull base lesion (arrow), compatible with a chondroid matrix tumor. Axial T2-weighted MRI (**b**) demonstrates multiple brain tumors, which represent astrocytomas

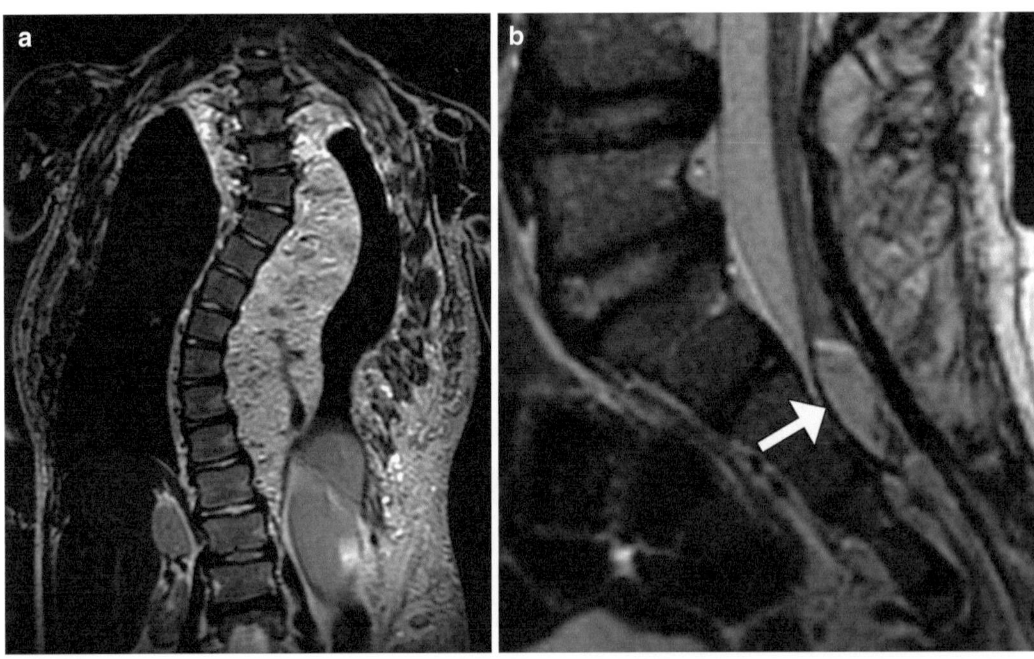

Fig. 7.37 CLOVES syndrome. Coronal (**a**) and sagittal (**b**) T2-weighted MRI images show scoliosis associated with extensive paraspinal and left chest and abdominal wall vascular malformations, as well as a low-lying tethered cord with an associated lipoma (arrow)

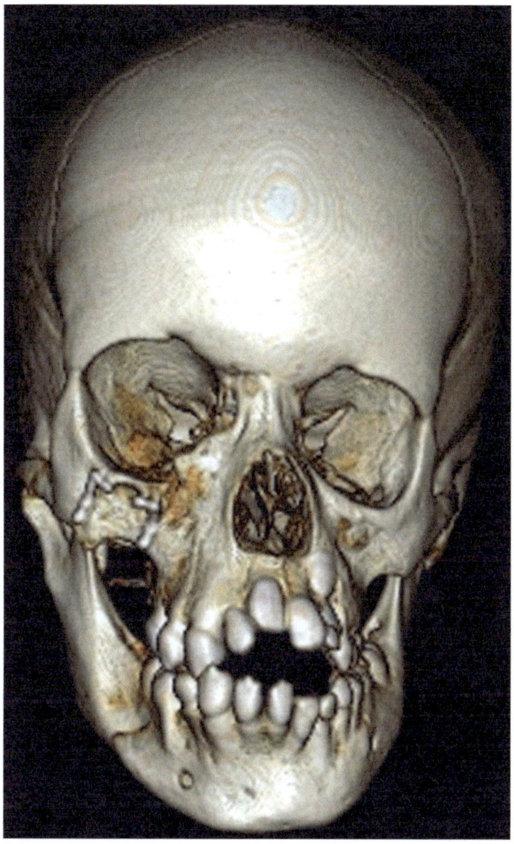

Fig. 7.38 Proteus syndrome. 3D CT image demonstrates hypoplasia of the left craniofacial skeleton

Coagulopathies and Hemoglobinopathies

Sickle Cell Disease

Overview

Sickle cell disease is a hemoglobinopathy caused by a mutation in the β-globin chain, which leads to polymerization of hemoglobin when deoxygenated. In turn, the polymerized hemoglobin causes red blood cells to assume a crescentic or sickle shape. The deformed and rigid erythrocytes tend to occlude arterioles, leading to hemolysis, ischemia, and inflammation.

Clinical Findings

There are numerous clinical manifestations of sickle cell disease, which can occur on an acute or chronic basis. Selected complications of sickle cell disease pertinent to the theme of this book include the following:

Primary central nervous system: silent cerebral infarcts, headache, ischemic and hemorrhagic stroke. Head, neck, and spine: labyrinthine hemorrhage, labyrinthitis ossificans, lacrimal gland swelling, orbital wall infarction, and subperiosteal hemorrhage or fluid, osteomyelitis, extramedullary hematopoiesis, bone marrow hyperplasia, iron deposition in bone marrow, as well as lymphoid hyperplasia, which may be a compensatory response for functional asplenia.

Cutaneous lesions: chronic ulcers from stagnant blood flow are common and usually involve the legs (Fig. 7.39). These typically appear "punched out," are painful, and may become infected.

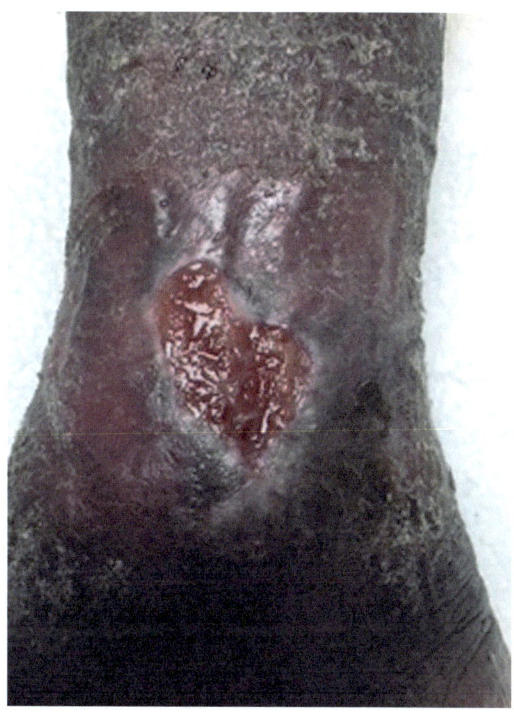

Fig. 7.39 Sickle cell disease. Photograph shows a leg ulcer. Courtesy of Ann Zmuda MD

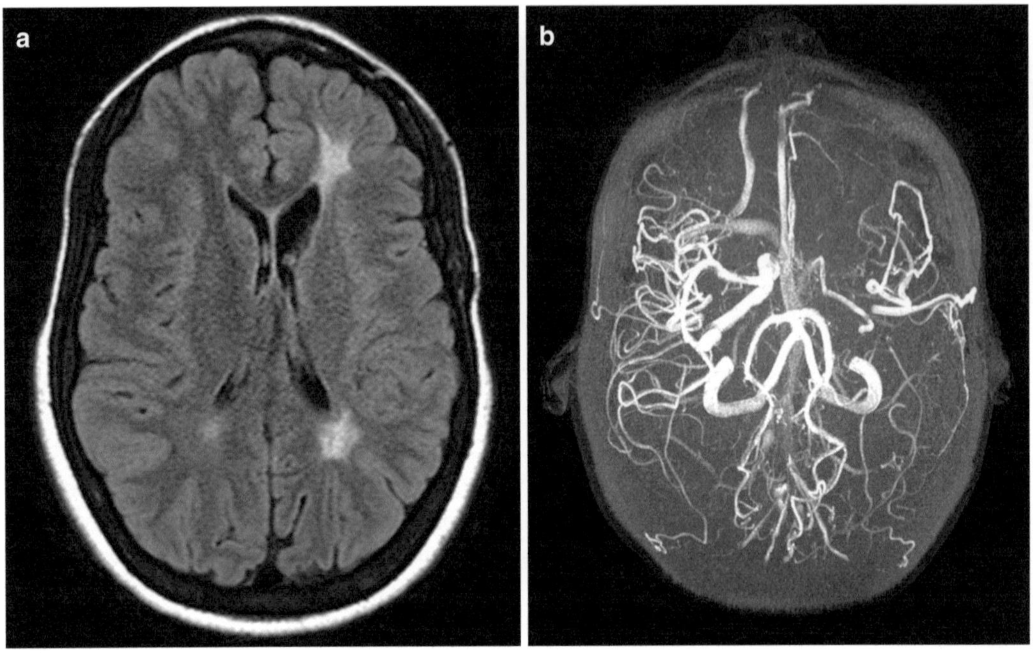

Fig. 7.40 Sickle cell disease. Axial T2-weighted FLAIR MRI (**a**) shows chronic ischemic lesions in the left cerebral hemisphere. The corresponding 3D MIP MRA image (**b**) shows extensive steno-occlusive disease at the circle of Willis, particularly on the left side

Imaging Findings

Neuroimaging is useful for evaluating sickle cell patients presenting with stroke. MRI and MRA are particularly suitable for depicting acute and chronic ischemic lesions in the brain and accompanying vasculopathy that often involves the anterior cerebral artery circulation with steno-occlusive disease (Fig. 7.40). Otherwise, CT is useful for screening for acute hemorrhagic strokes (Fig. 7.41). Orbital imaging with MRI or CT in sickle cell disease can be useful for evaluating patients with orbital crises. For example, orbital wall infarction can present with subperiosteal fluid collections (Fig. 7.42), as well as periorbital and orbital fat stranding and swelling. Head and neck imaging can reveal lymphadenopathy and enlarged tonsils and adenoids (Fig. 7.43). Osteonecrosis in the spine can lead to characteristic "H-shaped" vertebral bodies on sagittal images due to central endplate depressions (Fig. 7.44). Anemia in sickle cell disease manifests as low T1-weighted signal of the marrow (Fig. 7.44), as well as enlargement of the diploic space. The presence of extramedullary hematopoiesis can appear as masses, which are most commonly located in the paraspinal regions (Fig. 7.44).

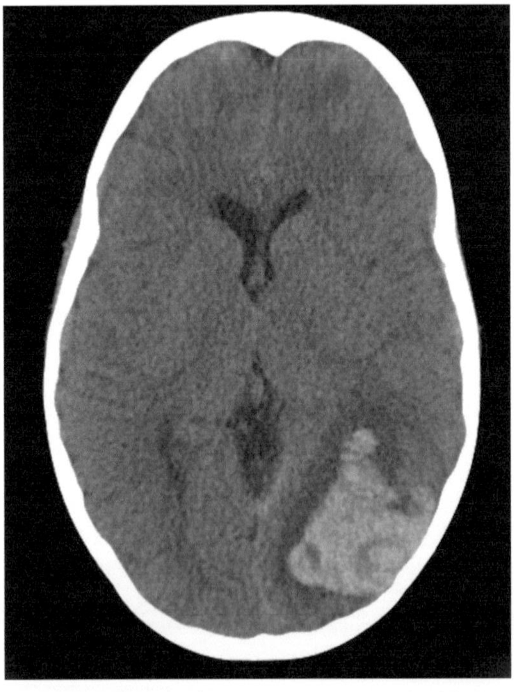

Fig. 7.41 Sickle cell disease. Axial CT image shows an acute hematoma in the left occipital lobe

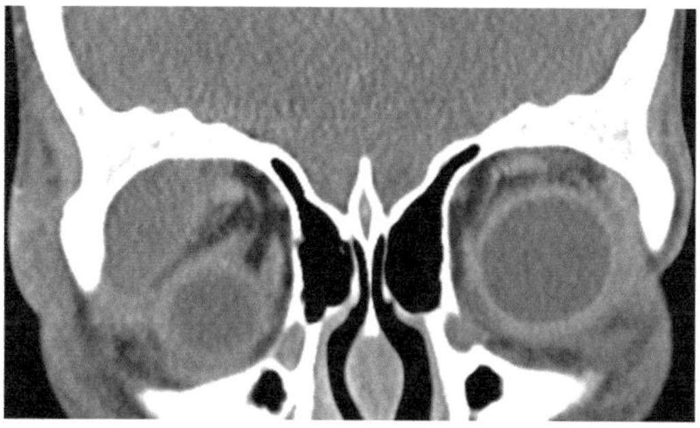

Fig. 7.42 Sickle cell disease. Coronal CT image in a patient with acute orbital crisis shows a right superolateral subperiosteal fluid collection

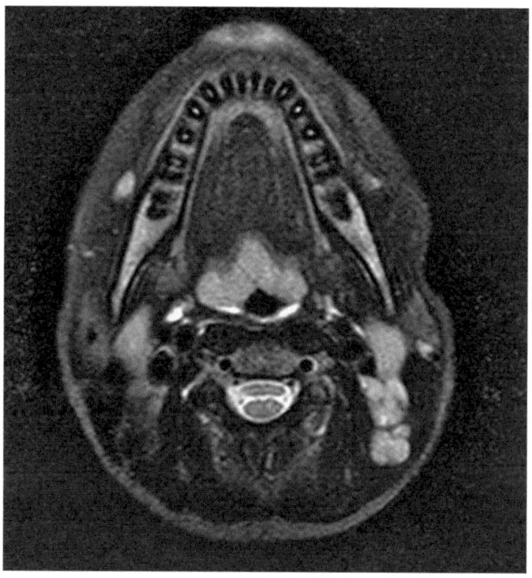

Fig. 7.43 Sickle cell disease. Axial fat-suppressed T2-weighted MRI shows enlarged lingual tonsils and cervical lymph nodes

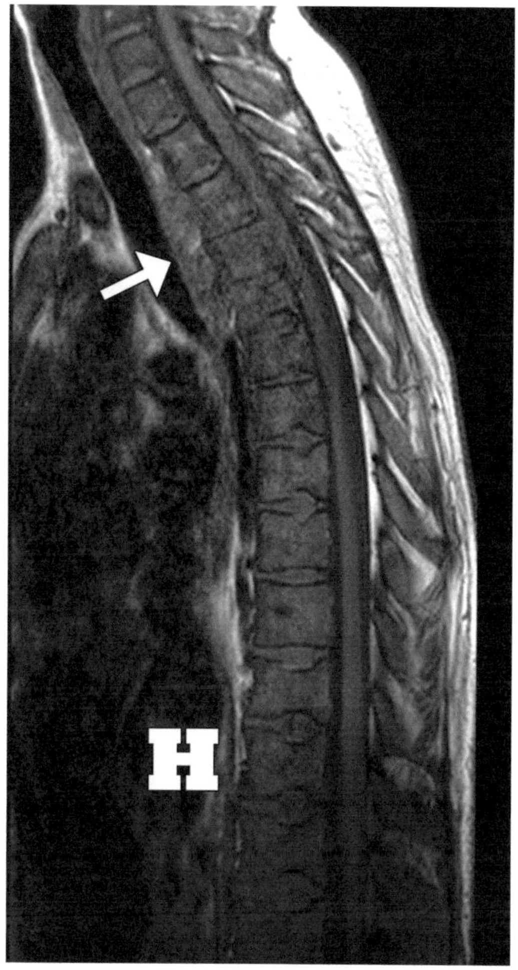

Fig. 7.44 Sickle cell disease. Sagittal T1-weighted MRI shows a thoracic paraspinal mass (arrow) related to extramedullary hematopoiesis, multiple vertebrae with superior and inferior endplate deformities (H), and diffusely low bone marrow signal

Disseminated Intravascular Coagulation

Overview

Disseminated intravascular coagulation (DIC) can result in extensive tissue damage. DIC may be initiated by a variety of insults, including sepsis, thermal burns over large surface, immunologic reactions, malignancy, venom, as well as vascular neoplasms such as kaposiform hemangioendotheliomas. In addition, localized coagulopathy can complicate vascular malformations that involve a venous component. The inhibitory mechanisms of clotting are blocked and there is temporary clotting of blood in the microcirculation, followed by consumption and depletion of platelets and plasma clotting factors. DIC is typically associated with decreased fibrinogen and increased fibrin degradation products (D-dimer). Skin biopsy demonstrates intravascular thrombi.

Clinical Findings

Cases of limited disseminated intravascular coagulation can manifest with focal areas of petechiae, purpuric papules, hemorrhagic bullae, and acral cyanosis, while extensive cases demonstrate widespread purpura and necrosis, occasionally leading to amputations (Fig. 7.45). Localized intravascular coagulopathy within venous malformations commonly presents with painful episodes in the affected body part and elevation of the D-dimer; pulmonary embolus can be a rare complication.

Imaging Findings

Disseminated intravascular coagulation can lead to thrombotic microangiopathy in the brain. This complication typically manifests as multifocal cortical and subcortical hemorrhagic infarctions (Fig. 7.46). Since the hemorrhage is often punctate, an initial CT may be negative. However, MRI is more sensitive for detecting intraparenchymal hemorrhage, particularly T2*-weighted or SWI sequences.

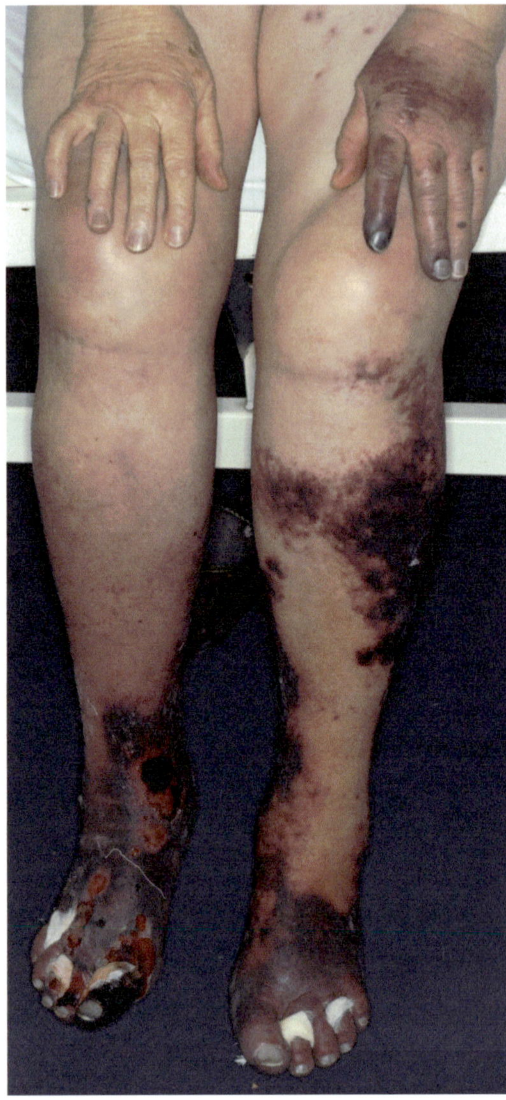

Fig. 7.45 Disseminated intravascular coagulation. Photograph shows extensive purpuric rashes in the extremities with areas of necrosis. Courtesy of Vesna Petronic-Rosic MD, MSc, MBA

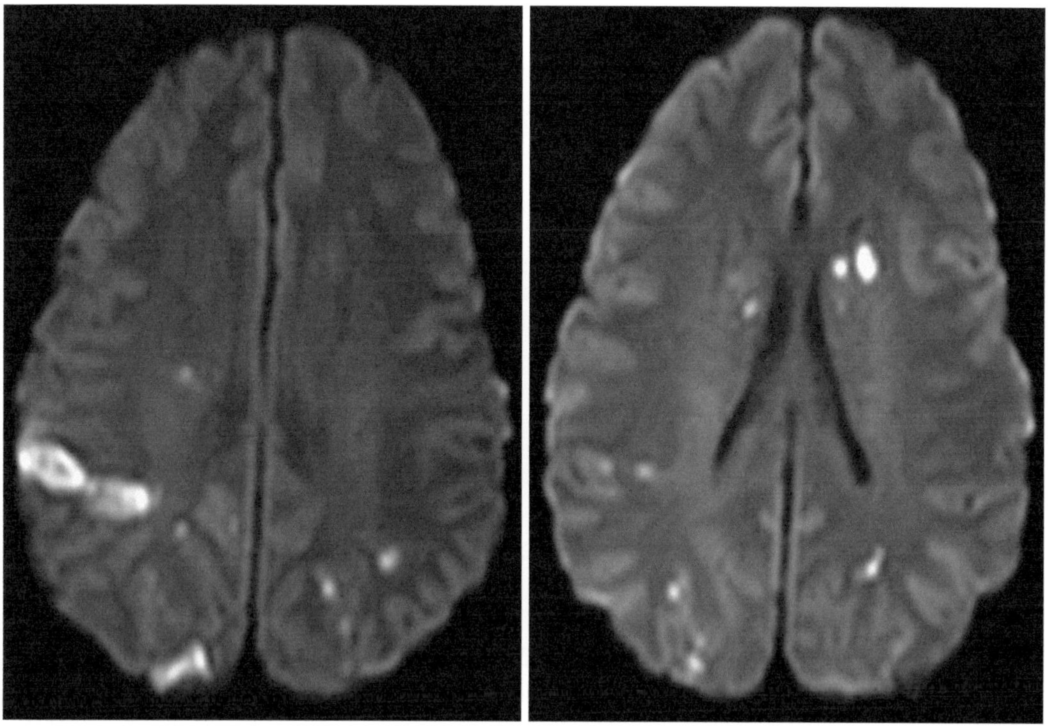

Fig. 7.46 Disseminated intravascular coagulation. Axial diffusion weighted images demonstrate numerous lesions with diffusion restriction in the cortex and subcortical cerebral white matter bilaterally, in a thromboembolic pattern

Suggested Reading

Alomari AI, Chaudry G, Rodesch G, Burrows PE, Mulliken JB, Smith ER, Fishman SJ, Orbach DB. Complex spinal-paraspinal fast-flow lesions in CLOVES syndrome: analysis of clinical and imaging findings in 6 patients. AJNR Am J Neuroradiol. 2011;32(10):1812–7.

Baker LL, Dillon WP, Hieshima GB, Dowd CF, Frieden IJ. Hemangiomas and vascular malformations of the head and neck: MR characterization. AJNR Am J Neuroradiol. 1993;14(2):307–14.

Bruch-Gerharz D, Gerharz CD, Stege H, Krutmann J, Pohl M, Koester R, Ruzicka T. Cutaneous lymphatic malformations in disappearing bone (Gorham-Stout) disease: a novel clue to the pathogenesis of a rare syndrome. J Am Acad Dermatol. 2007;56(2 Suppl):S21–5.

Buonanno FS, Cooper MR, Moody DM, Laster DW, Ball MR, Toole JF. Neuroradiologic aspects of cerebral disseminated intravascular coagulation. AJNR Am J Neuroradiol. 1980;1(3):245–50.

Certo M, Lopes L, Ramada J. Blue rubber bleb nevus syndrome: manifestations at computed tomography. Acta Radiol. 2007;48(9):962–6.

Ellchuk TN, Shah LM, Hewlett RH, Osborn AG. Suspicious neuroimaging pattern of thrombotic microangiopathy. AJNR Am J Neuroradiol. 2011;32(4):734–8.

Feldmeyer L, Baumann-Vogel H, Tournier-Lasserve E, Riant F, Jung HH, French LE, Kamarashev J. Hyperkeratotic cutaneous vascular malformation associated with familial cerebral cavernous malformations (FCCM) with KRIT1/CCM1 mutation. Eur J Dermatol. 2014;24(2):255–7.

Fisher-Jeffes ND, Domingo Z, Madden M, de Villiers JC. Arteriovenous malformations of the scalp. Neurosurgery. 1995;36(4):656–60; discussion 660.

Flors L, Leiva-Salinas C, Maged IM, Norton PT, Matsumoto AH, Angle JF, Hugo Bonatti M, Park AW, Ahmad EA, Bozlar U, Housseini AM, Huerta TE, Hagspiel KD. MR imaging of soft-tissue vascular malformations: diagnosis, classification, and therapy follow-up. Radiographics. 2011a;31(5):1321–40; discussion 1340–1.

Golden MJ, Morrison LA, Kim H, Hart BL. Increased number of white matter lesions in patients with familial cerebral cavernous malformations. AJNR Am J Neuroradiol. 2015;36(5):899–903.

Gurkanlar D, Gonul M, Solmaz I, Gonul E. Cirsoid aneurysms of the scalp. Neurosurg Rev. 2006;29(3):208–12.

Happle R. Capillary malformations: a classification using specific names for specific skin disorders. J Eur Acad Dermatol Venereol. 2015;29(12):2295–305.

Hoff SR, Rastatter JC, Richter GT. Head and neck vascular lesions. Otolaryngol Clin North Am. 2015;48(1):29–45.

Kassarjian A, Fishman SJ, Fox VL, Burrows PE. Imaging characteristics of blue rubber bleb nevus syndrome. AJR Am J Roentgenol. 2003;181(4):1041–8.

Kato GJ, Hebbel RP, Steinberg MH, Gladwin MT. Vasculopathy in sickle cell disease: biology, pathophysiology, genetics, translational medicine, and new research directions. Am J Hematol. 2009;84(9):618–25.

Kumar MS, Kumar MH, Sivakumar V, Kumar SH. A diagnostic challenge: pyogenic granuloma or oral focal mucinosis. BMJ Case Rep. 2015;2015.

Lee DG, Lee SK, Chang HW, et al. CT features of lobular capillary hemangioma of the nasal cavity. AJNR Am J Neuroradiol. 2010;31(4):749–54.

Maari C, Frieden IJ. Klippel-Trénaunay syndrome: the importance of "geographic stains" in identifying lymphatic disease and risk of complications. J Am Acad Dermatol. 2004;51(3):391–8.

Metry D, Heyer G, Hess C, et al. Consensus statement on diagnostic criteria for PHACE syndrome. Pediatrics. 2009;124(5):1447–56.

Minniti CP, Eckman J, Sebastiani P, Steinberg MH, Ballas SK. Leg ulcers in sickle cell disease. Am J Hematol. 2010;85(10):831–3.

Moake JL. Thrombotic microangiopathies. N Engl J Med. 2002;347:589–600.

Mulligan PR, Prajapati HJ, Martin LG, Patel TH. Vascular anomalies: classification, imaging characteristics and implications for interventional radiology treatment approaches. Br J Radiol. 2014;87(1035):20130392.

Nozaki T, Nosaka S, Miyazaki O, et al. Syndromes associated with vascular tumors and malformations: a pictorial review. Radiographics. 2013;33(1):175–95.

Olivieri B, White CL, Restrepo R, McKeon B, Karakas SP, Lee EY. Low-flow vascular malformation pitfalls: from clinical examination to practical imaging evaluation—part 2, venous malformation mimickers. AJR Am J Roentgenol. 2016;206(5):952–62.

Pavanello M, Melloni I, Antichi E, et al. Sinus pericranii: diagnosis and management in 21 pediatric patients. J Neurosurg Pediatr. 2015;15(1):60–70.

Ranger A, Szymczak A. Do intracranial neoplasms differ in Ollier disease and maffucci syndrome? An in-depth analysis of the literature. Neurosurgery. 2009;65(6):1106–13; discussion 1113–5.

Rodgers GP. Overview of pathophysiology and rationale for treatment of sickle cell anemia. Semin Hematol. 1997;34(3 Suppl 3):2–7.

Saito N, Nadgir RN, Flower EN, Sakai O. Clinical and radiologic manifestations of sickle cell disease in the head and neck. Radiographics. 2010;30(4):1021–34.

Sheu M, Fauteux G, Chang H, Taylor W, Stopa E, Robinson-Bostom L. Sinus pericranii: dermatologic considerations and literature review. J Am Acad Dermatol. 2002;46(6):934–41.

Steven A, Raghavan P, Rath TJ, Gandhi D. Neurologic and head and neck manifestations of sickle cell disease. Hematol Oncol Clin North Am. 2016;30(4):779–98.

Sun GH, Myer CM 3rd. Otolaryngologic manifestations of Maffucci's syndrome. Int J Pediatr Otorhinolaryngol. 2009;73(7):1015–8.

Takahashi S, Shinoda H, Nakano Y. Congenital stapedial fixation associated with Beckwith--Wiedemann syndrome: two cases of a woman and her brother. Am J Otol. 1996;17(1):111–4.

Thust SC, Burke C, Siddiqui A. Neuroimaging findings in sickle cell disease. Br J Radiol. 2014;87(1040):20130699.

Torregrosa A, Martí-Bonmatí L, Higueras V, Poyatos C, Sanchís A. Klippel-Trenaunay syndrome: frequency of cerebral and cerebellar hemihypertrophy on MRI. Neuroradiology. 2000;42(6):420–3.

Turner JT, Cohen MM Jr, Biesecker LG. Reassessment of the Proteus syndrome literature: application of diagnostic criteria to published cases. Am J Med Genet A. 2004;130A(2):111–22.

Ware RE, de Montalembert M, Tshilolo L, Abboud MR. Sickle cell disease. Lancet. 2017;390(10091):311–23.

Wassef M, Blei F, Adams D, et al. ISSVA board and scientific committee. Vascular anomalies classification: recommendations from the international society for the study of vascular anomalies. Pediatrics. 2015;136:e203–14.

White CL, Olivieri B, Restrepo R, McKeon B, Karakas SP, Lee EY. Low-flow vascular malformation pitfalls: from clinical examination to practical imaging evaluation—part 1, lymphatic malformation mimickers. AJR Am J Roentgenol. 2016;206(5):940–51.

Neuroimaging of Traumatic Skin Injuries and Associated Lesions

8

Tamari Miller, Marc Moisi,
and Daniel Thomas Ginat

Contents

Abstract

The skin, by virtue of being the largest organ in the human body and being exposed to the surroundings, is the generally first point of impact with trauma. Injury to the skin commonly is an indicator of trauma to underlying organs. Diagnostic imaging plays an important role in evaluating the extent of injury beyond the skin. This chapter reviews the clinical and imaging findings related to penetrating trauma, blunt trauma, thermal injury, and birth injury, non-accidental trauma, and associated complications involving the head and neck, such as fractures, intracranial hemor-

T. Miller
Pritzker School of Medicine, University of Chicago, Chicago, IL, USA

M. Moisi
Department of Neurosurgery, Wayne State University, Detroit, MI, USA

D. T. Ginat (✉)
Department of Radiology, University of Chicago, Pritzker School of Medicine, Chicago, IL, USA
e-mail: dtg1@uchicago.edu

D. T. Ginat (ed.), *Neuroradiological Imaging of Skin Diseases and Related Conditions*,
https://doi.org/10.1007/978-3-319-90931-8_8

rhage, brain injuries, retained foreign bodies, orbital injuries, infection, and vascular compromise.

Penetrating Trauma

Overview

Penetrating trauma is an injury that occurs when an object pierces the skin and/or underlying tissues, creating an open wound. There are five types of penetrating wounds, including abrasions, avulsions, incisions, lacerations, and punctures. An abrasion is no deeper than the epidermis caused by friction when the skin grazes or scrapes across a rough surface or object. An avulsion is characterized by a soft tissue flap. An incision is a cut with clean edges. A laceration is a cut in the skin and underlying soft tissues with jagged edges and is often contaminated with bacteria and debris. A puncture is caused by something sharp and pointed and is also prone to contamination. Furthermore, penetrating injuries can be broadly categorized based on mechanism as projectile, typically bullets, versus non-projectile, such as knives and other sharp objects, including sticks and broken glass.

In the head and neck, the location of penetrating injury has traditionally been divided into three zones by horizontal planes as follows:

- Zone 1 extends from the level of the clavicles and sternal notch to the cricoid cartilage. Critical structures within this zone include the great vessels, brachiocephalic veins, aortic arch, jugular veins, lung apices, esophagus, trachea, phrenic nerve, spinal cord, cervical nerve roots, and vagus nerve.
- Zone 2 extends from the level of the cricoid cartilage to the angle of the mandible. Critical structures within this zone include the carotid and vertebral arteries, jugular veins, pharynx, trachea, esophagus, cervical spine, spinal cord, and airway.
- Zone 3 extends from the level of the angle of the mandible to the base of the skull. Critical structures within this zone include the skull base, salivary and parotid glands, esophagus, jugular veins, cranial nerves IX–XII, carotid and vertebral arteries, and oropharynx.

Often times, while the entry wound is located in one zone, the path of the penetrating injury can traverse other zones. In addition, with high-velocity projectile injuries, tissue damage can be extensive and remote to the path of the projectile due to shock wave effects.

Clinical Findings

The different types of open skin injuries can present with variable degrees of pain and bleeding. Furthermore, depending on the particular location of the injury, patients may experience vision loss, neurological deficits, coma, and difficulty breathing and swallowing. Foreign bodies introduced in the wounds may or may not be fully visible on clinical exam (Fig. 8.1). Retained foreign bodies in the head and neck are particularly problematic in terms of function and infection. Unless a foreign body is projecting from the wound, it can be occult clinically.

Imaging Findings

CT without contrast is a suitable modality for evaluating suspected retained foreign bodies from penetrating trauma. Glass from broken windshields and bottles are often hyperattenuating on CT (Fig. 8.2). On the other hand, wood is often relatively radiolucent and can resemble soft tissue emphysema, which is also often associated with penetrating trauma. However, wood fragments tend to have more rectilinear margins (Fig. 8.3). Metal foreign bodies sometimes produce extensive streak artifact, which limits assessment on standard CT. In such cases, radiographs or scout images can provide a general overview of the depth of a foreign body (Fig. 8.4). Alternatively, dual-energy CT can be useful for minimizing metal beam hardening effects for more detailed assessment of the injury (Fig. 8.5). In particular, the artifact is less conspicuous on high-energy images.

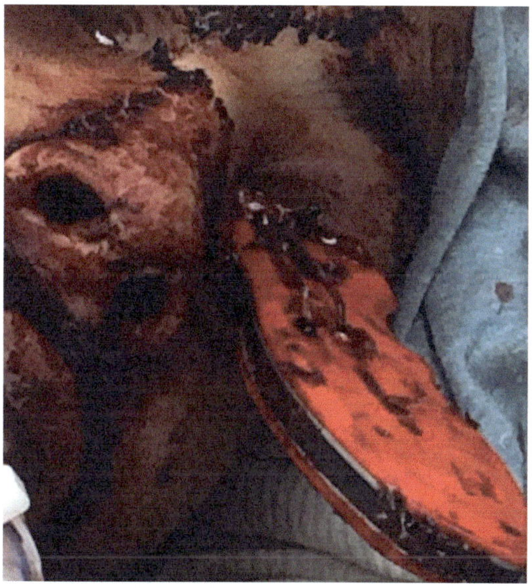

Fig. 8.1 Photograph shows a bloody stab wound with a knife that penetrates the left eye

Non-contrast CT is also suitable for evaluating for the presence of fractures and intracranial hemorrhage that can be associated with penetrating injuries (Fig. 8.6). In particular, bone fracture fragments and missile fragmentation can form secondary projectiles that cause additional injuries. Manifestations of intracranial injury that can be identified on non-contrast CT include intra- and extra-parenchymal hemorrhage, pneumocephalus, and cerebral edema.

CTA is the first-line imaging modality for evaluating suspected vascular injury related to penetrating trauma in the head and neck and has been shown to significantly reduce the number of negative surgical explorations. Stigmata of penetrating

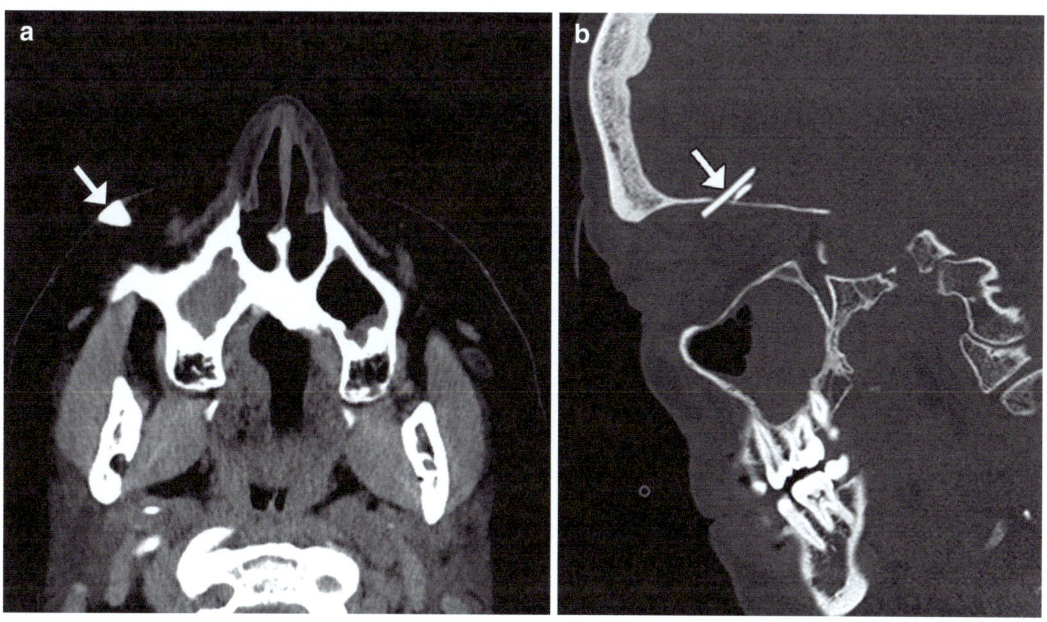

Fig. 8.2 Penetrating injury with retained glass foreign body. Axial (**a**) and coronal (**b**) CT images show hyperattenuating fragments in the right cheek and in the orbit with intracranal extension through an associated fracture of the orbital roof

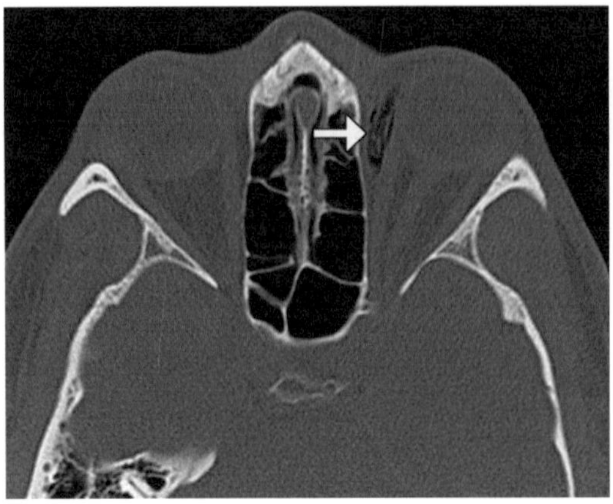

Fig. 8.3 Puncture wound with retained wood foreign body. Axial CT image show a low attenuation object in the medial right orbit (*arrow*)

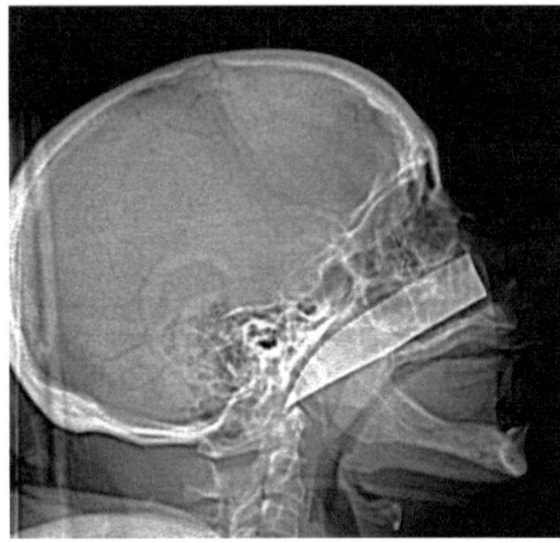

Fig. 8.4 Stab wound. The lateral scout image shows a knife that penetrates the face and traverses the sinonasal cavities

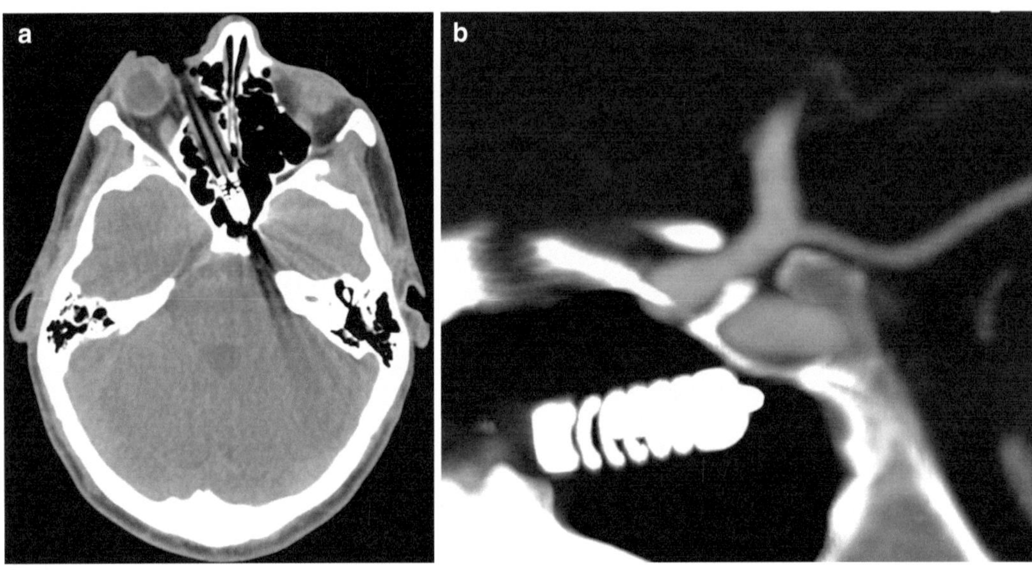

Fig. 8.5 Penetrating injury and dual energy CT. Axial CT image at 80 KVp (**a**) shows at pen that traverses the right orbit and paranasal sinuses with beam hardening artifact that obscures surrounding structures. CTA MIP image at 140 KVp (**b**) shows the pen and adjacent internal carotid artery with no significant artifact. Courtesy of Rajiv Gupta MD, PhD

injury to the head and neck arteries may include pseudoaneurysms and/or steno-occlusive lesions related to dissection or vasospasm (Fig. 8.7), which can be complicated by thrombus formation and cerebral infarction. Catheter angiography may be performed to further evaluate and treat vascular injuries in the head and neck.

MRI has no role in the imaging assessment of metallic projectile penetrating neck injury due to the presence of potentially ferromagnetic foreign body material. However, MRI is useful for evaluating non-projectile penetrating injury to the cervical spine or craniocervical junction. Other than potentially aiding in detecting foreign bodies,

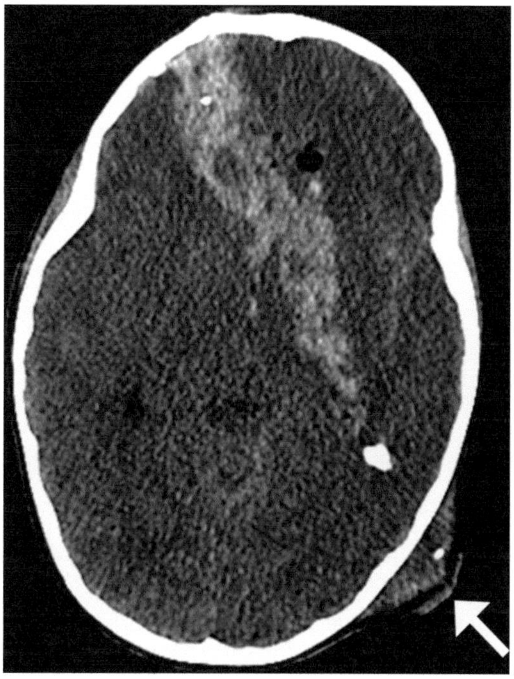

Fig. 8.6 Gunshot wound to the head with intracranial hemorrhage. Axial CT image shows hemorrhage in a linear trajectory traversing the brain along the path of a bullet that entered the left temporo-occipital scalp with a hematoma at the entry site (*arrow*)

ultrasound also has a limited role in penetrating neck injury, particularly given its inability to evaluate the upper aerodigestive tract and spine.

In the setting of suspected wound infections following penetrating trauma, contrast-enhanced CT can be performed, particularly if there is the possibility of retained metal foreign body. In the appropriate clinical setting, the presence of fat stranding suggests cellulitis and a rim-enhancing fluid collection suggests abscess (Fig. 8.8).

Blunt Trauma

Overview

In blunt or non-penetrating trauma, there may be an impact with a dull, firm surface or object, but the skin is not necessarily broken. Some of the main mechanisms of blunt trauma to the head, neck, and spine include motor vehicle accidents, direct assault, hanging, and sporting injuries. Blunt trauma often leads to some form of bleeding in the skin, which can manifest as one of the following depending upon the severity and extent:

- Bruise (contusion): minor hemorrhage within the skin, where disrupted vessels leak blood into the interstitial space.
- Petechia: A pinpoint, non-raised, perfectly round, purple-red spot caused by intradermal hemorrhage.
- Ecchymosis: A small hemorrhagic spot, larger than a petechia, in the skin or mucous membrane forming a non-elevated, rounded or irregular, blue-purple patch.
- Hematoma: A mass-like collection of blood, usually clotted, in an organ, space, or tissue, due to a break in the wall of a blood vessel.
- Hemorrhage: The escape of blood from the vessels, which can be retained in the interstitial space or extravasate outside the skin.

In the scalp, hemorrhage and hematomas can occur in the following spaces:

- Subcutaneous tissues: located between the skin and galea aponeurosis.
- Subgaleal space: located in the potential space between the galea aponeurosis and the periosteum of the skull.
- Subperiosteal space: located between the periosteum and the skull. Hemorrhage in this space is confined by the cranial sutures.

Skin manifestations of blunt trauma may be the tip of the iceberg of more extensive head and neck injury, which may include hemorrhage, brain and spinal cord contusions, fractures, airway compromise, vascular injury, and shear injury in the brain.

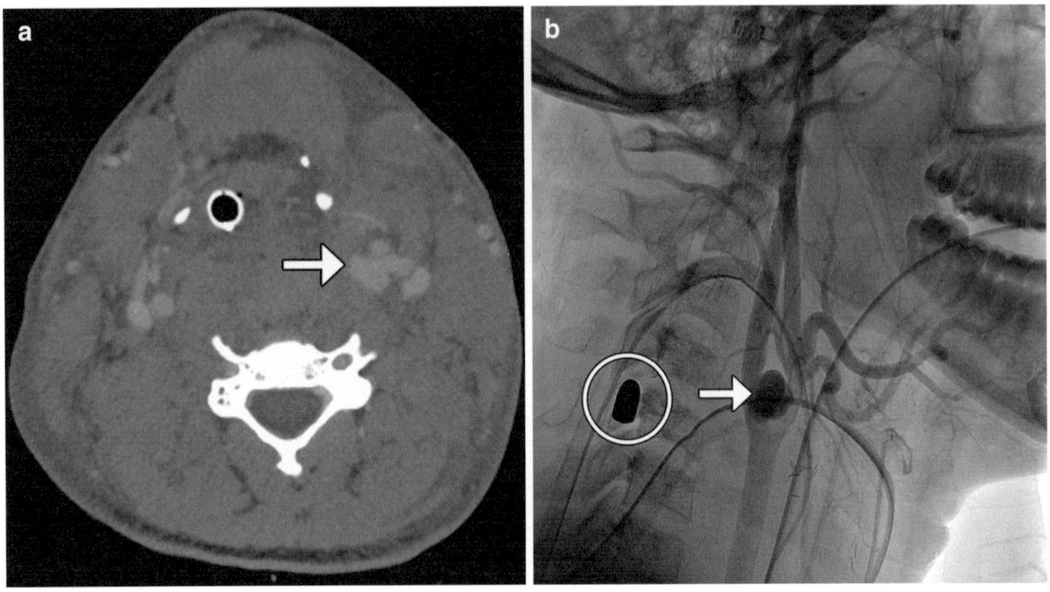

Fig. 8.7 Gunshot wound complicated by carotid pseudoaneurysm. Axial CTA image (**a**) shows a left caraotid bifurcation pseudoaneurysm (*arrow*) and extensive swelling of the surrounding neck soft tissues. Lateral catheter angiogram image (**b**) also shows the pseudoaneurysm (*arrow*) and nearby bullet (encircled)

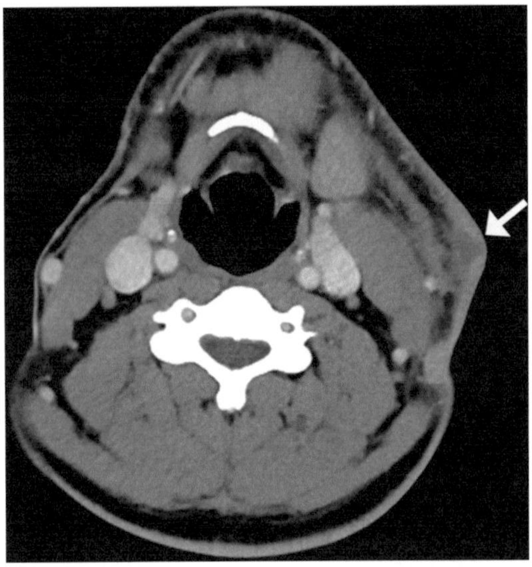

Fig. 8.8 Infected wound. The patient present with cellulitis following a shaving cut. Axial CT image with contrast shows a fluid collection with peripheral enhancement in the left lateral neck skin and subcutaneous tissues with associated fat stranding (*arrow*)

Clinical Findings

Blunt trauma to the head and neck may present with skin discoloration and swelling from the underlying hemorrhage in the acute setting. The skin lesions can have different patterns depending upon the mechanism of trauma. For example, bruising in the lower neck along the path of the seatbelt from motor vehicle collisions has a linear configuration across the lower neck and upper chest (Fig. 8.9) and can be a harbinger for injuries to the carotid artery, larynx, and cervical spine. Similarly, ecchymosis around the mastoid process (Battle's sign) represents leakage of blood behind the ear resulting from temporal bone fractures that communicated with the middle cranial fossa. The hematoma usually forms 1–2 days after trauma due to a disruption of the emissary veins traversing the postauricular soft tissue from the sigmoid sinus. Patients may also present with hearing loss from hemotympanum.

Other acute clinical findings that suggest major injury from blunt trauma and merit imaging include worsening level of consciousness, loss of consciousness for more than 5 min, focal neurological findings, seizure, failure of the mental status to improve over time, signs of a basal or depressed skull fracture, and confusion or aggression on examination.

A delayed sequela of blunt trauma to the cranium is an acquired encephalocoele, which

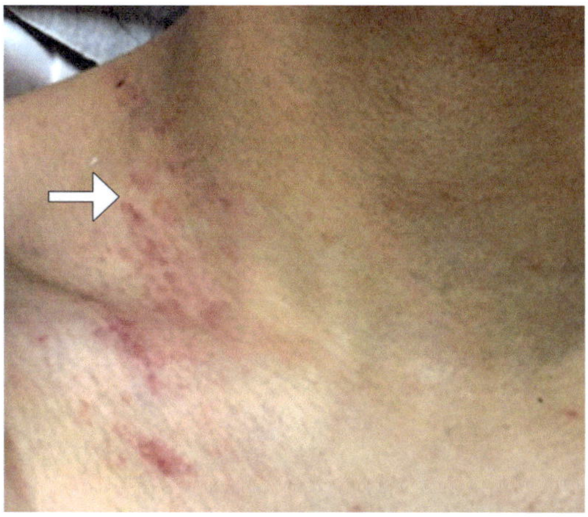

Fig. 8.9 Seatbelt sign. Photograph of a patient involved in a motor vehicle accident shows bruising along the path of a seatbelt strap in the right lower neck (*arrow*). Courtesy of Amy Ho MD

consists of herniation of intracranial contents through a growing fracture. Acquired encephalocoeles can present as a skin-covered bulge in the scalp that may fluctuate in size depending on the position of the patient. Patients with acquired encephaloceles may be prone to meningitis and can present with seizures.

Spine fractures are rather common with blunt trauma. Cervical spine injuries causing spinal cord trauma are rare in blunt trauma, yet can lead to severe morbidity and mortality. On the other hand, thoracolumbar burst fractures are associated with neurologic deficit in 65% of cases. Mechanical stability is an important consideration in the management of patients with traumatic spine injury. Spine stability is defined as the ability to prevent the development of neurologic injury and progressive deformity in response to physiologic loading and range of movement. Spine stability relies on the integrity of both bone and ligamentous components. Injury to either or both can result in spine instability that requires surgical stabilization.

Although uncommon, it is important to consider the possibility of laryngotracheal injury in patients with blunt trauma to the neck, such as through sports-related injuries, since this can lead to airway obstruction and dysphonia. Laryngotracheal injury can have a variety of manifestations, including endolaryngeal edema and hematoma, vocal cord injuries, fractures of the hyoid bone, epiglottis, and thyroid and cricoid cartilages, dislocations of the cricoarytenoid and cricothyroid joints, and laryngotracheal separation, which is the most immediately life-threatening laryngotracheal injury. Patients with blunt neck trauma can also present with neurological deficits from hypoxic ischemic injury due to protracted compression of the major vascular structures in the neck, such as from strangulation type injuries.

Imaging Findings

High-resolution non-contrast CT, including bone algorithm multiplanar reformatted images with up to 1 mm slice thickness is typically the modality of choice for evaluating patients with blunt maxillofacial trauma injuries since it can readily depict most bone and soft tissue injuries. Facial hemorrhage can appear as diffuse subcutaneous fat stranding and swelling or focal mass-like hematomas (Fig. 8.10). There can also be accompanying subcutaneous and orbital emphysema. While generally innocuous on its own, facial hemorrhage may represent the tip of the iceberg for more serious injury, including fractures (Table 8.1 and Fig. 8.11).

Beside fractures, blunt trauma in the region of the eyes can be associated with injuries to the orbital contents, such as globe rupture, lens dislocation, and hemorrhage (Fig. 8.12). Direct ophthalmic and ultrasound examination can be limited or even contraindicated in the setting of suspected globe rupture, and thus requires CT for evaluation of the orbital contents. Globe rupture can manifest as abnormal contours of the globe (flat-tire sign) or more subtle abnormal anterior chamber dimensions on CT. Alternatively, subluxation or dislocation of the lens appears as partial or complete detachment of the lens, usually posteriorly, and in rare cases can be predisposed by minor trauma in the setting of underlying connective tissue diseases, such as Marfan syndrome (Chap. 3). Traumatic cataracts can result from disruption of the lens, which appears relatively hypoattenuating on CT. Intraorbital hemorrhage is

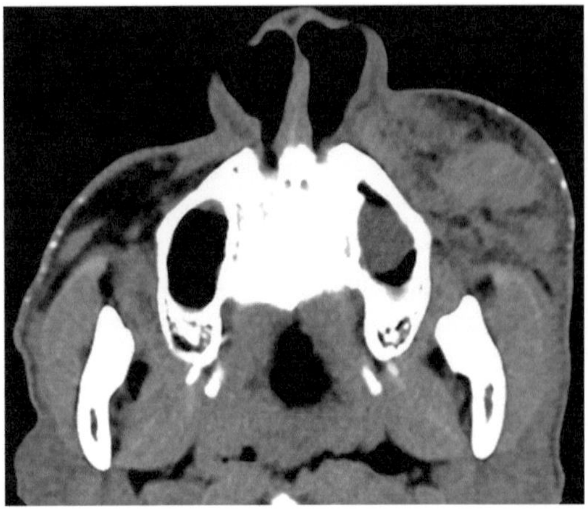

Fig. 8.10 Facial hemorrhage. Axial CT image shows mass-like hematomas and surrounding diffuse stranding and swelling of the left cheek subcutaneous fat

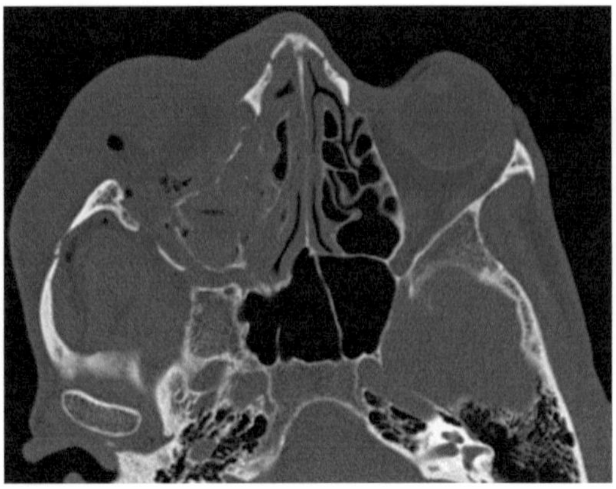

Fig. 8.11 Maxillofacial fractures. Axial CT image shows right facial swelling from hemorrhage and components of a right zygomaticomaxillary complex fracture with orbital emphysema and hemosinus

Table 8.1 Types of maxillofacial fractures

Type of fracture	Description
Nasal skeleton	May involve the nasal bone and/or frontal process of the maxilla
Naso-orbito-ethmoid	Midface fractures involving the orbital walls, ethmoid bone, and nasal skeleton
Orbital blow-out	Most commonly involve the lamina papyracea and/or orbital floor. There may be accompanying orbital fat and/or extraocular muscles, which can become entrapped. In rare cases, even the globe can herniate through the fracture site
Zygomaticomaxillary complex	Involves the zygomatic arch, lateral orbital wall, and walls of the maxillary sinus
LeFort	Type 1: floating palate Type 2: floating maxilla Type 3: floating face All three types generally include pterygoid plate fractures
Mandible	Fractures often occur in pairs as part of the ring theory. Otherwise, a single fracture may be accompanied by temporomandibular joint dislocation, which can be transient and not evident at the time of imaging

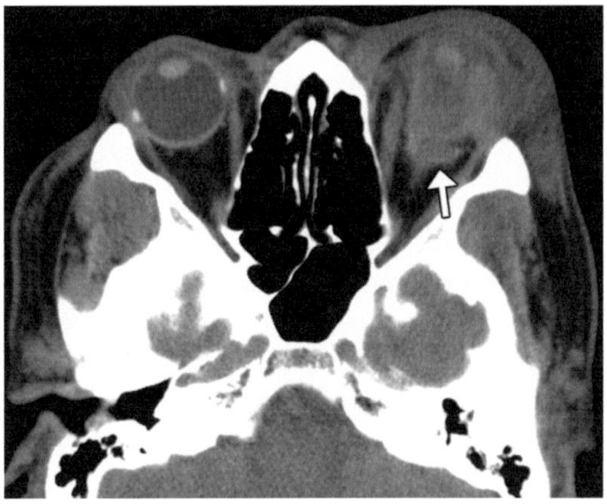

Fig. 8.12 Orbital injury. Axial CT image shows left preseptal hemorrhage, deformity of the left globe due to rupture with partial detachment and posterior displacement of the lens, as well as intraocular and retrobulbar hemorrhage (*arrow*) and swelling of the left medial rectus muscle

another potential complication of blunt trauma to the orbit that often accompanies orbital wall fractures. This mainly manifests as retrobulbar hemorrhage or subperiosteal hemorrhage. Ultimately, evaluation of orbital trauma on imaging should be approached systematically. For example, the "BALPINE" mnemonic can be helpful and includes bones, anterior chamber, lens, posterior globe structures, intraconal orbit, neurovascular structures, and extraocular muscles/extraconal orbit.

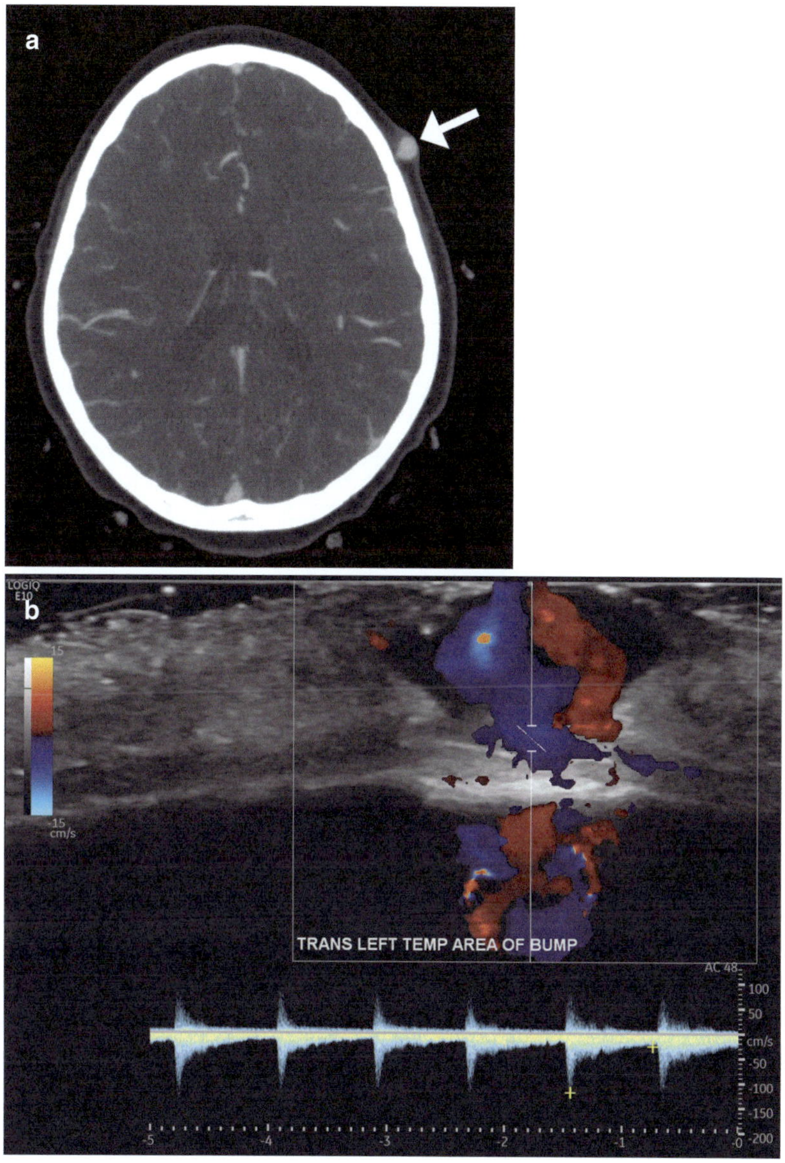

Fig. 8.13 Scalp injury with arterial pseudoaneurysm. Axial CTA (**a**) shows a small rounded collection of contrast in the left scalp (*arrow*). The corresponding Doppler ultrasound image (**b**) shows blood flow with a to-and-fro waveform and "yin & yang" color pattern

Scalp hematomas are often encountered as isolated findings on imaging performed to evaluate for underlying skull fractures and intracranial injury in patients with acute blunt head trauma. The scalp hematomas can occur in the various layers of the scalp, as described subsequently in the birth trauma section. On occasion, dedicated vascular imaging may be warranted to assess rapidly enlarging scalp hematomas due to arterial injury. Imaging findings indicative of active hemorrhage include the spot sign, which represents extraluminal pooling of contrast, or the presence of pseudoaneurysm (Fig. 8.13).

Non-contrast head CT is considered to be the first-line of imaging modality for evaluating intracranial injury associated with blunt head trauma, while MRI may be useful in specific situations. A classic pattern of intracranial injury related to blunt head trauma is coup-contre-coup injury, which can manifest with skull fracture, brain contusion, and/or hemorrhage underlying the site of impact (coup) and brain contusion and/or hemorrhage opposite to the site of impact (Fig. 8.14), as well as lens dislocations on rare occasions. The severity of the contre-coup injury is often more pronounced than the coup injury.

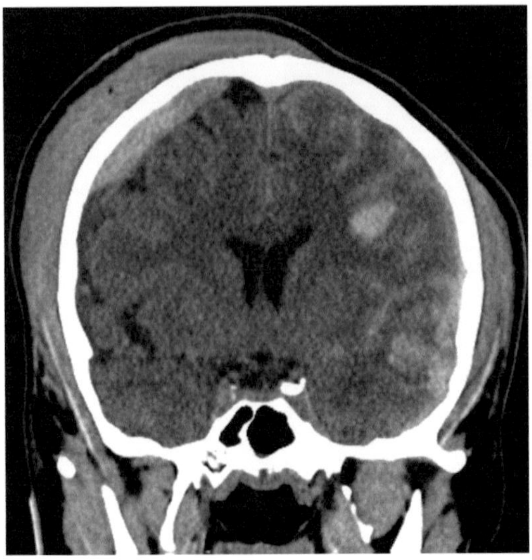

Fig. 8.14 Scalp hematoma with contre-coup intracranial injury. Axial CT image shows a right scalp hematoma with underlying epidural hemorrhage and contralateral hemorrhagic contusions, subarachnoid hemorrhage, and subdural hemorrhage

The detection rate of contusions is 36% by CT and 57% by MRI. In addition to contusions, blunt trauma associated with high deceleration forces can lead to shearing with diffuse axonal injury in the brain. The grey-white matter junctions of the cerebral hemispheres, corpus callosum, and brainstem are sites of predilection for diffuse axonal injury, in increasing order of severity. Imaging can demonstrate edema, which may display restricted diffusion acutely, and microhemorrhages at the site of diffuse axonal injury (Fig. 8.15). The detection rate of hemorrhagic diffuse axonal injury is 22% by CT and 47% by MRI.

It is important to describe the degree to which skull fractures are depressed since surgical repair may be warranted if there is displacement by more than the thickness of the calvarium. Ping pong fractures are a particular form of depressed fractures that can occur in neonates and infants in which the bone is deformed without actual breakage from the rest of the skull (Fig. 8.16). On the other hand, diastatic fractures can enlarge and lead to brain herniation and/or cerebrospinal fluid leakage through the skull defect, which is known as growing skull fracture or craniocerebral erosion. This complication is readily depicted on MRI, whereby the herniated brain is often gliotic (Fig. 8.17). Furthermore, skull base fractures from blunt trauma can lead to cerebrospinal fluid leakage, which can be suggested by the presence of pneumocephalus on CT and accompanying sinonasal or otomastoid fluid, which is otherwise nonspecific (Fig. 8.18).

Spine fractures and subluxation can be associated with blunt trauma to the head, neck, or trunk. High-resolution multiplanar CT is the modality of choice for screening for cervical spine and thoracolumbar fractures. Spine injuries often occur at sites remote from the actual point of impact and may involve multiple levels. In particular, approximately 20% of patients with a spinal column fracture will have a noncontiguous fracture. In addition, there is a risk of vertebral artery injury with cervical spine trauma, particularly with foramen transversarium involvement, and/or subluxation at the C1 to C3 levels. In such cases, CTA should also be performed, which may demonstrate paucity of vertebral artery opacification if there is occlusion, dissection, thrombus, intimal damage, or transection (Fig. 8.19), versus increased opacification if there is pseudoaneurysm or rupture, and early opacification of surrounding vein if there is arteriovenous fistula formation. MRI is more useful than CT for evaluating spinal cord injury, ligamentous injury, hematomas, disc herniation, and perhaps facet joint involvement and should be performed in patients with neurological deficits when possible. In particular, acute spinal cord injury can manifest as deformity due to retropulsed bone or hemorrhage within the spinal canal with or without associated edema with high T2 signal (Fig. 8.20). If the vascular supply of the spinal cord is compromised, acute infarction can occur, which can be depicted on diffusion weighted imaging.

Finally, high-resolution CT is the modality of choice for evaluating suspected laryngotracheal injury from blunt trauma and the degree of associated airway narrowing (Fig. 8.21). Imaging findings may include direct signs, such as deformity and dislocation of the laryngeal cartilages,

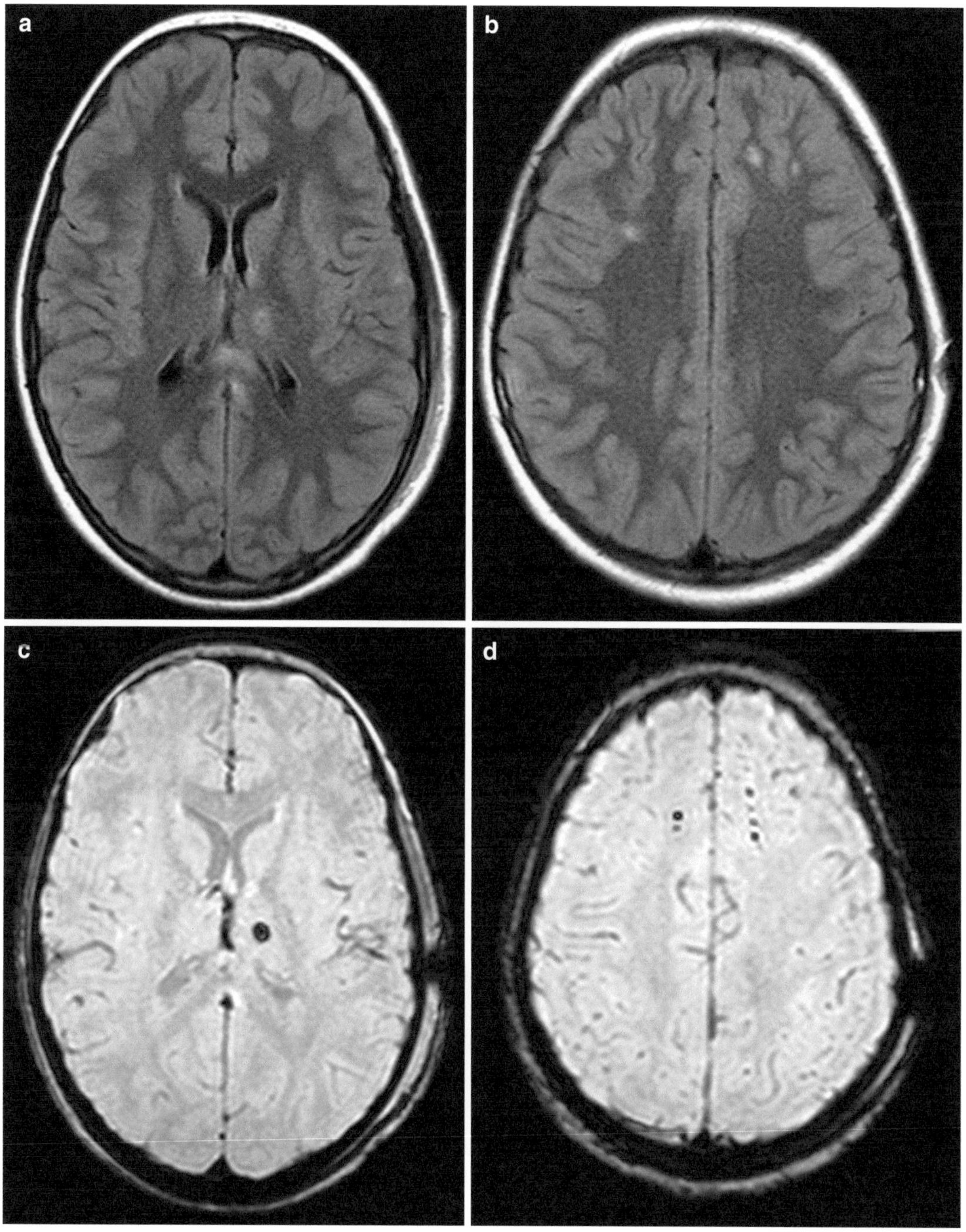

Fig. 8.15 Blunt head trauma with diffuse axonal injury. The patient was involved in a high-speed motor vehicle collision. Axial T2-weighted FLAIR (**a**, **b**) and SWI (**c**, **d**) MR images show edema in the posterior corpus callosum, left thalamus, and at the grey-white interfaces of the bilateral frontal lobes with associated punctate hemorrhages, with associated restricted diffusion in some of the affected areas (**e**, **f**). There is left scalp swelling

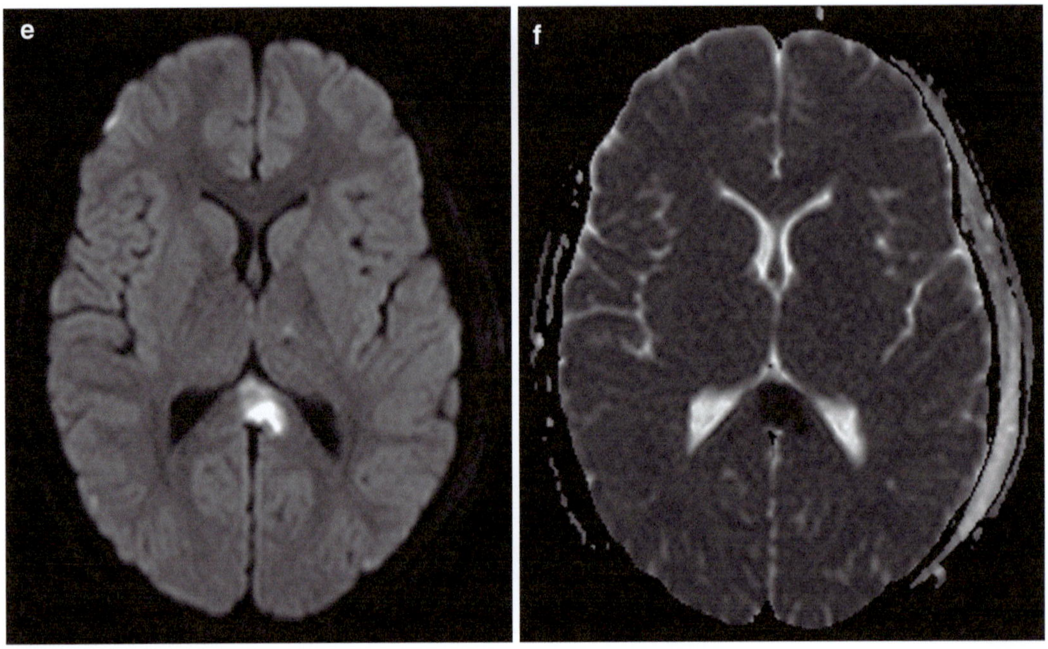

Fig. 8.15 (continued)

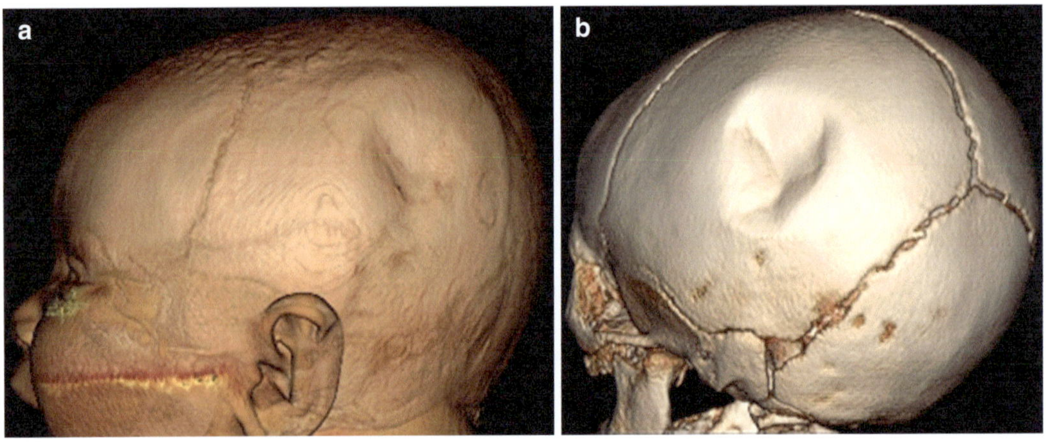

Fig. 8.16 Ping pong fracture. A television set fell on this infant's head. 3D skin (**a**) and bone (**b**) CT images show crater-like right parietal scalp and calvarial depression without actual cortical disruption

or indirect signs, such as soft tissue swelling and subcutaneous emphysema. Blunt injury to the neck can also result in intracranial injuries due to hypoxic ischemia, which can result from airway or vascular compromise, especially through strangulation, such as from hanging. This can manifest as diffuse effacement of the cerebrospinal fluid spaces and loss grey-white matter differentiation on CT and diffuse restricted diffusion and swelling, primarily involving the grey matter structures (Fig. 8.22). On occasion, strangulation injury can also lead to intracranial hemorrhage secondary to venous hypertension from jugular vein compression.

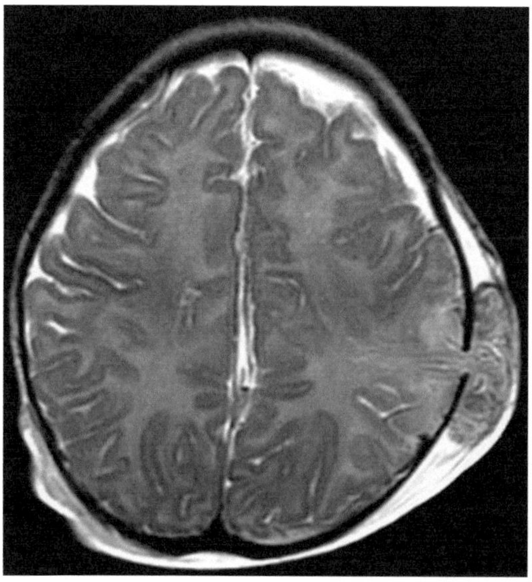

Fig. 8.17 Acquired encephalocoele from a growing fracture. Axial T2-weighted MRI shows gliotic brain tissue and cerebrospinal fluid herniating through the fracture site on the left side with elevation of the overlying scalp

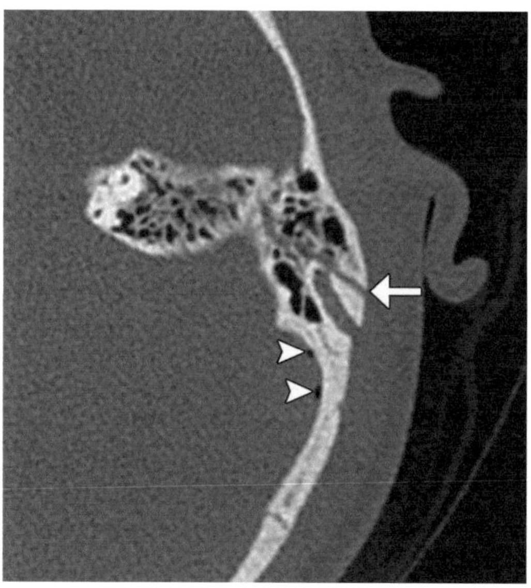

Fig. 8.18 Skull base fracture complicated by cerebrospinal fluid leakage. Axial CT image show a fracture (*arrow*) that traverses the mastoid bone with opacification of the mastoid air cells and pneumocephalus (*arrowheads*)

Thermal Injuries

Overview

Thermal injuries in the head and neck regions can occur through various mechanisms, such as fire, hot objects, electricity, and frostbite. Exposed structures in the face, such as the ears and nose are most vulnerable. Burns to the head and neck region may be accompanied by inhalation injury and associated and compromised airways. Prompt treatment is important in order to minimize complications, such as infection and necrosis. Furthermore, Marjolin ulcer is a delayed complication of burn scars that consists of malignant degeneration, most commonly in the form of squamous cell carcinoma, but basal cell carcinoma and sarcomas can also occur.

Clinical Findings

Burns are classified on a tier system based on the layers of the skin that are affected. First-degree burns affect the epidermis; second-degree burns penetrate to the dermis; and third-degree burns reach the subcutaneous adipose tissue. Painful, erythematous, and edematous skin lesions are characteristic of first-degree burns. Second-degree burns may form blisters and the skin may appear white or splotchy. The skin may appear charred or white and have a leathery, moist appearance in third-degree burns (Fig. 8.23). An analogous range of skin lesions can result from frostbite, in which superficial frostbite involves the skin and subcutaneous tissues, manifesting as mild swelling, paleness, sometimes with clear blisters, but the skin usually remains pliable and soft. In contrast, deep frostbite injury affects structures underneath the subcutaneous tissues and presents with hyperesthesia and loss of cold

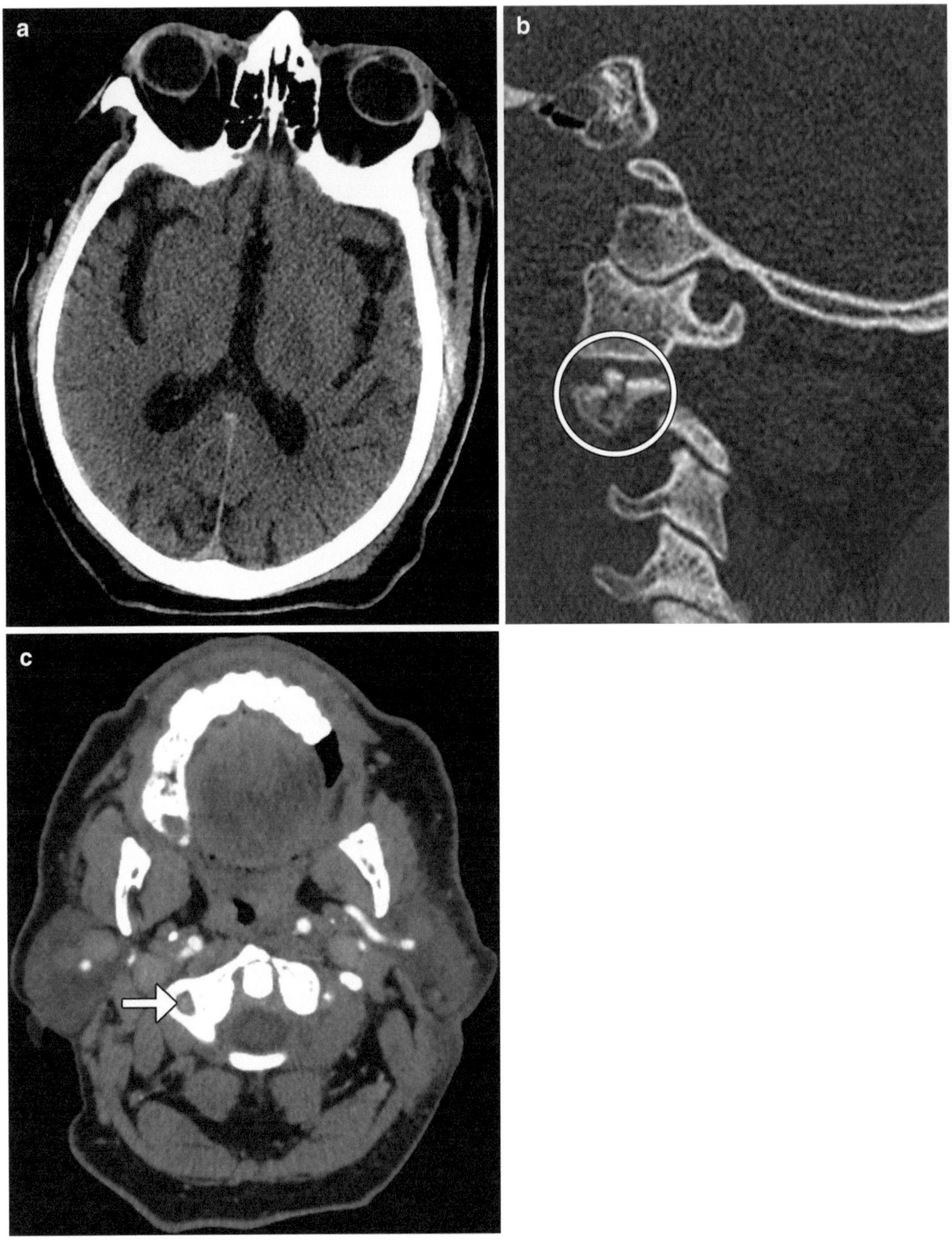

Fig. 8.19 Blunt trauma with cervical spine and vertebral artery injury. Axial CT of the head shows left temporal scalp hemorrhage (**a**). Sagittal cervical spine CT image (**b**) shows a comminuted and displaced fracture of the right lateral mass of C2 (encircled). Axial CTA image (**c**) shows paucity of opacification of the right vertebral artery (*arrow*)

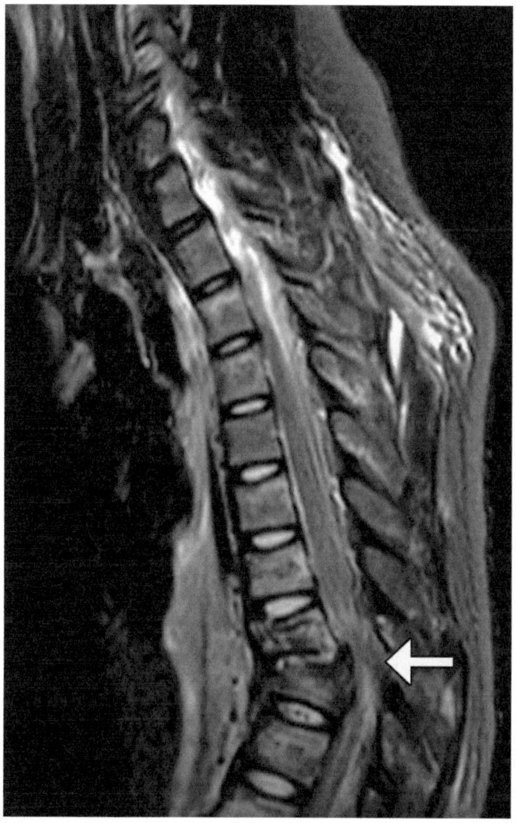

Fig. 8.20 Blunt spine trauma with fracture and spinal cord injury. The patient experienced bilateral lower extremity paralysis after being hit in the back by a large tree branch. Sagittal STIR MRI shows edema in the upper back soft tissues and a Chance fracture at the thoracolumbar junction with retropulsion and compression of the spinal cord (*arrow*)

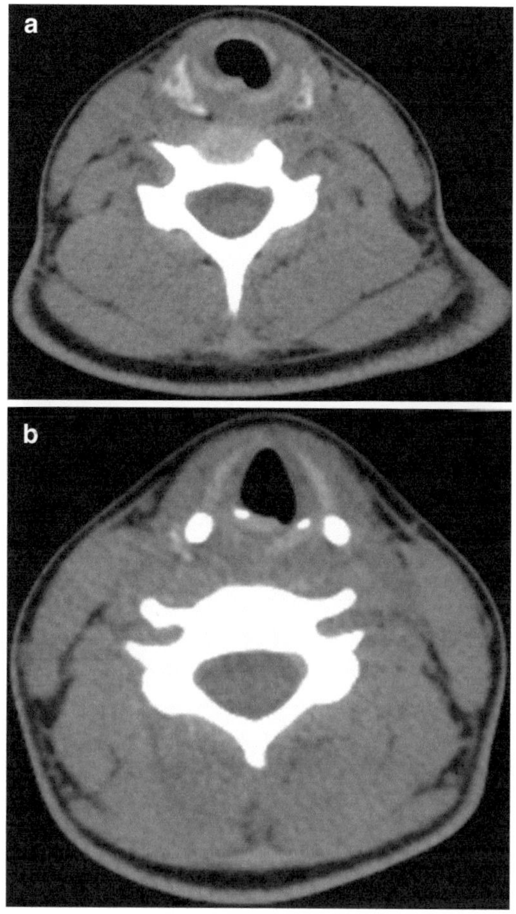

Fig. 8.21 Laryngeal fracture. The patient experienced dysphonia after being struck by a football in the neck. Axial CT images (**a**, **b**) show a displaced fracture of the posterior cricoid and associated soft tissue swelling and contour deformity of the subglottic lumen

sensation, and the skin appears dark and hard, with occasional hemorrhagic blisters. Furthermore, thermal injuries can be complicated by infection and osteonecrosis. Over time, thermal injuries can lead to scarring, which can appear as deformity and abnormal texture of the skin. Growth of the burn scars may indicate malignant transformation.

Imaging Findings

In the acute setting, there can be swelling of the affected soft tissue from burn injuries, with corresponding subcutaneous fat stranding visible on imaging in more severe cases (Fig. 8.24). CT can be useful for evaluating the extent of osteonecrosis in calvarial burn injuries for preoperative planning and manifests as delayed osteolysis (Fig. 8.25). CT imaging can also be useful for evaluating scar tissue formation that obliterates the external auditory canal and results in hearing loss (Fig. 8.26). In addition, CT or MRI may be useful for evaluating the extent of malignancies arising from burn scars. While most of these neoplasms may have nonspecific imaging features, cutaneous osteosarcomas can contain calcifications.

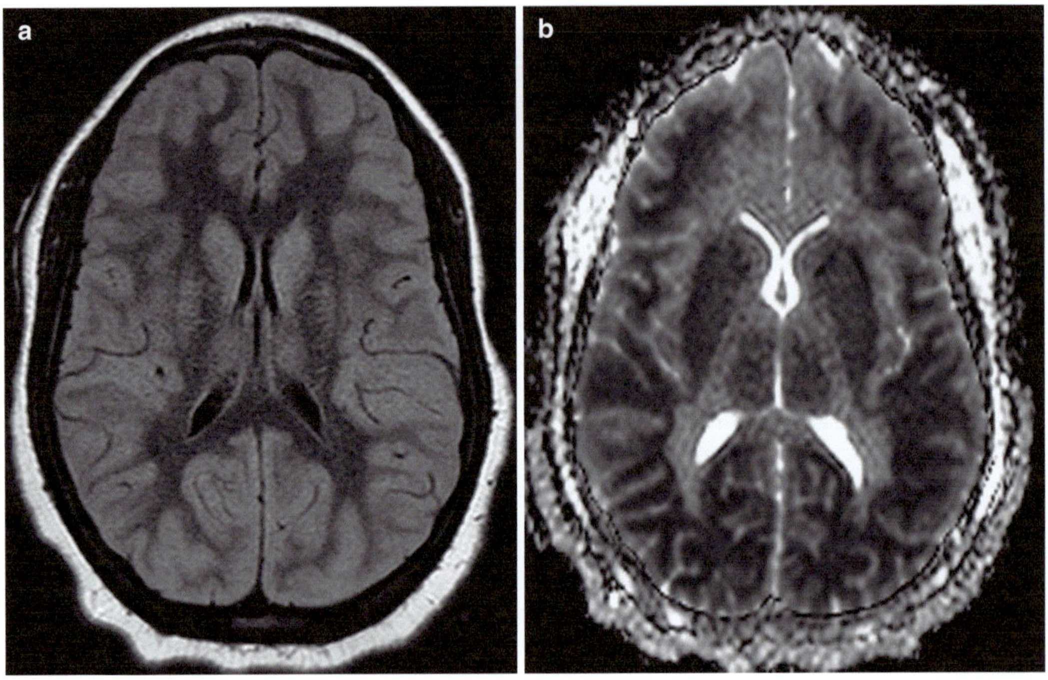

Fig. 8.22 Strangulation from hanging with diffuse hypoxic ischemic injury. Axial FLAIR (**a**) and ADC map (**b**) show extensive diffuse restricted diffusion and swelling of the bilateral cerebral hemispheres in a hypoxic-ischemic pattern

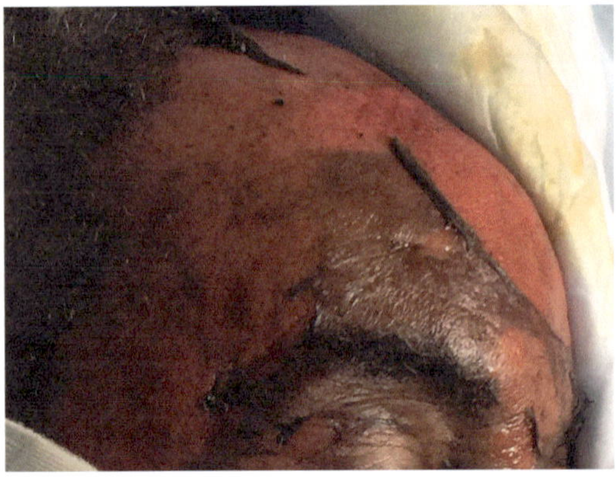

Fig. 8.23 Thermal injury. The patient suffered a second degree burn to the head, with erythema and sloughing of the skin. Courtesy of Lawrence Gottlieb, MD

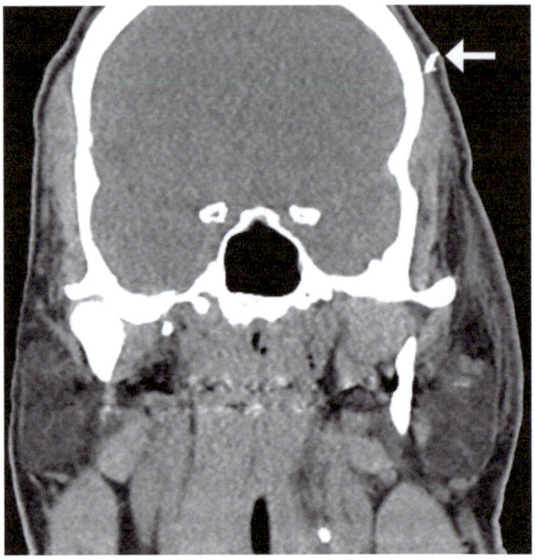

Fig. 8.24 Thermal injury. Coronal CT image shows edema in the left facial soft tissues secondary to a burn after being struck by a firework with a firework fragment embedded in the scalp (*arrow*)

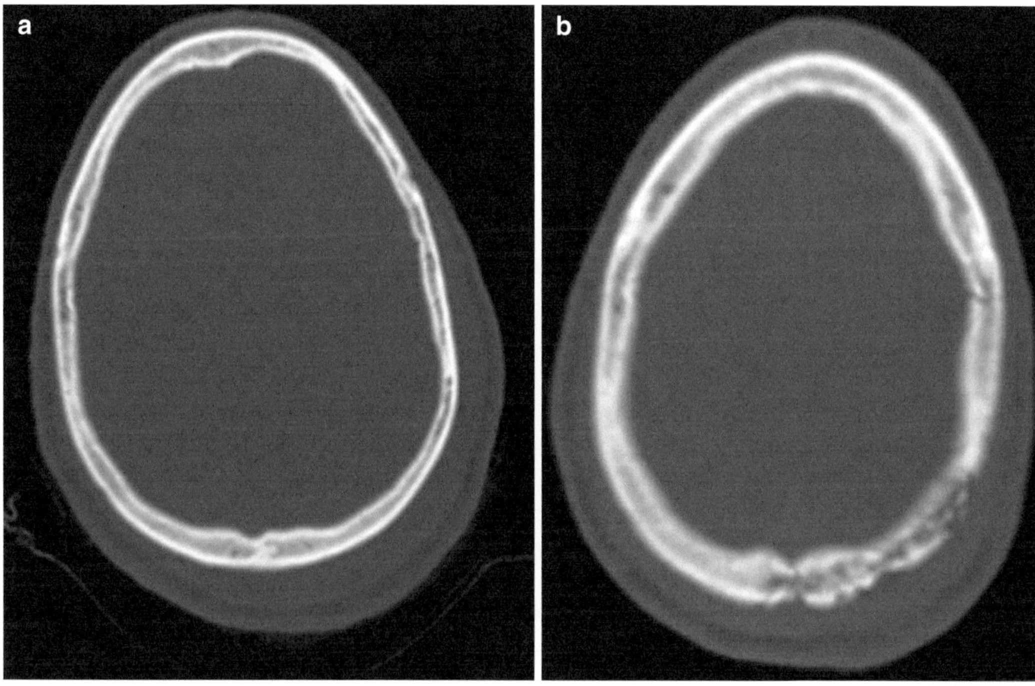

Fig. 8.25 Thermal injury with osteonecrosis. Axial CT image (**a**) at initial presentation shows posterior scalp swelling, but an intact calvarium. Axial CT image (**b**) obtained several months later shows osteolysis in the left parietal bone underlying the area of prior scalp injury

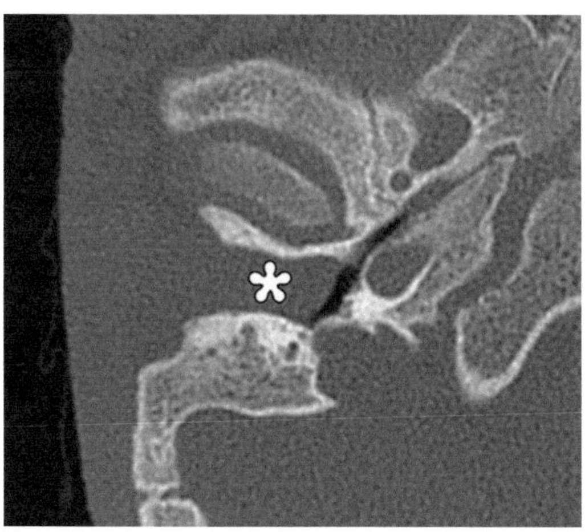

Fig. 8.26 Thermal injury with scar tissue formation. The patient incurred an electrical burn to the right side of the body, resulting in loss of the auricle, extensive scarring, and hearing loss. Axial CT image shows soft tissue material filling the right external auditory canal (*)

Birth Trauma

Overview

Birth-related injury is defined as traumatic/ischemic event sustained during delivery. Scalp lesions incurred during birth include the following:

- Abrasions and lacerations: typically minor and tend to occur mainly after vacuum extraction and forceps delivery.
- Caput succedaneum: serosanguinous collection within the subcutaneous fibrofatty space between the skin and the adjacent galea aponeurotica. It is caused by the mechanical trauma of the fetal cranium pushing through the cervix.

- Subgaleal hemorrhage: located between the galea aponeurosis and the calvarial periosteum. This space extends from the orbital margins anteriorly, to the nuchal ridge posteriorly, and the temporal fascia laterally and normally contains loose connective tissue and small blood vessels. Subgaleal hemorrhage is most often associated with vacuum extraction and forceps delivery.
- Cephalohematoma: subperiosteal hemorrhage that accumulates between the calvarial periosteum and the adjacent outer table of the skull and would be deep to the temporalis muscle. It is also associated with vacuum extraction, forceps, and breech delivery.

Other birth-related injuries to the head and neck region that are beyond the scope of this section include intracranial hemorrhage, which is not rare even in asymptomatic infants, brain contusions, shear force, diffuse axonal injury, hypoxia-ischemic injury, suture diastasis, skull fracture, peripheral nerve injury, particularly involving the brachial plexus, and fibromatosis coli.

Clinical Findings

Cephalohematomas can present as soft tissue swelling with purpura/ecchymosis over the affected part of the scalp. These typically extend across suture lines and usually resolve within a few days without treatment.

Subgaleal hematomas can present as firm or fluctuant swelling of the scalp across suture lines. The loose connective tissue in this space can permit massive bleeding, which can result in hemorrhagic shock. Treatment is mainly supportive.

Cephalohematomas can present as firm scalp swelling confined by the sutures. Thus, these are often unilateral and are not associated with skin discoloration. The subperiosteal hemorrhage often accumulates gradually and may only be apparent a few days after birth. Significant blood loss is rare. Cephalohematomas rarely calcify, which may lead to a cosmetic deformity. Seldomly the cephalohematoma requires evacuation for cosmetic purposes if it does not resorb on its own.

Imaging Findings

Ultrasound, CT, or MRI may be implemented for more precisely localizing birth-related scalp hemorrhage and the possibility of associated intracranial injuries. MRI in particular can readily demonstrate the depth of birth-related scalp injuries, as well as any associated intracranial hemorrhagic and ischemic lesions. The different layers of the scalp are especially conspicuous when separated by hemorrhage, with the galea aponeurotica appearing as a low signal membrane that extends across suture lines and the periosteum as a low signal membrane that is confined to suture lines (Fig. 8.27). In addition,

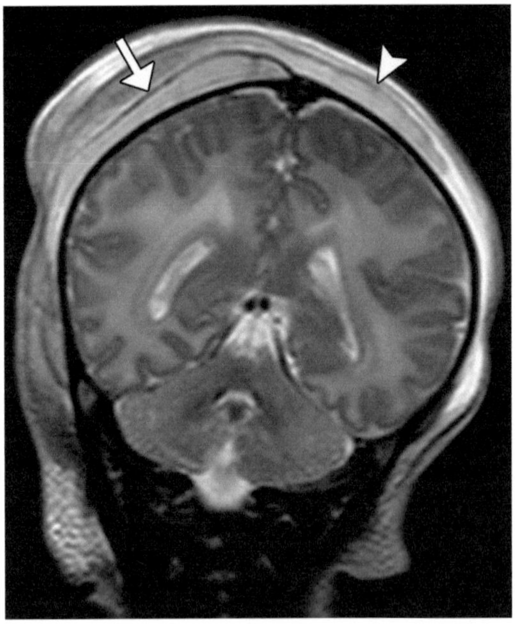

Fig. 8.27 Birth injury of the scalp. Coronal T2-weighted MRI shows a right cephalohematoma deep to the periosteum (*arrow*), which is bounded in the midline to the sagittal suture, a subgaleal hematoma, which crosses the midline and is bounded by the galea aponeurotica (*arrowhead*), as well as subcutaneous fluid, compatible with caput succedaneum

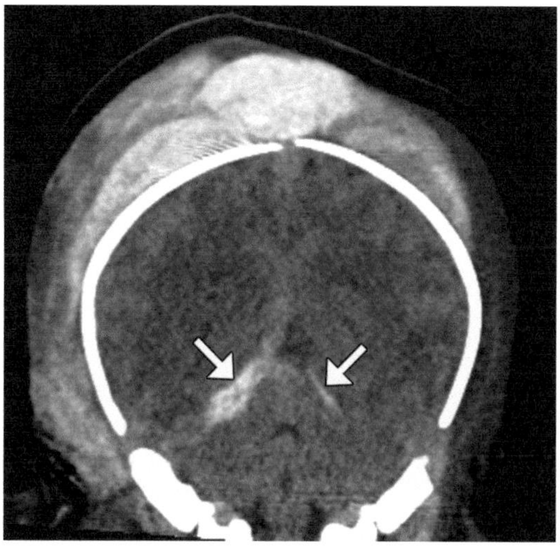

Fig. 8.28 Birth-related injury with scalp and intracranial hemorrhage. Coronal CT image shows extensive bilateral cephalohematomas and subgaleal hematomas, as well as subdural hemorrhages along the tentorial leaflets bilaterally (*arrows*)

unlike cephalohematoma, subgaleal hemorrhage is superficial to the temporal muscle. Despite the ionizing radiation exposure, CT is often preferred over MRI if there is respiratory and/or hemodynamic instability due to the relative rapidity of the scan. CT is also better than ultrasound for detecting posterior fossa abnormalities, especially retrocerebellar and tentorial subdural hemorrhages in the setting of birth-related injuries (Fig. 8.28), as well as skull fractures, which are often linear and usually affect the parietal bones (Fig. 8.29).

Non-accidental Trauma

Overview

Non-accidental trauma, or child abuse, is the intentional infliction of pain and suffering on children. Significant injuries that can result from non-accidental trauma in general include rib fracture, metaphyseal fracture, interhemispheric subdural hemorrhage, shear-type brain and spinal cord injury, hypoxic ischemic injury, vertebral compression fracture, retinal hemorrhage, and small bowel hematoma and laceration. Shaking has been implicated as a major causative mechanism in abusive head and neck injury (shaken baby syndrome). Blunt trauma, strangulation, and suffocation are other important causes of brain injury in the setting of non-accidental trauma.

Ultimately, substantiating non-accidental trauma typically requires a multidisciplinary approach and gathering comprehensive history. It is the responsibility of healthcare professionals to detect cases of abuse and intervene appropriately to prevent further harm. Thus, it is important to be able to recognize findings attributable to child abuse and differentiate these from accidental injury.

Clinical Findings

Skin lesions may be the leading sign of physical abuse. The most common dermatologic signs of child abuse are bruises and abrasions followed by lacerations, scratches, soft tissue edema, strap marks, hematomas, burns, and bites. Bruises are the most common of these injuries and those that occur in protected areas or in non-ambulatory children are suspicious for non-accidental trauma (Fig. 8.30). Furthermore, multiple bruises in clusters, with a defined pattern, or different stages of healing are strongly suggestive of abuse. The mechanisms of abuse and corresponding skin findings are listed in Table 8.2.

Imaging Findings

Although CT has generally been the recommended as the first-line screening imaging modality for suspected non-accidental head trauma, MRI consisting of T1-weighted, T2-weighted, gradient-recalled echo or susceptibility-weighted imaging, and diffuse-weighted imaging sequences has many advantages, including no exposure to

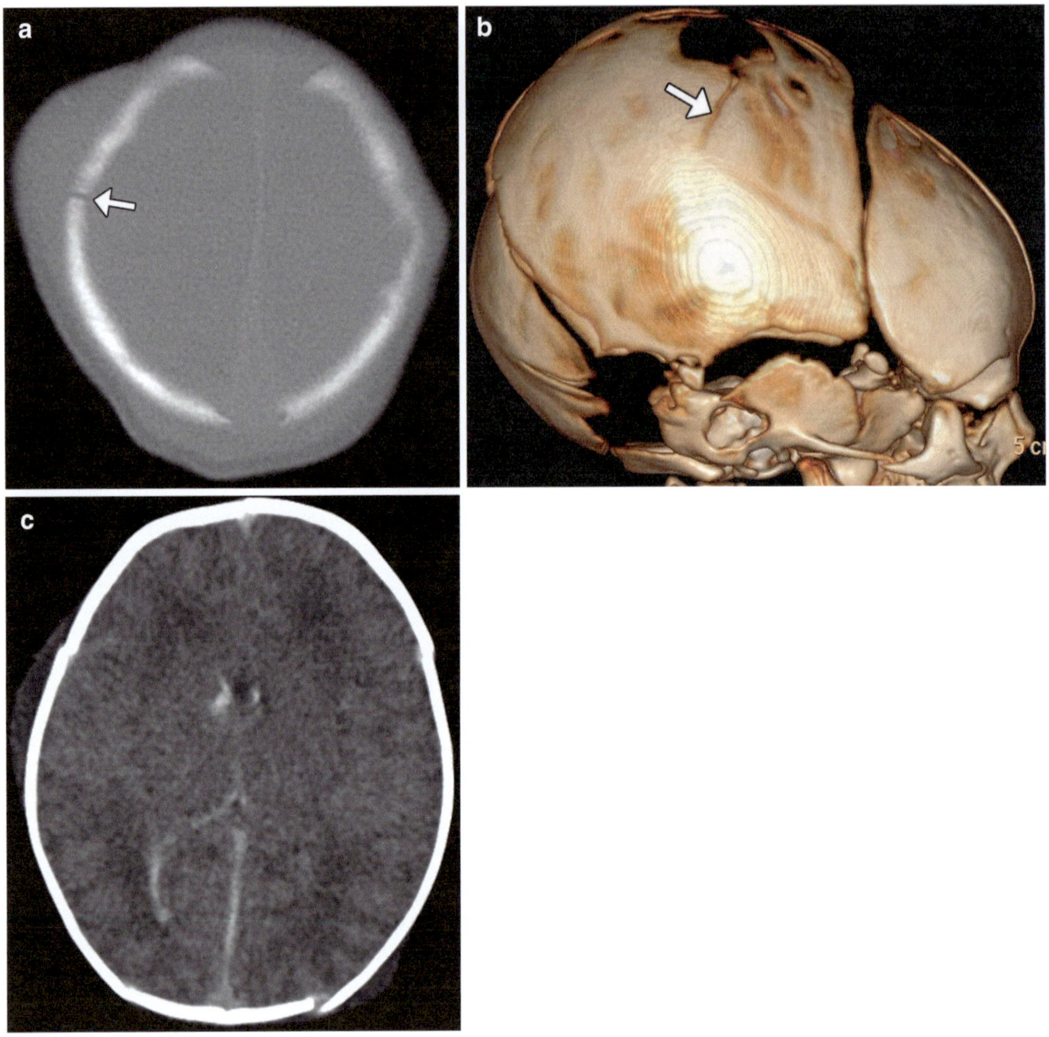

Fig. 8.29 Forceps delivery with scalp injury and skull fracture. Axial (**a**) and 3D (**b**) CT bone window and axial soft tissue window (**c**) CT images show orthogonally situated scalp hematoma, as well as an underlying right parietal bone fracture (*arrows*) and intracranial hemorrhage. Courtesy of Kayleen Jahangir MD

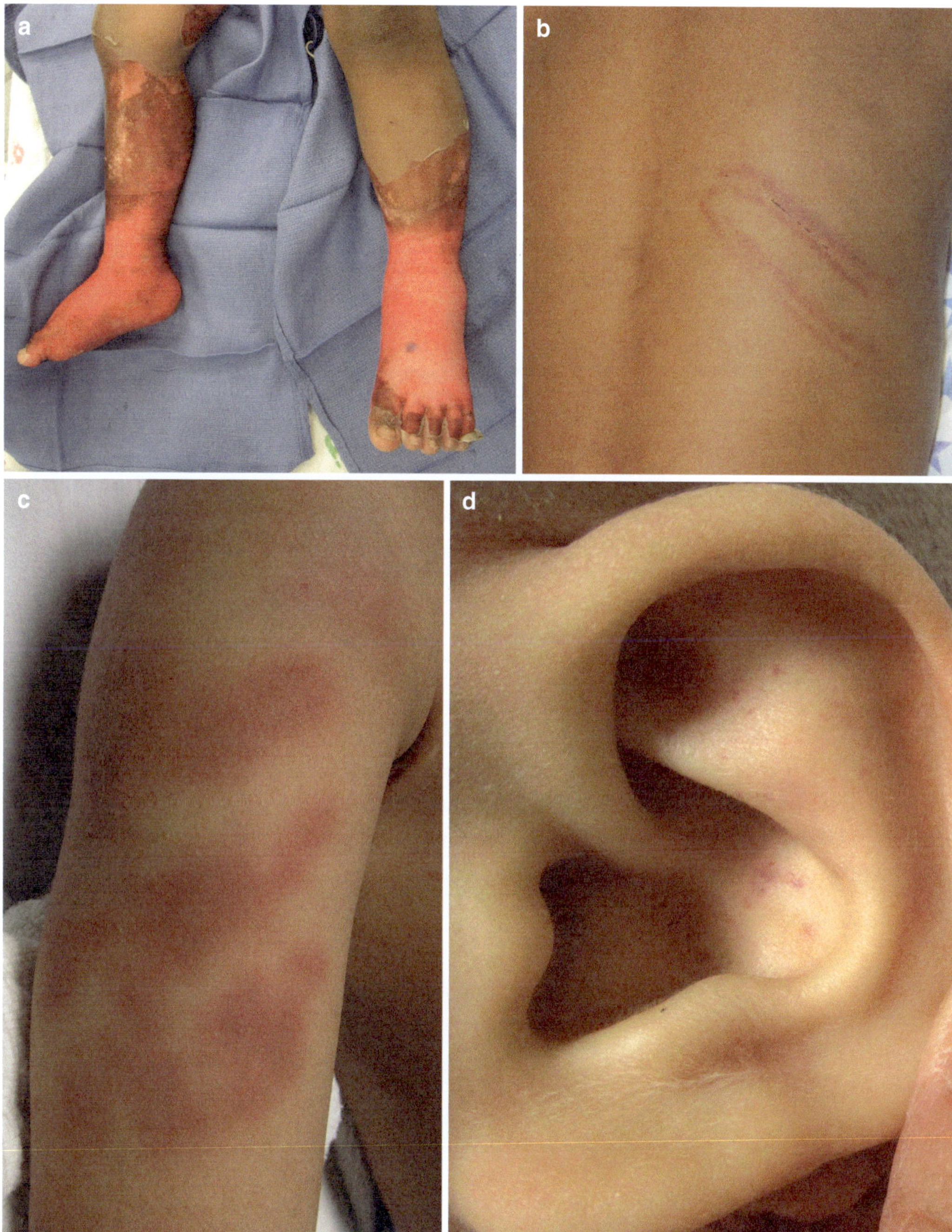

Fig. 8.30 Non-accidental trauma. Photographs of different patients show burn injury involving the bilateral legs (**a**), loops marks on the back (**b**), multiple bruises in the arm (**c**), and ecchymoses in the ear (**d**). Courtesy of Veena Ramaiah MD

ionizing radiation, better depiction of shear injuries, hypoxic ischemic insult, and the ability to more precisely date hemorrhages.

The appearance of intracranial hemorrhage on CT and MRI evolves over time. On CT, acute hemorrhage typically appears as hyperattenuating acutely and gradually becomes isoattenuating to cerebrospinal fluid chronically. Although there may be some degree of variability, especially if there is recurrent bleeding at the same site, the typical appearances of intracranial hematomas on MRI as they progress tend to have fairly well-defined signal characteristics, as denoted in Table 8.3 and exemplified in (Fig. 8.31). If there is layering within the hematoma, dating is more accurate when estimated

Table 8.2 Patterns of skin lesions for selected types of abusive injury

Form of injury	Appearance of corresponding skin lesion
Hands	Marks shaped like the hand or oval fingertips or pinchmarks; linear excoriations from fingernail scratches
Belt	Elongated, wide bands of ecchymoses with markings in the shape of the belt buckle, sometimes with puncture wounds; often in the back or buttocks region
Cords	Linear or looped ecchymosis; often in the back or buttocks region
Burns	Scalding immersion pattern with involvement of the back and posterior head and buttocks with central sparing, or in a stocking-like distribution, but sparing of flexure creases, shapes such as cigarette tips, fork tines, light bulbs, irons, and grills, particularly if second or third degree

Table 8.3 Temporal appearance of intracranial hematomas on MRI

Age of the hemorrhage	MRI
Acute (1–3 days after injury)	Hypointense on T1-weighted images and hypointense on T2-weighted images
Early subacute (3–7 days)	Hyperintense on T1-weighted images and becomes hypointense on T2-weighted images
Late subacute (8–14 days)	Hyperintense on both T1- and T2-weighted images
Chronic (beyond 14 days)	Hypointense on T1-weighted images and hypointense on T2-weighted images

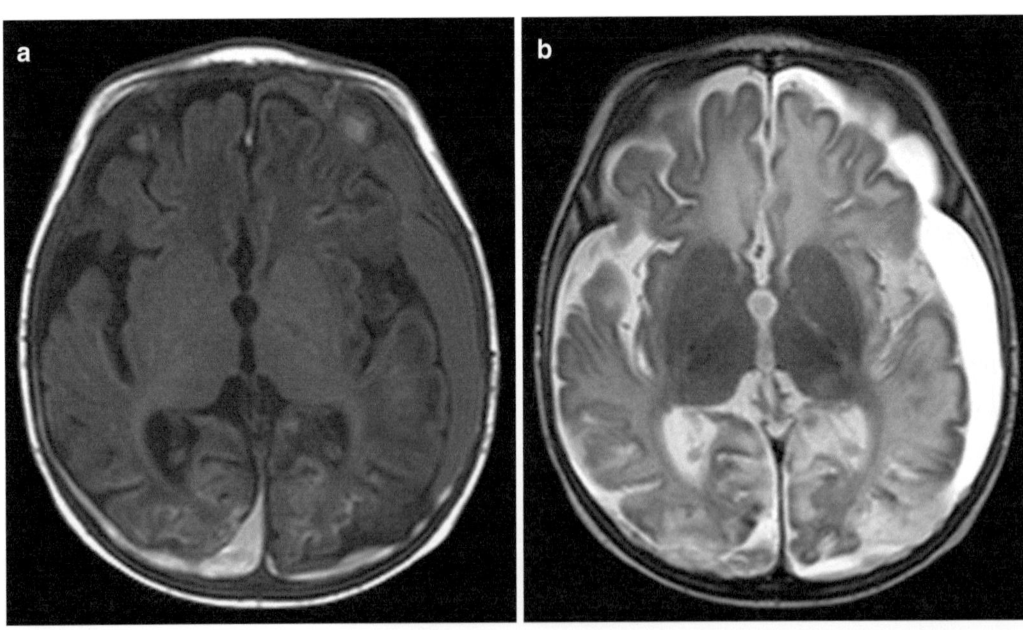

Fig. 8.31 Non-accidental trauma with intracranial hemorrhages of different ages. Axial T1-weighted (**a**) and T2-weighted (**b**) MR images show bilateral cerebral convexity subdural fluid collections with varying signal characteristics. There is also encephalomalacia in the bilateral occipital lobes related to prior infarction

based on the layering component. Subdural hematomas can be associated with a bridging vein rupture, which appears as a linear intravascular clot connected to relatively globular perivascular thrombus at the site of vessel rupture, which can have the configuration of a "tadpole" or "lollipop" on imaging (Fig. 8.32).

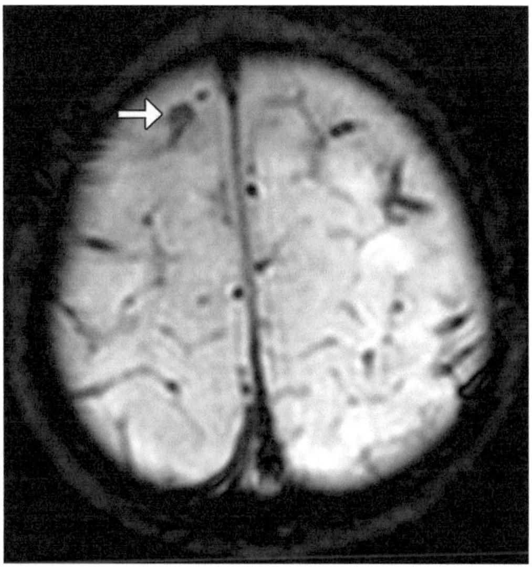

Fig. 8.32 Non-accidental trauma with vessel rupture. Axial SWI MRI sequence shows an area of susceptibility effect adjacent to a cortical vein along the right frontal convexity with a "tadpole' configuration (*arrow*)

Diffuse parenchymal injury can be associated with subdural hemorrhage, retinal hemorrhage, or cervicomedullary junction injury, but can also manifest as an isolated process secondary to asphyxiation or strangulation. Diffuse parenchymal injury in infant abusive is the imaging feature most predictive of outcome and is most commonly attributable to hypoxic ischemic injury and less often diffuse axonal injury. In either case, DWI is the most sensitive sequence for detecting the post-traumatic cytotoxic injury since the T2 prolongation of cerebral edema is otherwise inconspicuous in relatively unmyelinated brain (Fig. 8.33). Abusive hypoxic ischemia injury is often associated with craniocervical junction injuries, including spinal canal hemorrhage, spinal cord injury, nerve root avulsions, and ligamentous and paraspinal soft tissue injuries, which are also best depicted on MRI.

Multiple, complex, and diastatic skull fractures imply a high-energy mechanism that is

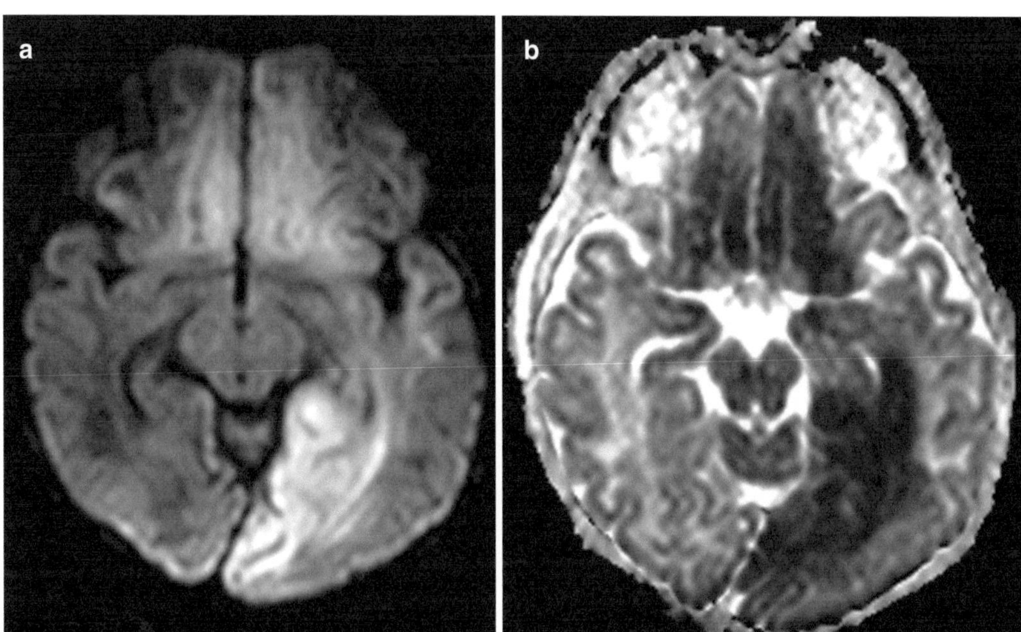

Fig. 8.33 Non-accidental trauma with acute cerebral infarction. Axial DWI (**a**) and ADC map (**b**) show restricted diffusion in multiple vascular territories

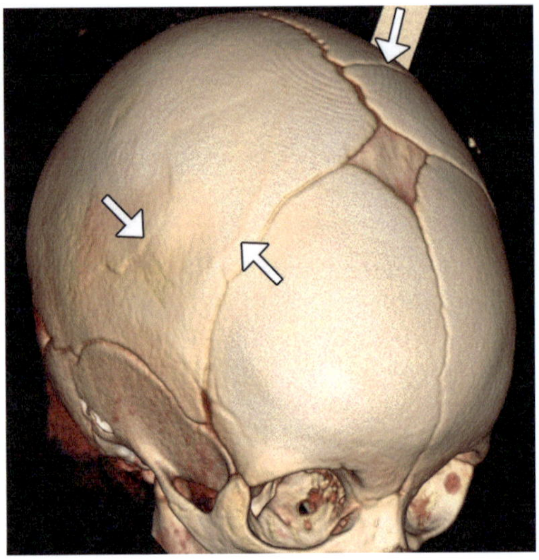

Fig. 8.34 Non-accidental trauma with skull fractures. 3D CT image shows multiple skull fractures (*arrows*)

concerning for abuse, particularly in the absence of a suitable explanation (Fig. 8.34). Alternatively, ping pong type fractures tend to occur in infants, as detailed previously. Multiplanar reconstructions and volume-rendered bone CT images are particularly useful for detecting fractures. However, there is generally poor correlation of skull fracture with intracranial hemorrhage or brain injury. Furthermore, dating of skull fractures on CT is imprecise.

Suggested Reading

Aras MH, Miloglu O, Barutcugil C, Kantarci M, Ozcan E, Harorli A. Comparison of the sensitivity for detecting foreign bodies among conventional plain radiography, computed tomography and ultrasonography. Dentomaxillofac Radiol. 2010;39(2):72–8.

Betts AM, O'Brien WT, Davies BW, Youssef OH. A systematic approach to CT evaluation of orbital trauma. Emerg Radiol. 2014;21(5):511–31.

Bray PW, Mahoney JL, Campbell JP. Sensitivity and specificity of ultrasound in the diagnosis of foreign bodies in the hand. J Hand Surg. 1995;20(4):661–6.

Burns EC, Grool AM, Klassen TP, Correll R, Jarvis A, Joubert G, Bailey B, Chauvin-Kimoff L, Pusic M, McConnell D, Nijssen-Jordan C, Silver N, Taylor B, Osmond MH, Pediatric Emergency Research Canada (PERC) Head Injury Study Group. Scalp hematoma characteristics associated with intracranial injury in pediatric minor head injury. Acad Emerg Med. 2016;23(5):576–83.

Dreizin D, Letzing M, Sliker CW, Chokshi FH, Bodanapally U, Mirvis SE, Quencer RM, Munera F. Multidetector CT of blunt cervical spine trauma in adults. Radiographics. 2014;34(7):1842–65.

Ersahin Y, Gülmen V, Palali I, Mutluer S. Growing skull fractures (craniocerebral erosion). Neurosurg Rev. 2000;23(3):139–44.

Ginat DT, Mayich M, Daftari-Besheli L, Gupta R. Clinical applications of dual-energy CT in head and neck imaging. Eur Arch Otorhinolaryngol. 2016;273(3):547–53.

Gumussoy M, Ugur O, Cukurova I, Uluyol S. Recurrent meningitis and frontal encephalocele as delayed complications of craniofacial trauma. J Craniofac Surg. 2014;25(2):529–30.

Huang CY, Feng CH, Hsiao YC, Chuang SS, Yang JY. Burn scar carcinoma. J Dermatolog Treat. 2010;21(6):350–6.

Kaviani F, Javad Rashid R, Shahmoradi Z, Gholamian M. Detection of foreign bodies by spiral computed tomography and cone beam computed tomography in maxillofacial regions. J Dent Res Dent Clin Dent Prospects. 2014;8(3):166–71.

Kemp AM, Jaspan T, Griffiths J, Stoodley N, Mann MK, Tempest V, Maguire SA. Neuroimaging: what neuroradiological features distinguish abusive from non-abusive head trauma? A systematic review. Dis Child. 2011;96(12):1103–12.

Khurana B, Sheehan SE, Sodickson A, Bono CM, Harris MB. Traumatic thoracolumbar spine injuries: what the spine surgeon wants to know. Radiographics. 2013;33(7):2031–46.

Lupetin AR, Hollander M, Rao VM. CT evaluation of laryngotracheal trauma. Semin Musculoskelet Radiol. 1998;2(1):105–16.

Maier H, Tisch M, Lorenz KJ, Danz B, Schramm A. [Penetrating injuries in the face and neck region. Diagnosis and treatment]. HNO. 2011;59(8):765–82.

Mendis D, Anderson JA. Blunt laryngeal trauma secondary to sporting injuries. J Laryngol Otol. 2017;131(8):728–35.

Nachtergaele P, Van Calenbergh F, Lagae L. Craniocerebral birth injuries in term newborn infants: a retrospective series. Childs Nerv Syst. 2017;33(11):1927–35.

Nelson DW, Martin MJ, Martin ND, Beekley A. Evaluation of the risk of noncontiguous fractures of the spine in blunt trauma. J Trauma Acute Care Surg. 2013;75(1):135–9.

Osguthorpe JD. Head and neck burns. Evaluation and current management. Arch Otolaryngol Head Neck Surg. 1991;117(9):969–74.

Peterson JJ, Bancroft LW, Kransdorf MJ. Wooden foreign bodies: imaging appearance. AJR Am J Roentgenol. 2002;178(3):557–62.

Reichard R. Birth injury of the cranium and central nervous system. Brain Pathol. 2008;18(4):565–70.

Sixta S, Moore FO, Ditillo MF, Fox AD, Garcia AJ, Holena D, Joseph B, Tyrie L, Cotton B, Eastern Association for the Surgery of Trauma. Screening for thoracolumbar spinal injuries in blunt trauma: an Eastern Association for the Surgery of Trauma practice management guideline. J Trauma Acute Care Surg. 2012;73(5 Suppl 4):S326–32.

Spies M, McCauley RL, Mudge BP, Herndon DN. Management of acute calvarial burns in children. J Trauma. 2003;54(4):765–9.

Ssenyonga PK, Le Feuvre D, Taylor A. Head and neck neurovascular trauma: clinical and angiographic correlation. Interv Neuroradiol. 2015;21(1):108–13.

Swerdlin A, Berkowitz C, Craft N. Cutaneous signs of child abuse. J Am Acad Dermatol. 2007;57(3):371–92.

Tekes A, Pinto PS, Huisman TA. Birth-related injury to the head and cervical spine in neonates. Magn Reson Imaging Clin N Am. 2011;19(4):777–90; viii.

Vázquez E, Delgado I, Sánchez-Montañez A, Fábrega A, Cano P, Martín N. Imaging abusive head trauma: why use both computed tomography and magnetic resonance imaging? Pediatr Radiol. 2014;44(Suppl 4):S589–603.

Watanabe K, Kida W. Battle's sign. N Engl J Med. 2012;367(12):1135.

Wintermark M, Sanelli PC, Anzai Y, Tsiouris AJ, Whitlow CT, American College of Radiology Head Injury Institute. Imaging evidence and recommendations for traumatic brain injury: advanced neuro- and neurovascular imaging techniques. AJNR Am J Neuroradiol. 2015;36(2):E1–E11.

Wright JN. CNS injuries in abusive head trauma. AJR Am J Roentgenol. 2017;208(5):991–1001.

Zakrison TL, Williams BH. Cervical spine evaluation in the bluntly injured patient. Int J Surg. 2016;33(Pt B):246–50.

Neuroimaging of Post-treatment and Iatrogenic Conditions Related to the Skin and Subcutaneous Tissues

9

Andrew Kuhn, Charles J. Schatz, Daniel Haraf, and Daniel Thomas Ginat

Contents

A. Kuhn
Department of Radiology, Yale University Medical Center, New Haven, CT, USA

C. J. Schatz
Department of Radiology, Beverly Tower Wilshire Advanced Imaging, University Southern California, Keck School of Medicine, Los Angeles, CA, USA

D. Haraf
Department of Radiation Oncology, University of Chicago, Chicago, IL, USA

D. T. Ginat (✉)
Department of Radiology, University of Chicago, Pritzker School of Medicine, Chicago, IL, USA
e-mail: dtg1@uchicago.edu

D. T. Ginat (ed.), *Neuroradiological Imaging of Skin Diseases and Related Conditions*,
https://doi.org/10.1007/978-3-319-90931-8_9

Abstract

Various treatment effects and implants related to the skin and subcutaneous tissues can be encountered on neuroimaging. Examples include staples, tissue expanders, Mohs micrographic surgery, grafts, radiation therapy, cosmetic and reconstructive fillers and implants, and complications that can result, such as tumor recurrence, as well as Gadolinium-based contrast agents and nephrogenic systemic fibrosis. This chapter reviews the imaging findings of these particular topics.

Skin Staples

Overview

Narrow skin defects from trauma or surgery can be expeditiously closed using metallic staples (Fig. 9.1). The staples are usually removed after 1–2 weeks once the skin heals.

Imaging Findings

Skin staples are frequently encountered on imaging performed during the early postoperative

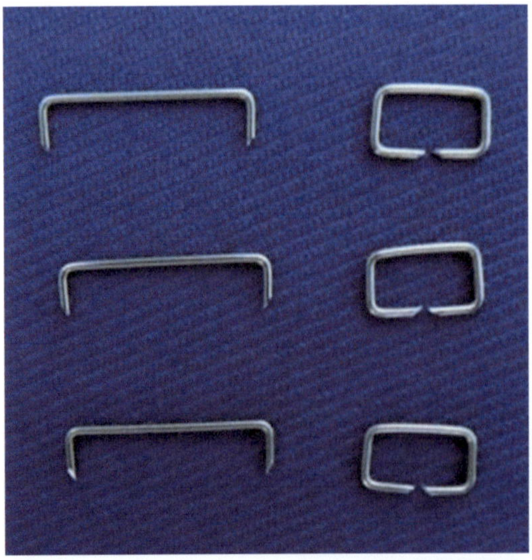

Fig. 9.1 Photograph of skin staples. Courtesy of Triangle Exim

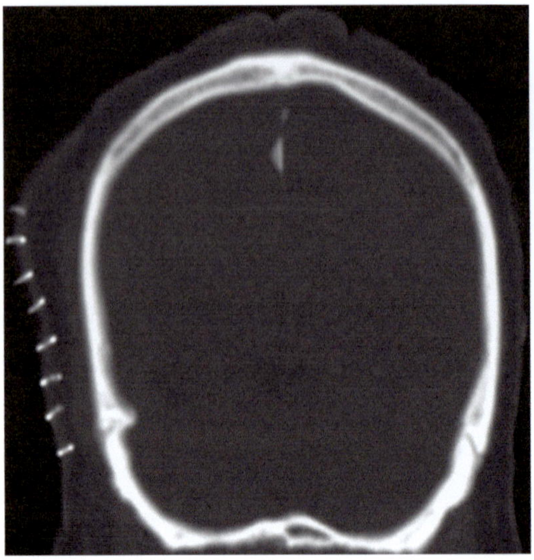

Fig. 9.2 Skin staples. Coronal CT image shows a row of several skin staples in the right scalp

period. Although composed of metal, staples typically do not produce significant beam-hardening artifacts on CT (Fig. 9.2). Surgical staples do not increase skin surface temperature or change in position after MRI and the presence of stainless steel surgical staples appear to be safe at 3T.

Tissue Expanders

Overview

Tissue expanders are used in the scalp for reconstruction of defects caused by trauma, thermal or electric burns, resection of benign or malignant tumors, congenital defects, resection of nevi, infections, and osteoradionecrosis. Although smaller scalp defects can heal via secondary intention without the need for tissue expansion, this may result in skin contracture and limited or absent hair growth. Tissue expansion exploits the ability of skin to be stretched under continuous tensions. This can be accomplished using a silicon balloon inserted under the skin that can be progressively filled with saline (Fig. 9.3).

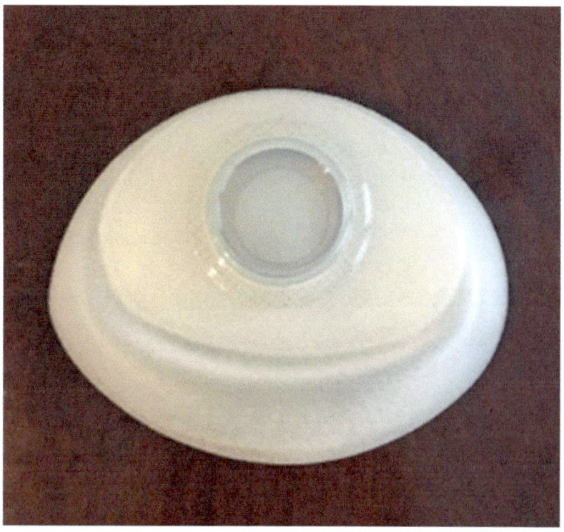

Fig. 9.3 Photograph of an unfilled tissue expander. Courtesy of Melissa Guilbeau

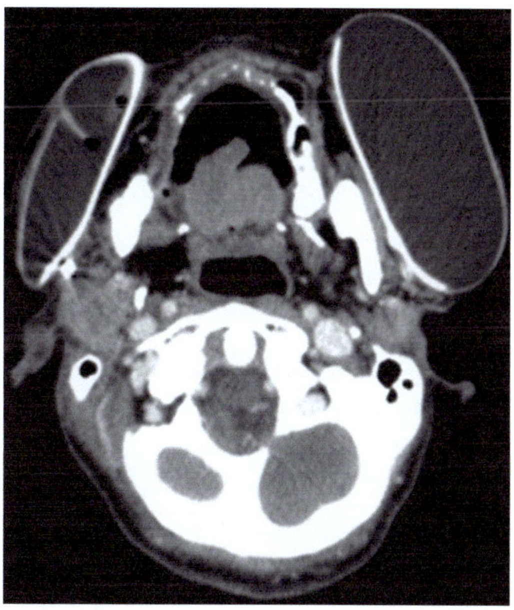

Fig. 9.4 Tissue expander. Axial CT image shows the fluid-filled silicone sacs in the bilateral cheeks

Imaging Findings

On imaging, tissue expanders appear as fluid-filled sacs located beneath the skin and have variable sizes, depending on how much saline has been injected (Fig. 9.4). The devices can be encountered incidentally on imaging, in the vicinity of the area requiring the skin coverage.

Mohs Micrographic Surgery

Overview

Mohs micrographic surgery is a tissue-sparing technique that allows for excision of skin cancers alongside direct microscopic examination of the resected specimen in order to maximize preservation of normal tissues while achieving complete tumor resection. Thin sections of tissue are removed sequentially and the process is repeated until the surgical margins are free of tumor. Following complete clearance of the tumor, reconstruction of the surgical defect is performed. This can be accomplished using a variety of techniques, including complex linear closures, skin flaps, and skin grafts. Alternatively, delayed repair or healing by secondary intention can be implemented, which can be associated with inflammation and scarring (Fig. 9.5).

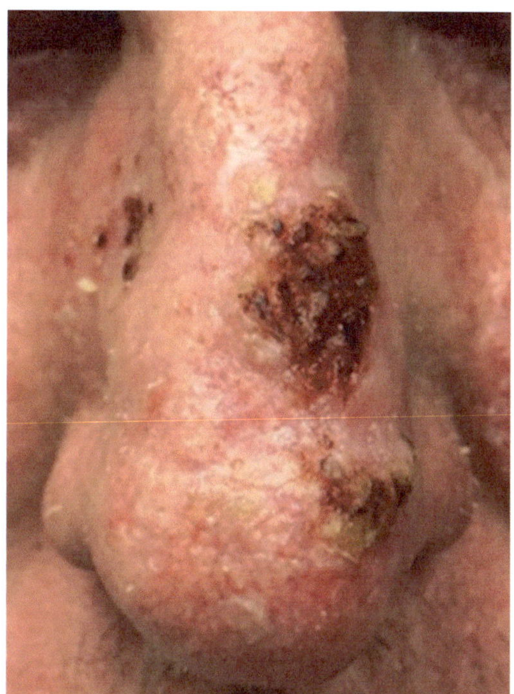

Fig. 9.5 Mohs micrographic surgery. Photograph shows healing skin defects with erythema and scar tissue along the dorsum of the nose

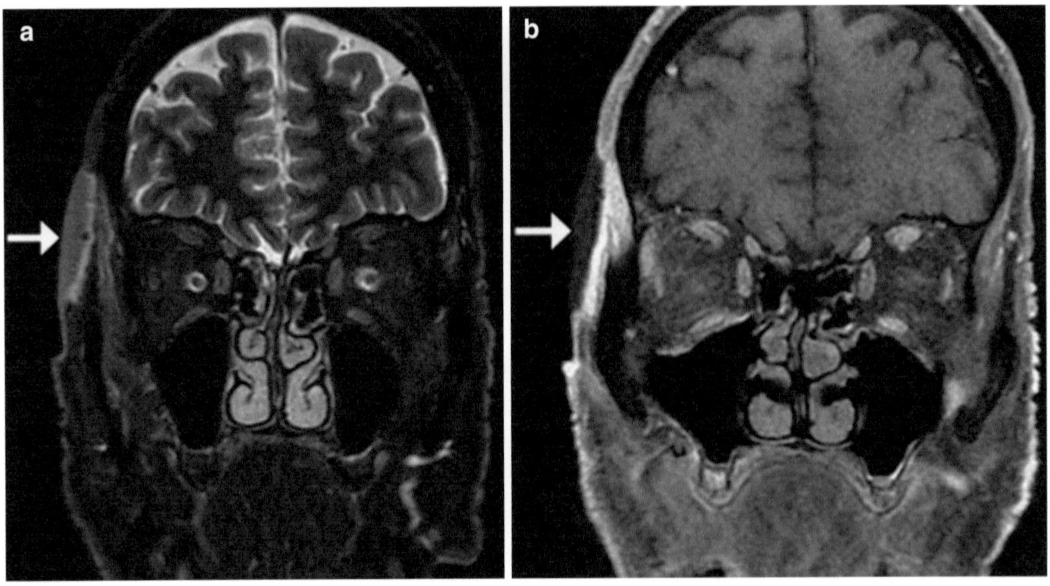

Fig. 9.6 Mohs micrographic surgery. Coronal STIR (**a**) and fat-suppressed post-contrast T1-weighted (**b**) MR images show a right frontotemporal scalp defect (*arrow*) with an overlying dressing and diffuse enhancement of the underlying soft tissues

Imaging Findings

MRI may be obtained after Mohs micrographic surgery in order to assess for residual or recurrent tumor. During the first few weeks to months after surgery, diffuse enhancement from inflammation or granulation tissue beneath the defect can be demonstrated on imaging (Fig. 9.6), which can render assessment for residual or recurrent tumor challenging.

Skin and Myocutaneous Grafts

Overview

The use of skin grafts has increased the ability of surgeons to perform reconstructive surgery by improving outcomes including quality of life for patients suffering from trauma, burns, and cancer. Donor sites are selected based on the desired thickness, texture, and color. They are also selected to minimize discomfort and cosmetic disfigurement at the donor site. The scalp is often used as a donor site because it heals quickly, is associated with low complication rates, and has desirable cosmetic properties.

Split thickness skin grafts consist of transfers of epidermis and some, but not all of the dermis from the donor site, thereby enabling the site of the donor tissue to heal. Full thickness skin grafts utilize the complete layer of skin, involving both the epidermis and entire dermis. Full thickness grafts exhibit less contraction in general and are desirable for facial grafts for aesthetic reasons and for joints or finger tips for the functional advantages associated with minimal contraction. Conversely, split thickness skin grafts are favored for patients with truncal and head and neck defects because the increased wound contraction minimizes scarring (Fig. 9.7).

Myocutaneous grafts are used for filling larger defects (Fig. 9.8). These flaps are either pedicled or free. Pedicle flaps are local or regional muscles that are attached by a vascular supply and rotated into the defect, where they are configured for the particular purpose. On the other hand, free flaps or microvascular free tissue transfer are distant units of tissue that are harvested with a vascular pedicle. The entire flap is transferred with or without the overlying skin to the head and neck defect, where they are revascularized by microsurgical anastomosis to recipient site vessels. Graft failure can be caused by formation of a hematoma/seroma, infection, excessive mechanical tension, and/or inadequate perfusion.

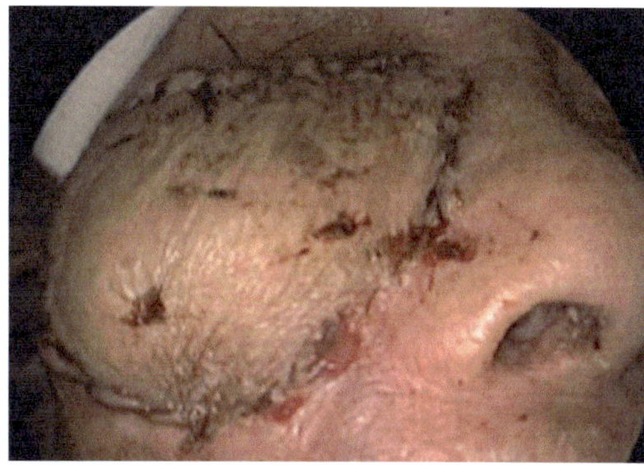

Fig. 9.8 Myocutaneous flap. Photograph shows a flap filling an orbital exenteration and maxillectomy defect

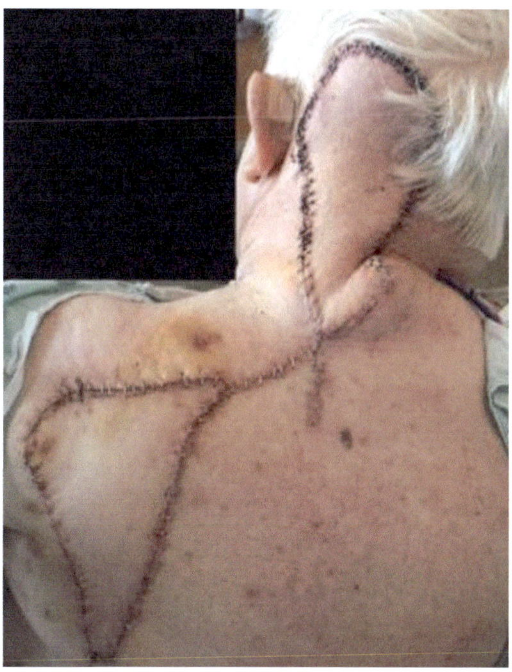

Fig. 9.7 Skin graft. Photograph shows donor and recipient skin graft sites in the back and neck/scalp regions, which are secured by skin staples

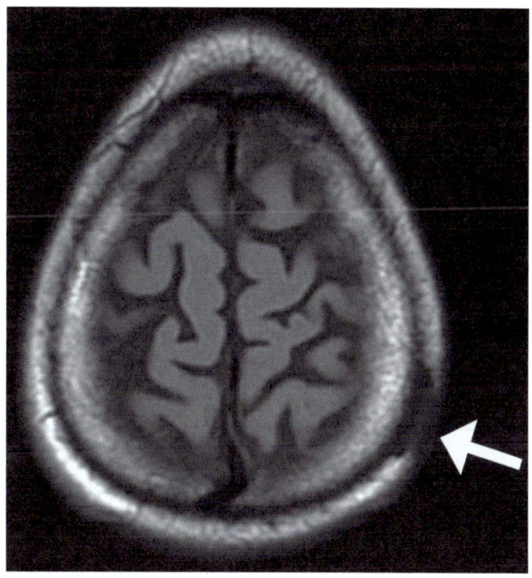

Fig. 9.9 Skin graft. Axial T1-weighted MRI shows a hypointense area (*arrow*) at the site where a scalp tumor was resected

Imaging Findings

Split-thickness and full-thickness skin grafts are often indistinguishable from normal skin on routine radiological imaging, aside from paucity of subcutaneous fat in some cases (Fig. 9.9). On the other hand, myocutaneous flaps can be recognized by the presence of skin and subcutaneous fat components overlying muscle and sometimes bone, particularly for reconstructing the mandible. The muscular components of flaps typically demonstrate enhancement on MRI (Fig. 9.10), which should not be misinterpreted as tumor. Rather, recurrent tumor appears as a focal mass, usually along the margins of the flaps. Effacement of the fat in or around the flap can be an indirect finding associated with recurrence.

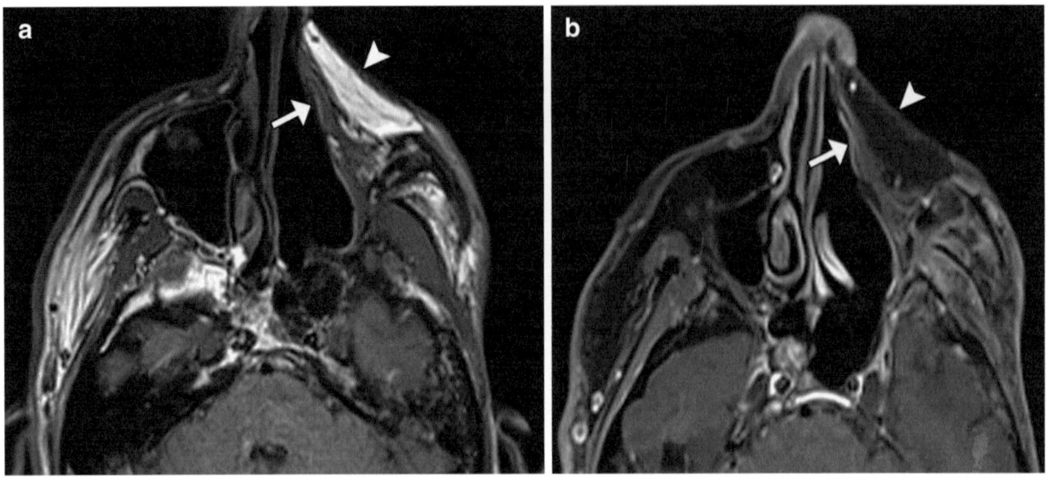

Fig. 9.10 Myocutaneous flap. Axial T1-weighted (**a**) and fat-suppressed post-contrast T1-weighted (**b**) MR images show the cutaneous (arrowheads) and enhancing muscle (*arrows*) components of a flap used to reconstruct a left maxillectomy defect

Radiation Therapy Effects

Overview

The effects of radiation therapy on the skin include acute radiation dermatitis, chronic radiation dermatitis, and radiation recall. Patients receiving radiotherapy for cancer may develop radiation dermatitis. Risk factors for radiation dermatitis include radiation dose, body habitus, proximity of tumor to skin and prior sun exposure. Other complications of radiation therapy include fibrosis, nonhealing ulcers, fistulas, lymphedema, plexopathy, and radionecrosis. In particular, osteoradionecrosis is a condition in which irradiated bone becomes devitalized and exposed through the overlying skin or mucosa and persists without healing for at least 3 months.

Acute radiation dermatitis is dose-dependent, initially appearing as diffuse erythema of the skin and edema in the subcutaneous fat due to inflammation (Fig. 9.11). With increasing dose, the reaction can progress to dry and eventually moist desquamation. Chronic radiation dermatitis, on the other hand, constitutes fibrotic change of the tissue that was irradiated months or years earlier and is caused by inflammatory cytokines and tissue factors. Like acute radiation dermatitis, chronic radiation dermatitis is dose dependent.

Radiation recall is an inflammatory reaction to a chemotherapeutic drug that occurs in patients who have previously received radiation therapy. The chemotherapeutic drug generates an acute dermatitis in the region where the patient had been previously exposed to radiation. These drugs include, but are not limited to anthracyclines like doxorubicin, daunorubicin, and idarubicin, as well as methotrexate, paclitaxel, and cyclophosphamide. Radiation recall typically occurs several years after undergoing radiation therapy.

Necrosis of the skin and underlying tissues can lead to ulceration with exposure of critical structures and are prone to superimposed infection (Fig. 9.12). In particular, fistulas are tracts that form through necrosed tissues, connecting the skin to an underlying cavity, such as pharyngocutaneous or orocutaneous fistulas (Fig. 9.13).

Patients who have been exposed to previous head and neck radiation have an increased risk of necrosis and fistula formation because irradiated tissue displays hypovascularity at baseline, which is believed to impair the postoperative healing process. Both fistula formation and skin necrosis can occur at doses as low as 60 Gy and tend to manifest 6–12 months after radiation therapy.

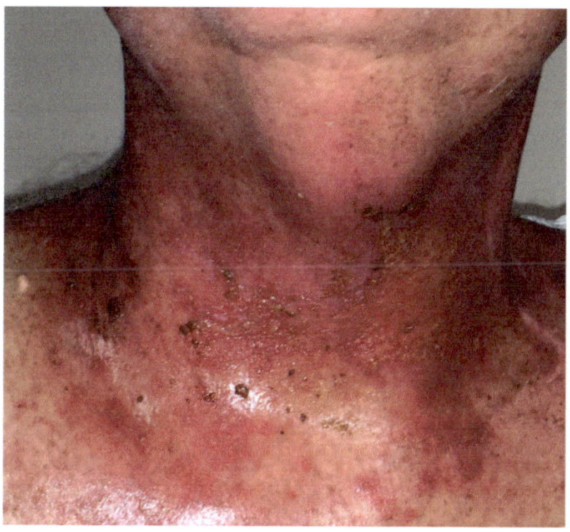

Fig. 9.11 Radiation dermatitis. Clinical photograph of radiation dermatitis shows diffuse erythema in the neck of a patient treated for head and neck cancer

Imaging Findings

Early findings related to radiation therapy that can be encountered on CT and MRI include thickening of the skin and platysma, stranding of the subcutaneous fat, retropharyngeal edema, increased enhancement and atrophy of the major salivary glands, and thickening and increased enhancement of the pharyngeal soft tissues (Fig. 9.14). In chronic radiation dermatitis, there is development of diffuse fibrosis of the involved tissues, which may cause a diagnostic dilemma due to the inability to clearly discern lymph nodes or tumors.

Imaging is useful for evaluating the extent of radiation necrosis in the head and neck. When severe, there can be skin and underlying soft tissue defects that are sometimes accompanied by osteonecrosis and infection (Fig. 9.15). Osteonecrosis can appear as a focal lytic lesion with cortical destruction, sequestrum formation, and loss of the trabeculation on CT and abnormal bone marrow

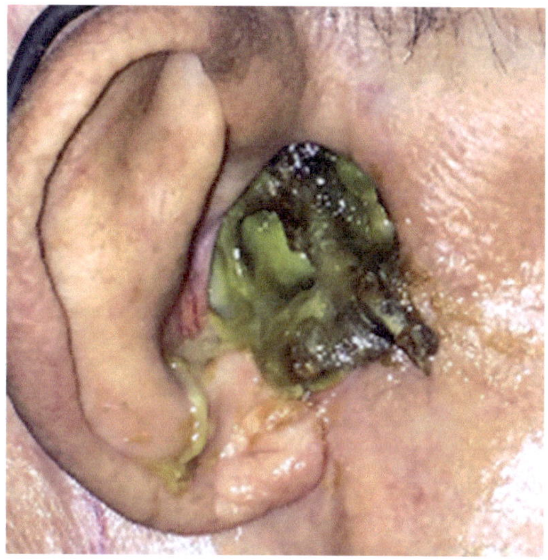

Fig. 9.12 Skin necrosis and infection. Photograph shows a large preauricular skin defect with purulent material and exposure of the mandibular condyle in a patient treated for squamous cell carcinoma

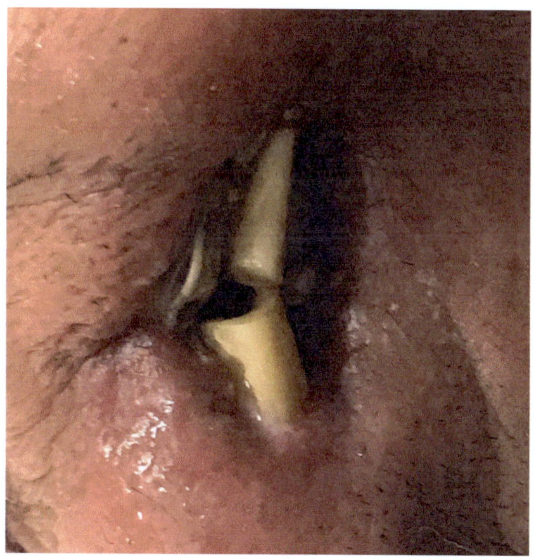

Fig. 9.13 Fistula. Photograph shows a lower face skin defect that communicates with the oral cavity, with exposure of the fibular bone grafts used to reconstruct the mandible

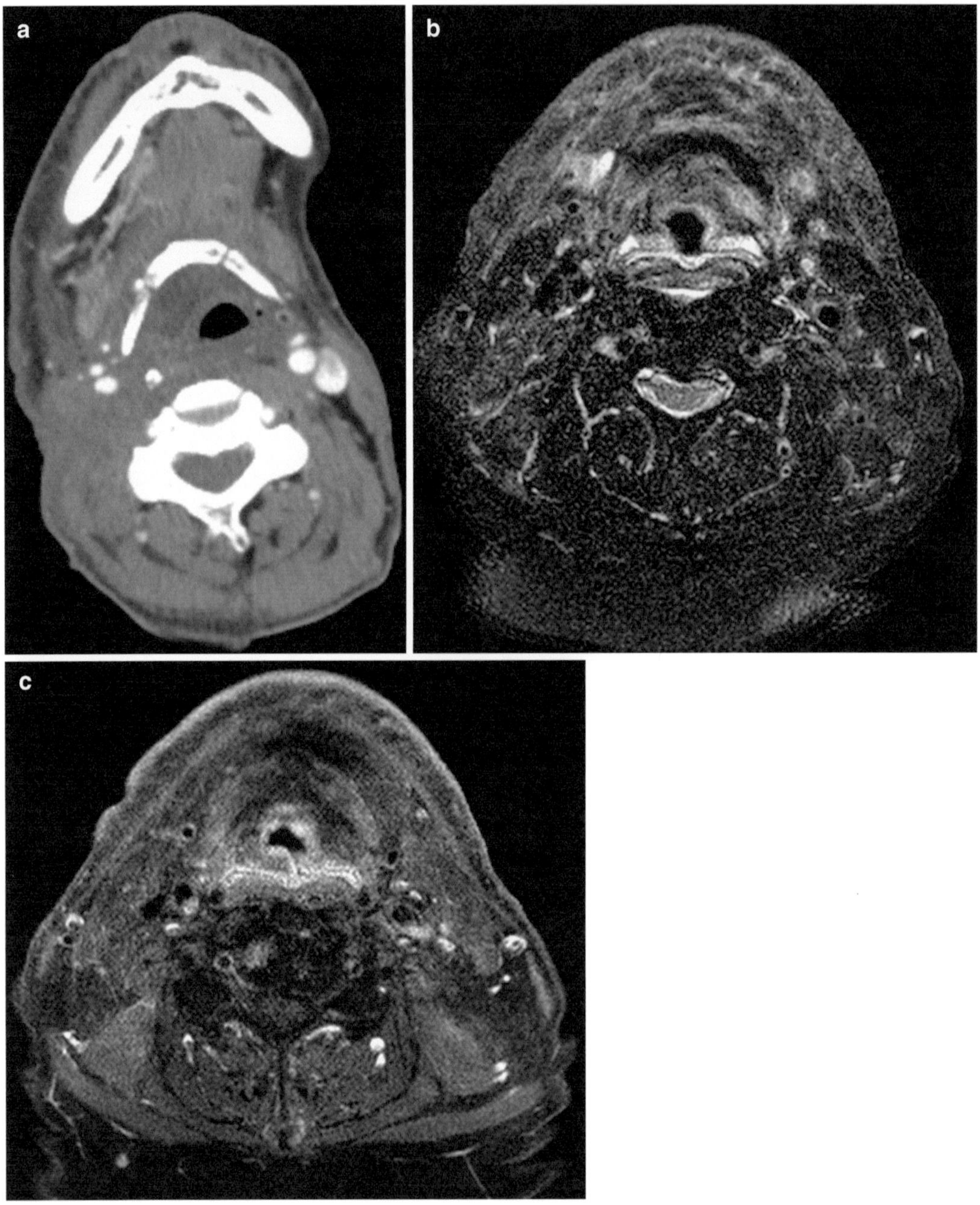

Fig. 9.14 Radiation dermatitis and associated findings. Axial CT image (**a**) shows diffuse stranding of the right neck subcutaneous tissues, thickening of the platysma, pharyngeal edema, atrophy and hyperattenuation of the submandibular glands, and narrowing of the carotid artery, suggestive of radiation vasculopathy. Axial fat-suppressed T2-weighted (**b**) and post-contrast T1-weighted (**c**) MR images in a different patient show diffuse swelling and reticulation of the anterior neck soft tissues and edema and mucositis in the pharynx

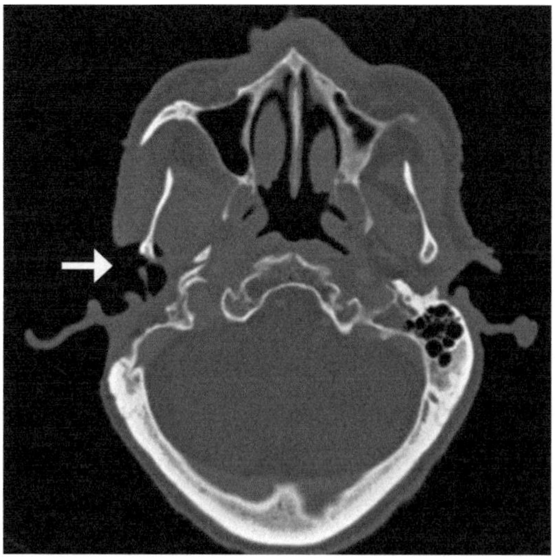

Fig. 9.15 Skin and osteonecrosis. The axial CT image shows the depth of the right preauricular skin defect (*arrow*) with exposure and partial lysis of the mandibular condyle in the same patient as shown in Fig. 9.12

signal on MRI, which can resemble infection. Recurrent tumors in the radiation field can predispose to skin ulceration and fistula formation. In patients with suspected orocutaneous or pharyngocutaneous fistulas, CT with contrast is the preferred imaging modality due to the ability to delineate the fistulous channel and generally adequate ability to detect tumor (Fig. 9.16). Otherwise, MRI or ^{18}FDG-PET can aid in detecting recurrent tumor. However, ^{18}FDG-PET performed less than 10–12 weeks after completion of radiation therapy can lead to false-positive results due to the presence of post-radiation inflammation.

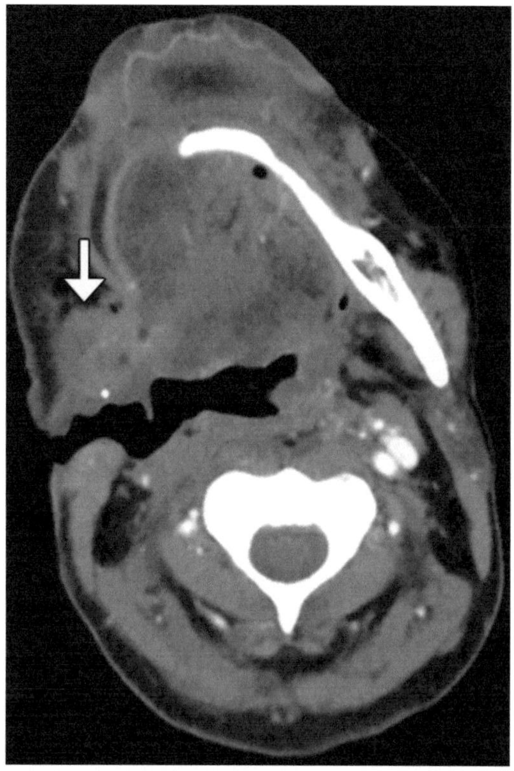

Fig. 9.16 Pharyngocutaneous fistula and tumor recurrence. Axial CT image shows a wide defect that extends from the skin of the right neck to the oropharynx, adjacent to a mass (*arrow*)

Incision Site Tumor Recurrence

Overview

Tumor seeding following head and neck and cranial surgery can result in tumor recurrence at the skin incision site. This complication can occur even with deep tumors that do not initially involve the skin, such as brain tumors, due to disruption of natural anatomical boundaries and seeding during surgery. While the recurrent tumor at the incision site may be apparent on clinical exam as an exophytic skin mass (Fig. 9.17), there may be additional recurrent tumor that grows deep into the underlying skin and subcutaneous tissues, which may not be as evident on clinical examination. Indeed, it has been reported that although residual tumor was clinically observed in only 12% of patients at incision sites, histologically apparent tumor was present in 69% of cases!

Imaging Findings

Imaging may be obtained in patients with suspected incision site tumor recurrence in order to assess the extent of the tumor and identify any additional sites of tumor recurrence or metasta-

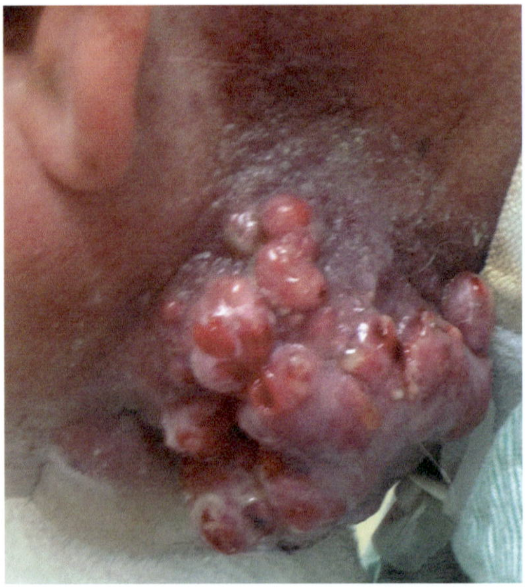

Fig. 9.17 Incision site tumor recurrence. Photograph shows an exophytic, fungating mass along the neck incision plane in a patient with an aerodigestive tract squamous cell carcinoma with lymph node metastases

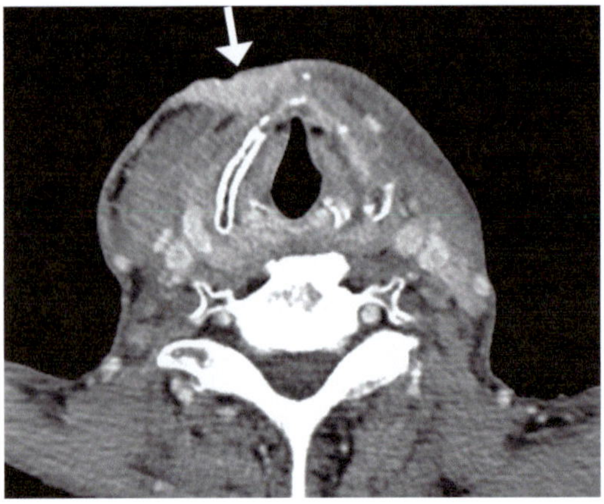

Fig. 9.18 Incision site tumor recurrence. Axial CT image shows an enhancing mass (arrow) involving the skin along the surgical approach performed for glossectomy in a patient with a history of oral squamous cell carcinoma. There are also findings related to radiation therapy in the surrounding soft tissues

ses. While the imaging features may vary depending upon the particular type of tumor, the incision site tumor recurrences tend to be bulkier and more irregular than the usual scar tissue that may otherwise be encountered (Fig. 9.18). Enlargement of the lesion on serial imaging is

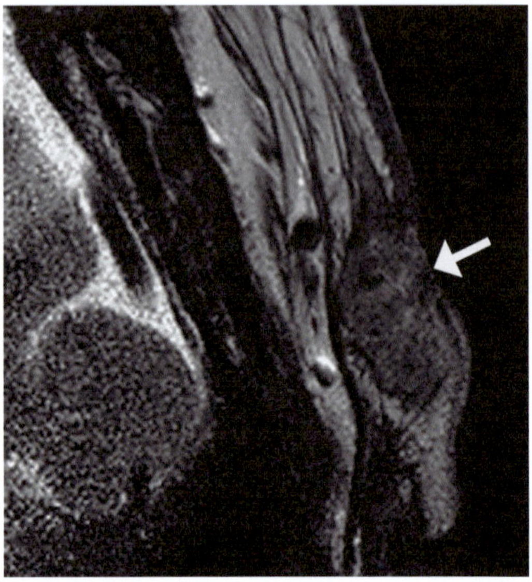

Fig. 9.19 Incision site tumor recurrence. Axial T2-weighted MRI obtained with high-resolution microscopy coil shows a mass that represents recurrent squamous cell carcinoma (*arrow*) beneath the skin surgical site with extension into the underlying subcutaneous tissues

also suggestive of recurrent tumor rather than a benign, transient post-treatment process, such as seroma. A keloid can certainly enlarge over time, but the clinical features tend to be sufficiently distinctive. MRI with diffusion-weighted imaging can be helpful for early detection of small incision site recurrences, which often stand out as brighter than the surrounding tissues. MRI with high-resolution microscopy coil imaging can also be useful for precisely delineating the depth of recurrent tumors in the cutaneous tissues (Fig. 9.19).

It is also important to focus on other areas that may have been disrupted by the surgery. For example, pleomorphic adenoma has a tendency to seed into the parapharyngeal space in addition to the parotidectomy bed and dermal incision plane, with multiple lesions that can have a bunch of grapes appearance on imaging. Furthermore, with neck dissection, the altered lymphatic drainage can lead to lymph node metastases at relatively unconventional locations, such as the retropharyngeal lymph nodes. Finally, after resection of extensive malignant scalp neoplasms that involved craniectomy or

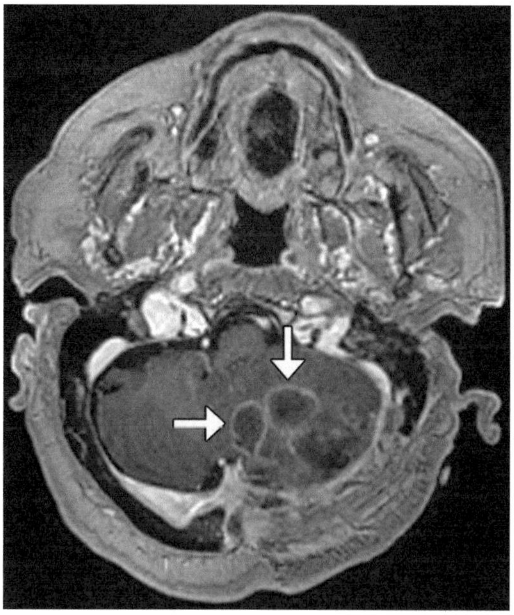

Fig. 9.20 Recurrent tumor with intracranial extension. Axial post-contrast T1-weighted MRI shows peripherally enhancing tumors (*arrows*) in the left cerebellar hemisphere following craniectomy and scalp reconstruction for skin squamous cell carcinoma resection

cranioplasty, intracranial spread of recurrent tumor is a potential complication and is best evaluated via MRI (Fig. 9.20).

Cosmetic Fillers

Overview
Cosmetic filler treatments are performed not only for rejuvenation of facial wrinkles, but also for pathological entities, including HIV-associated lipoatrophy, acne scars, and acquired facial asymmetry from trauma or conditions that lead to hemifacial atrophy including progressive hemifacial atrophy syndrome and scleroderma. A wide variety of cosmetic filler agents have been used, including those comprised of hyaluronic acid, calcium hydroxylapatite, collagen, and liquid silicone, for example.

Imaging Findings

The imaging features of cosmetic fillers depend upon the type of filler material as follows:

- *Calcium hydroxylapatite* is a biodegradable filler. It is approved for use for moderate to severe facial folds, as well as for HIV-induced lipoatrophy. The filler stimulates the production of collagen. It appears as high attenuation linear streaks or clumps on CT, with attenuation values between 280 and 700 HU (Fig. 9.21). On MRI, it appears as low-to-intermediate signal intensity on both T1- and T2-sequences. Since calcium hydroxylapatite is resorbed slowly, these effects are often demonstrated over 2 years after its original injection, leaving behind soft tissue attenuation fibrosis. There is often associated hypermetabolism on ^{18}FDG-PET, presumably related to inflammatory cell infiltration and neofibrogenesis.
- *Hyaluronic acid* is a reversible agent that dissipates over time. On CT, the hyaluronic acid gel can appear as clumps or streaks of fluid attenuation. On MRI, the high fluid content of the gel confers T2 hyperintensity, but there can be associated enhancement that can last at least several months (Fig. 9.22).

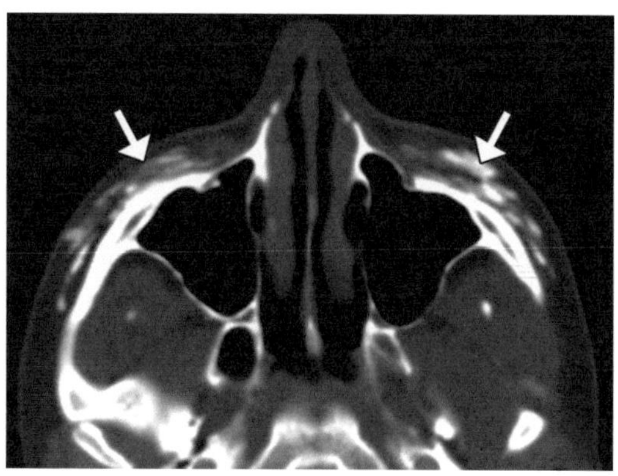

Fig. 9.21 Calcium hydroxylapatite filler. Axial CT image shows streaky calcifications in the bilateral cheeks (*arrows*)

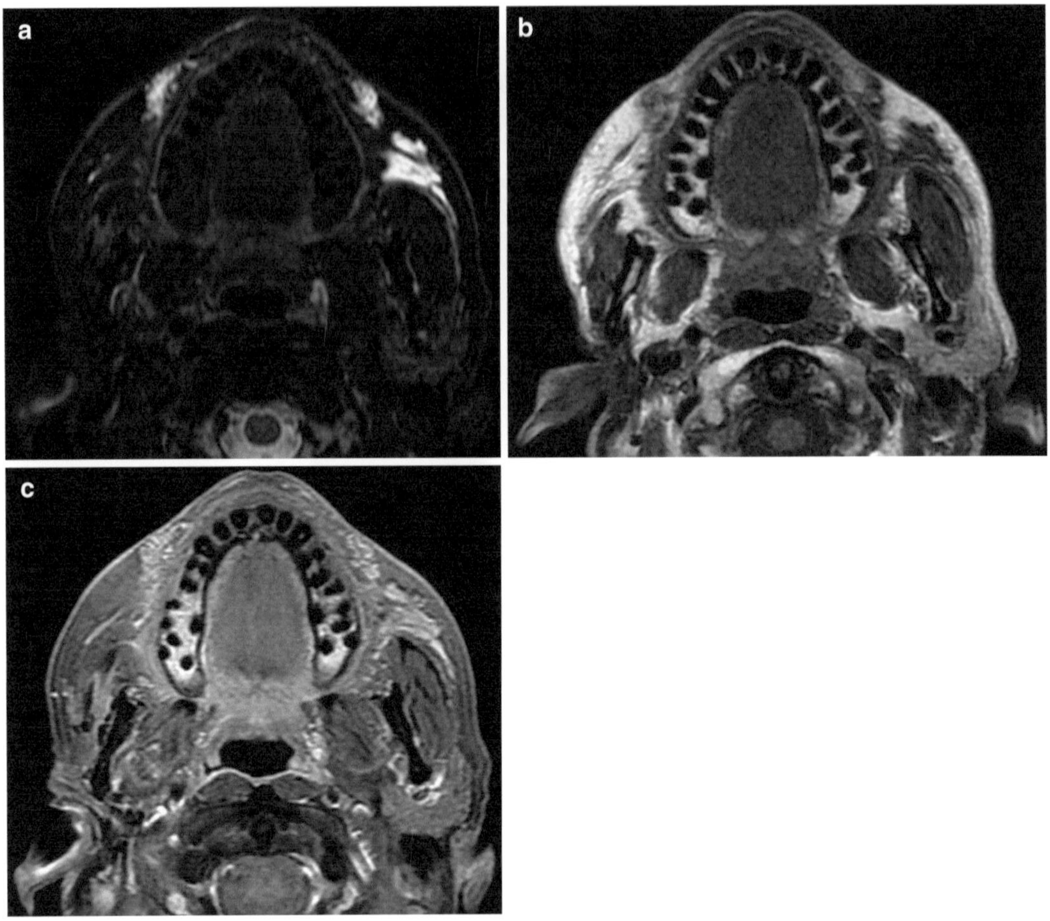

Fig. 9.22 Hyaluronic acid filler. Axial fat-suppressed T2-weighted (**a**), T1-weighted (**b**), and post-contrast fat-suppressed T1-weighted (**c**) MR images show enhancement of the gel located within the bilateral nasolabial folds and left cheek

- *Liquid silicone*, also known as silicone oil, has been used for both facial rejuvenation and treating acne scars. The filler displays attenuation similar to soft tissue on CT. Compared to the other filler agents, complications, such as granulomas tend to be more frequent and may be severe and irreversible (Fig. 9.23).

Many complications can occur with facial fillers and some of these can be depicted on radiological imaging. For example, filler migration is the spontaneous movement of filler material away from the intended site of injection and occurs in a small percentage of patients. This can create discomfort, a cosmetically distressing appearance, and dysfunction of affected tissue, such as the inability to close the eyelids. Treatment includes local corticosteroid injections, hyaluronidase injections for hyaluronic acid, or excision of the filler. Inflammation begins soon after placement of the filler and typically subsides quickly, although a severe chronic inflammatory response may also occur. Predisposing risk factors include underlying inflammatory diseases, dental caries, and sinusitis. On imaging, there may be diffuse swelling and contrast enhancement of surrounding tissues. Granuloma formation is a foreign body response that is most commonly associated with silicone oil, but can occur with other agents and can appear as a soft tissue nodule (Fig. 9.24), which is not necessarily contiguous with the filler material. Infections occur in a small proportion of patients, with *Staphylococcus aureus* representing the most frequent organism involved. On imaging, infection appears as diffuse enhancement and stranding of subcutaneous tissues adjacent to the filler. Otherwise, there can be a peripherally enhancing fluid collection if an abscess develops (Fig. 9.25).

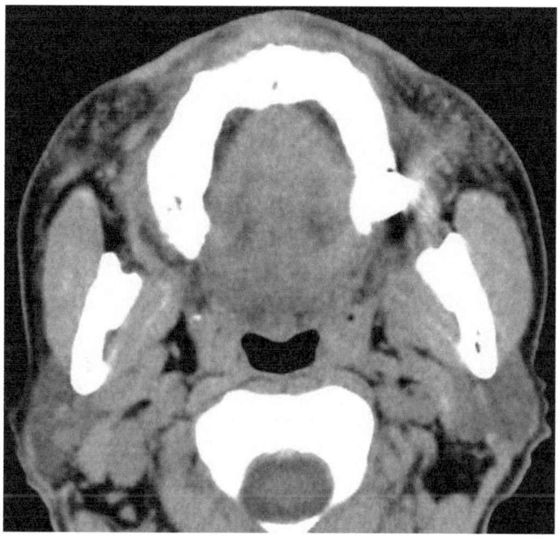

Fig. 9.23 Liquid silicone. Axial CT image shows scattered foci of soft tissue attenuation in the subctaneous tissues of the bilateral cheeks

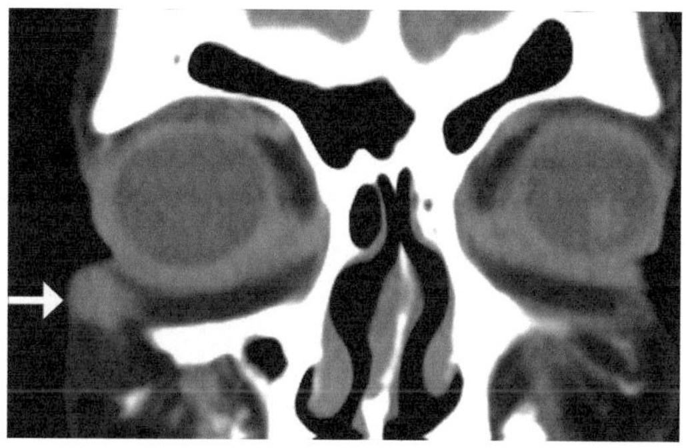

Fig. 9.24 Injection granuloma. Coronal CT image shows a soft tissue noduar lesion in the right lateral periorbital region and calcium-based filler material in the right cheek

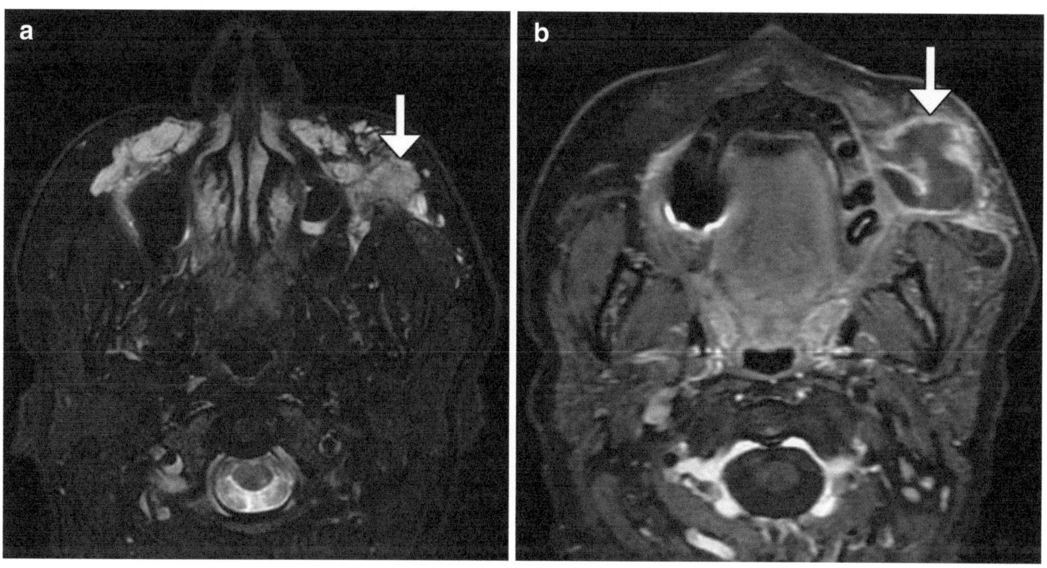

Fig. 9.25 Filler with abscess. Axial fat-suppressed T2-weighted (**a**) and fat-suppressed post-contrast T1-weighted (**b**) MR images show filler material in the bilateral cheeks, as well as a rim-enhancing fluid collection in the left cheek (*arrows*). Courtesy of Lawrence Ginsberg MD

Cosmetic and Reconstructive Implants

Overview

Many facial reconstruction and augmentation procedures involve the use of implants. For example, crescent-shaped silicone rubber implants inserted into the subperiosteal space are a popular choice for cosmetic facial augmentation. Maxillofacial fracture reconstruction implants can also be composed of silicone, as well as several other types of synthetic materials, such as titanium and porous polyethylene. Various complications can be associated with facial implants. In particular, those that affect the skin include implant displacement with skin indentation or extrusion, inclusion cyst formation, and sinocutaneous fistula formation with sinusitis (Figs. 9.26 and 9.27).

Imaging Findings

Diagnostic imaging is useful for evaluating the position of most facial implants and related complications. For example, the commonly used silicone implants appear hyperattenuating on CT, but are less conspicuous on MRI due to their low signal, particularly when juxtaposed with air or bone. The complications associated with displaced or extruding implants, such as peri-prosthetic soft tissue infection, sinusitis, and inclusion cyst formation can be adequately delineated via high-resolution CT (Figs. 9.28 and 9.29).

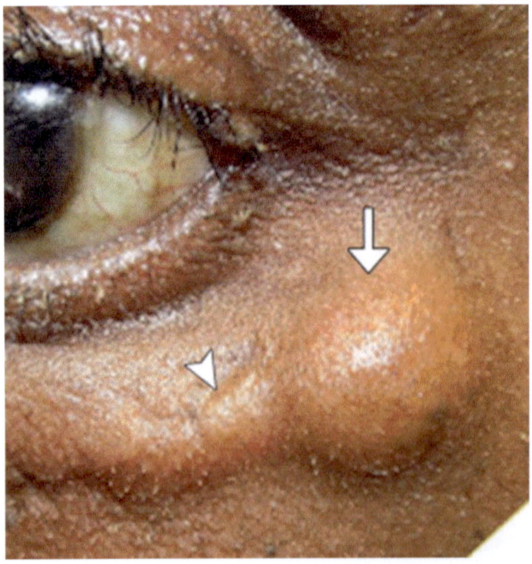

Fig. 9.26 Photograph shows indentation of the skin from a displaced orbital floor reconstruction implant (arrowhead) and an adjacent inclusion cyst (arrow)

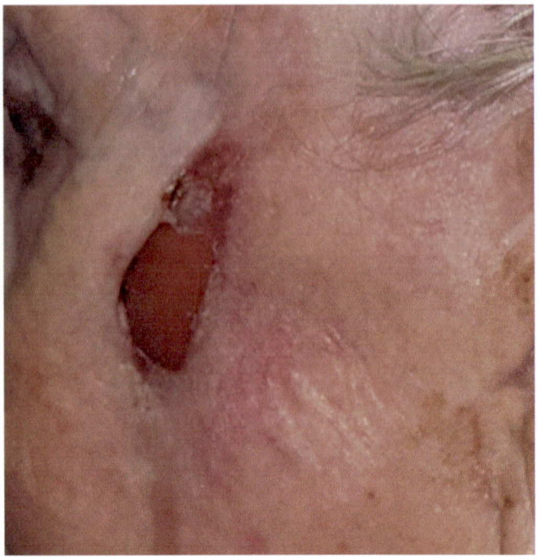

Fig. 9.27 Implant extrusion. Photograph shows a skin defect in the cheek with exposure of a silicone implant. Courtesy of Ryan Salvador, MD

Keloids

Overview

Keloids represent benign, but exuberant fibrous tissue proliferation that can form at surgical incision sites and beyond in individuals with a predisposition. These lesions appear as flesh-colored or reddish nodules or plaques that can cause cosmetic concerns (Fig. 9.30). Treatment of keloids consists not only of the injectable medications triamcinolone and 5-fluorouracil, but also may include post-excisional radiation therapy to prevent re-growth. In particular, linear acceleration electron beam therapy or Co-60 teletherapy yield the lowest recurrence rates following keloid resection than other radiation techniques at the same radiation doses.

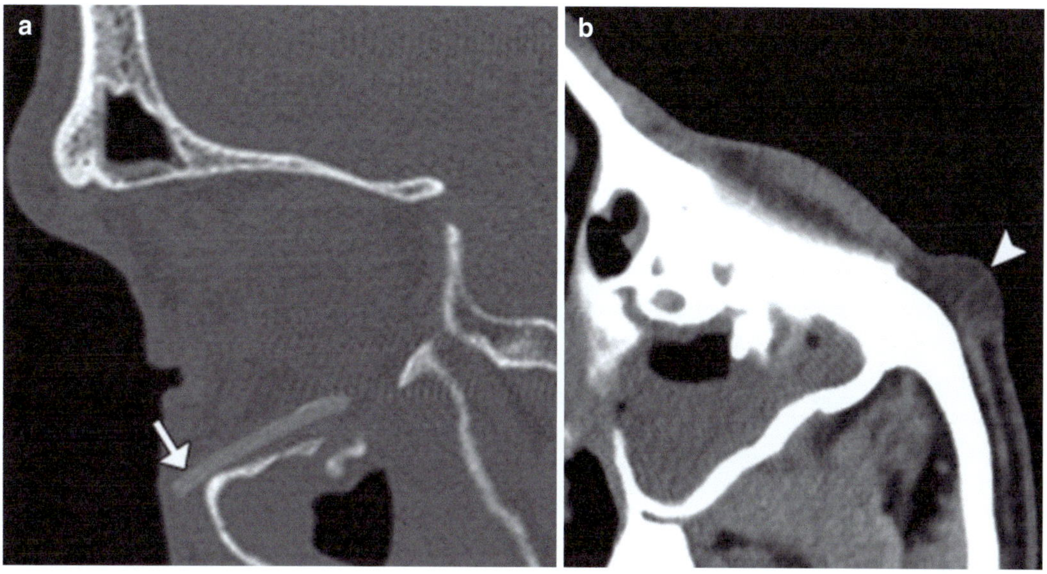

Fig. 9.28 Implant displacement with inclusion cyst. Sagittal CT image (**a**) shows an anteriorly displaced silicone orbital floor reconstruction plate (*arrow*) that indents the skin. Axial CT image (**b**) shows a cystic lesion (*arrowhead*) in the skin adjacent to the implant, which corresponds to an acquired inclusion cyst in the same patient shown in Fig. 9.26

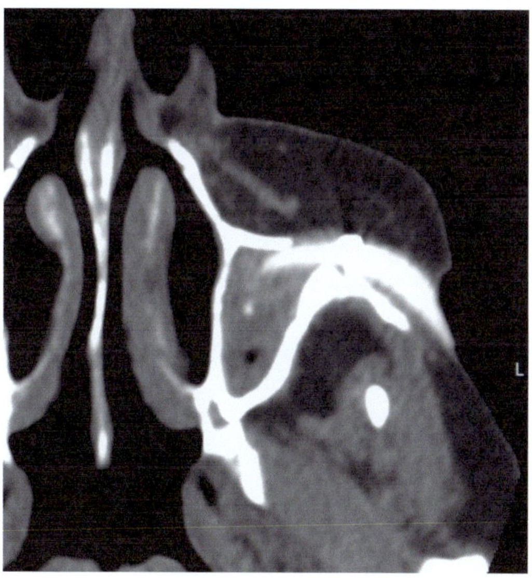

Fig. 9.29 Implant extrusion and sinocutaneous fistula. Axial CT image shows a left cheek skin defect overlying the displaced left cheek silicone implant, which has also eroded into the maxillary sinus, with associated sinusitis

Imaging Findings

On CT, keloids appear as well-circumscribed, sometimes lobulated soft tissue tumors

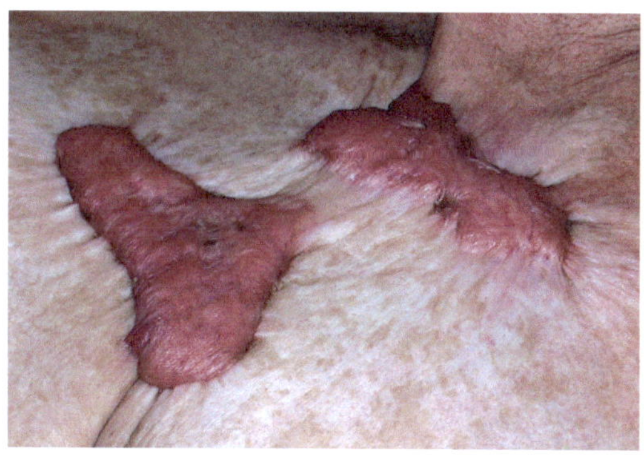

Fig. 9.30 Keloid. Photograph shows two reddish plaques along a surgical incision site. Courtesy of Lawrence Gottlieb, MD

(Fig. 9.31). On MRI sequences, keloids exhibit low signal intensity on all pulse sequences due to their high collagen composition. Keloids often exhibit greater ^{18}FDG uptake on PET than surrounding tissue due to increased metabolic activity from the relatively large population of macrophages relative to normal skin. This phenomenon may be attributable to hyperplasia of the extracellular matrix, the production of which requires increased cellular metabolism.

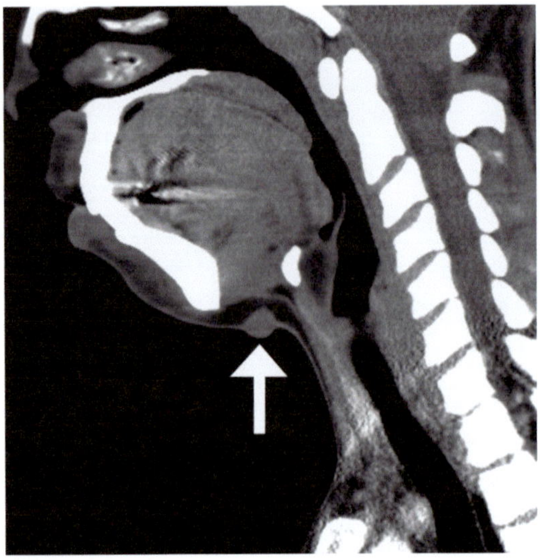

Fig. 9.31 Keloid. Sagittal CT image shows a nodular soft tissue skin lesion (arrow) after resection of a root of tongue dermoid cyst

Gadolinium-Based Contrast Agents and Nephrogenic Systemic Fibrosis

Overview

Nephrogenic systemic fibrosis (NSF) is a rare delayed complication of GBCA administration that occurs in patients with severe renal failure. This condition has been associated with linear contrast agents, such as Omniscan, Magnevist, and OptiMARK, and is related to the release of gadolinium from the chelating agents. NSF predominantly affects the liver, lungs, heart, and skin. In particular, the skin involvement in NSF typically manifests as bilateral symmetric epidermal atrophy and hair loss in the legs (Fig. 9.32). There can also be hyperpigmentation and skin induration or wrinkling. No new cases have been reported in literature in recent years, likely due to increased awareness of the condition leading to restricted use of GBCA in patients with low GFR. Gadolinium retention in tissue is a cumulative, dose-dependent phenomenon; however, the level of gadolinium deposition in tissues and associated symptoms of NSF can wane over time. Besides NSF, Gadolinium deposition can occur in neural tissues after GBCA administration, even in the setting of intact blood–brain barrier and normal renal function. However, the clinical significance of such deposits remains unclear.

Imaging Findings

On brain MRI the accumulation of Gd appears as high signal intensity on T1-weighted images in the dentate nucleus, globus pallidus, and pulvinar region of the thalamus (Fig. 9.33). The signal approximately correlates with the number of previous GBCA administrations. Since the risks associated with these Gd deposits are unknown, exposure to GBCA should be kept to a minumum, with preferential use of macrocyclic chelates, which seem to be deposited at lower concentrations.

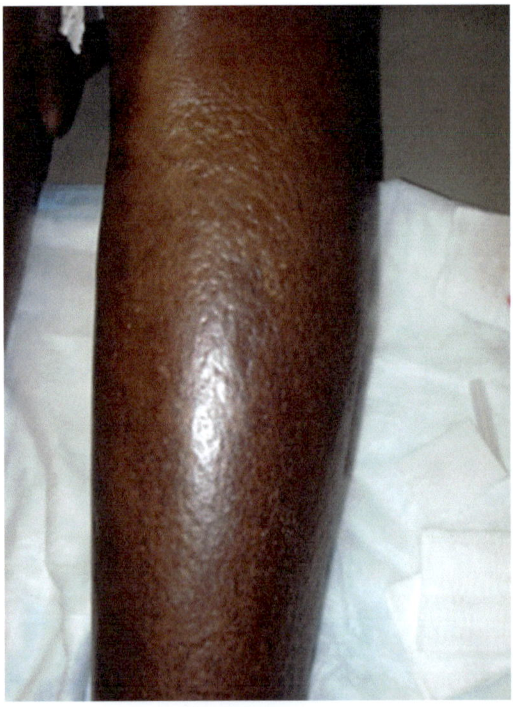

Fig. 9.32 Nephrogenic systemic fibrosis. Photograph shows epidermal atrophy and hairlessness in the legs. Courtesy of Vesna Petronic-Rosic MD

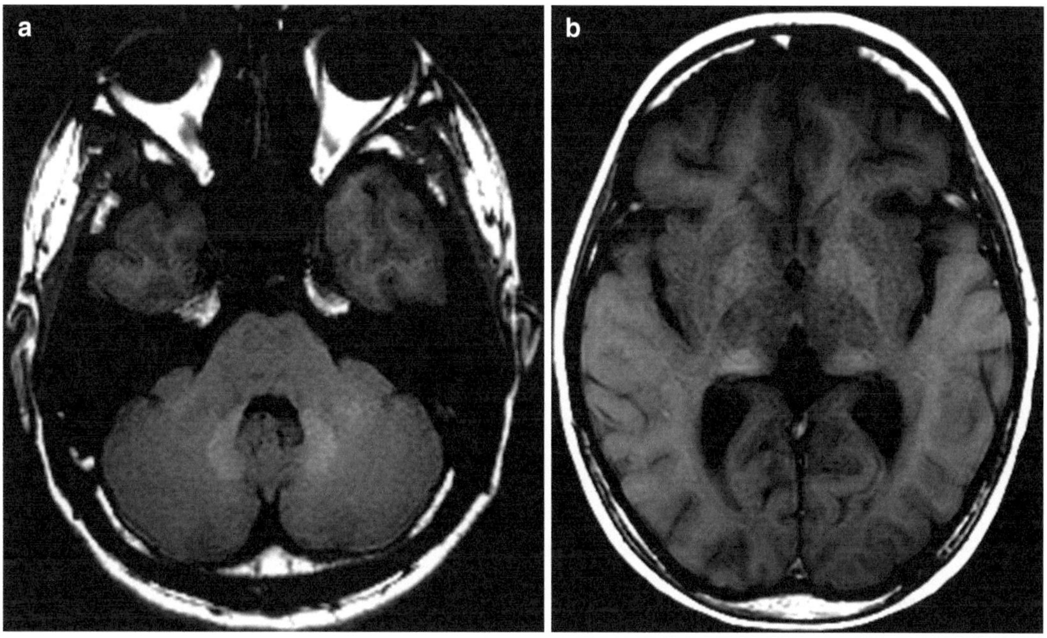

Fig. 9.33 Gadolinium brain deposition. Axial T1-weighted MR images (**a** and **b**) show hyperintensity in the bilateral dentate nuclei, globus pallidi, and pulvinar regions of the thalami in a patient who had undergone several MRI exams with linear Gadolinium-based agents

Suggested Reading

Batra J, Bekal RK, Byadgi S, Attresh G, Sambyal S, Vakade CD. Comparison of skin staples and standard sutures for closing incisions after head and neck cancer surgery: a double-blind, randomized and prospective study. J Maxillofac Oral Surg. 2016;15(2):243–50.

Blackmon J, Machan M, Rajpara A, Beatty R. Recurrent basal cell carcinoma with intracranial invasion: a case report and literature review. Dermatol Online J. 2014;20(7). pii: 13030/qt11t0g5h8.

Chan RJ, Larsen E, Chan P. Re-examining the evidence in radiation dermatitis management literature: an overview and a critical appraisal of systematic reviews. Int J Radiat Oncol Biol Phys. 2012;84, 357(3):–62.

Chong J, Chan LL, Langstein HN, Ginsberg LE. MR imaging of the muscular component of myocutaneous flaps in the head and neck. AJNR Am J Neuroradiol. 2001;22(1):170–4.

Conen K, Mosna-Firlejczyk K, Rochlitz C, Wicki A, Itin P, Arnold AW, Gross M, Zimmerman F, Zippelius A. Vemurafenib-induced radiation recall dermatitis: case report and review of the literature. Dermatology. 2015;230(1):1–4.

Dedivitis RA, Aires FT, Cernea CR, Brandao LG. Pharyngocutaneous fistula after total laryngectomy: systematic review of risk factors. Head Neck. 2015;37(11):1691–7.

Di Girolamo M, Mattei M, Signore A, Grippaudo FR. MRI in the evaluation of facial dermal fillers in normal and complicated cases. Eur Radiol. 2015;25(5):1431–42.

Funt D, Pavicic T. Dermal fillers in aesthetics: an overview of adverse events and treatment approaches. Clin Cosmet Investig Dermatol. 2013;6:295–316.

Ginat DT, Schatz CJ. Imaging features of midface injectable fillers and associated complications. Am J Neuroradiol. 2013a;34(8):1488–95.

Ginat DT, Schatz CJ. Imaging of silastic cheek implant penetration into the maxillary sinus. JAMA Otolaryngol Head Neck Surg. 2013b;139(2):199–201.

Ginat DT, Kelly HR, Schaefer PW, Davidson CJ, Curry W. Recurrent scalp metastasis from glioblastoma following resection. Clin Neurol Neurosurg. 2013;115(4):461–3.

Glastonbury CM, Parker EE, Hoang JK. The post-radiation neck: evaluating response to treatment and recognizing complications. Am J Roentgenol. 2010;195(2):W164–71.

Gurlek A, Alaybeyoglu N, Demir C, Aydogan H, Bilen B, Aezturk A. Aesthetic reconstuction of large scalp defects by sequential tissue expansion without interval. Aesthet Plast Surg. 2005;28(4):245–50.

Hafner MF, Fetzner L, Hassel JC, Debus J, Potthof K. Prophylaxis of acute radiation dermatitis with an innovative FDA-approved two-step skin care system in a patient with head and neck cancer undergoing a platin-based radiochemotherapy: a case report and review of the literature. Dermatology. 2013;227(2):171–4.

Hudgins PA. Flap reconstruction in the head and neck: expected appearance, complications, and recurrent disease. Eur J Radiol. 2002;44(2):130–8.

Kanegaye JT, Vance CW, Chan L, Schonfeld N. Comparison of skin stapling devices and standard sutures for pediatric scalp lacerations: a randomized study of costs and time benefits. J Pediatr. 1997;130(5):808–13.

Lin S, Hanasono M, Skoracki R. Scalp and calvarial reconstruction. Semin Plast Surg. 2008;22(4):281–93.

Makitie A, Irish J, Gullane P. Pharyngocutaneous fistula. Curr Opin Otolaryngol Head Neck Surg. 2003;11(2):78–84.

Mansouri B, Bicknell LM, Hill D, Walker GD, Fiala K, Housewright C. Mohs micrographic surgery for the management of cutaneous malignancies. Facial Plast Surg Clin North Am. 2017;25(3):291–301.

McDonald R, McDonald J, Kallmes D, Jentoft M, Murray D, Thielen K, Williamson E, Eckel L. Intracranial gadolinium deposition after contrast-enhanced MR imaging. Radiology. 2015;275(3):772–82.

McDonald RJ, McDonald JS, Kallmes DF, Jentoft ME, Paolini MA, Murray DL, Williamson EE, Eckel LJ. Gadolinium deposition in human brain tissues after contrast-enhanced MR imaging in adult patients without intracranial abnormalities. Radiology. 2017;27:161595.

Mehrara B, Disa J, Pusic A. Scalp reconstruction. J Surg Oncol. 2006;94:504–8.

Minton TJ. Contemporary Mohs surgery applications. Curr Opin Otolaryngol Head Neck Surg. 2008;16(4):376–8.

Moore MG, Lin DT, Deschler DG, Wang JJ, Chan AW. Risk of incisional recurrence after midface and anterior skull base surgery in sinonasal malignancies. Skull Base. 2011;21(2):87–92.

Mundada P, Kohler R, Boudabbous S, Toutous Trellu L, Platon A, Becker M. Injectable facial fillers: imaging features, complications, and diagnostic pitfalls at MRI and PET CT. Insights Imaging. 2017;8(6):557–72.

Saito N, Nadgir RN, Nakahira M, Takahashi M, Uchino A, Kimura F, Truong MT, Sakai O. Posttreatment CT and MR imaging in head and neck cancer: what the radiologist needs to know. Radiographics. 2012;32(5):1261–82; discussion 1282–4.

Schad S, Heitland P, Kuhn-Velten W, Gross G, Jonas L. Time-dependent decrement of dermal gadolinium deposits and significant improvement of skin symptoms in a patient with nephrogenic systemic fibrosis after temporary renal failure. J Cutan Pathol. 2013;40(11):935–44.

Schatz CJ, Ginat DT. Imaging features of rhinoplasty. Am J Neuroradiol. 2014;35(2):216–22.

Winkler AA, Soler ZM, Leong PL, Murphy A, Wand TD, Cook TA. Complications associated with alloplastic implants in rhinoplasty. Arch Facial Plast Surg. 2012;14(6):437–41.

MIX
Papier aus verantwortungsvollen Quellen
Paper from responsible sources
FSC® C105338

If you have any concerns about our products,
you can contact us on
ProductSafety@springernature.com

In case Publisher is established outside the EU,
the EU authorized representative is:
Springer Nature Customer Service Center GmbH
Europaplatz 3, 69115 Heidelberg, Germany

Printed by Libri Plureos GmbH
in Hamburg, Germany